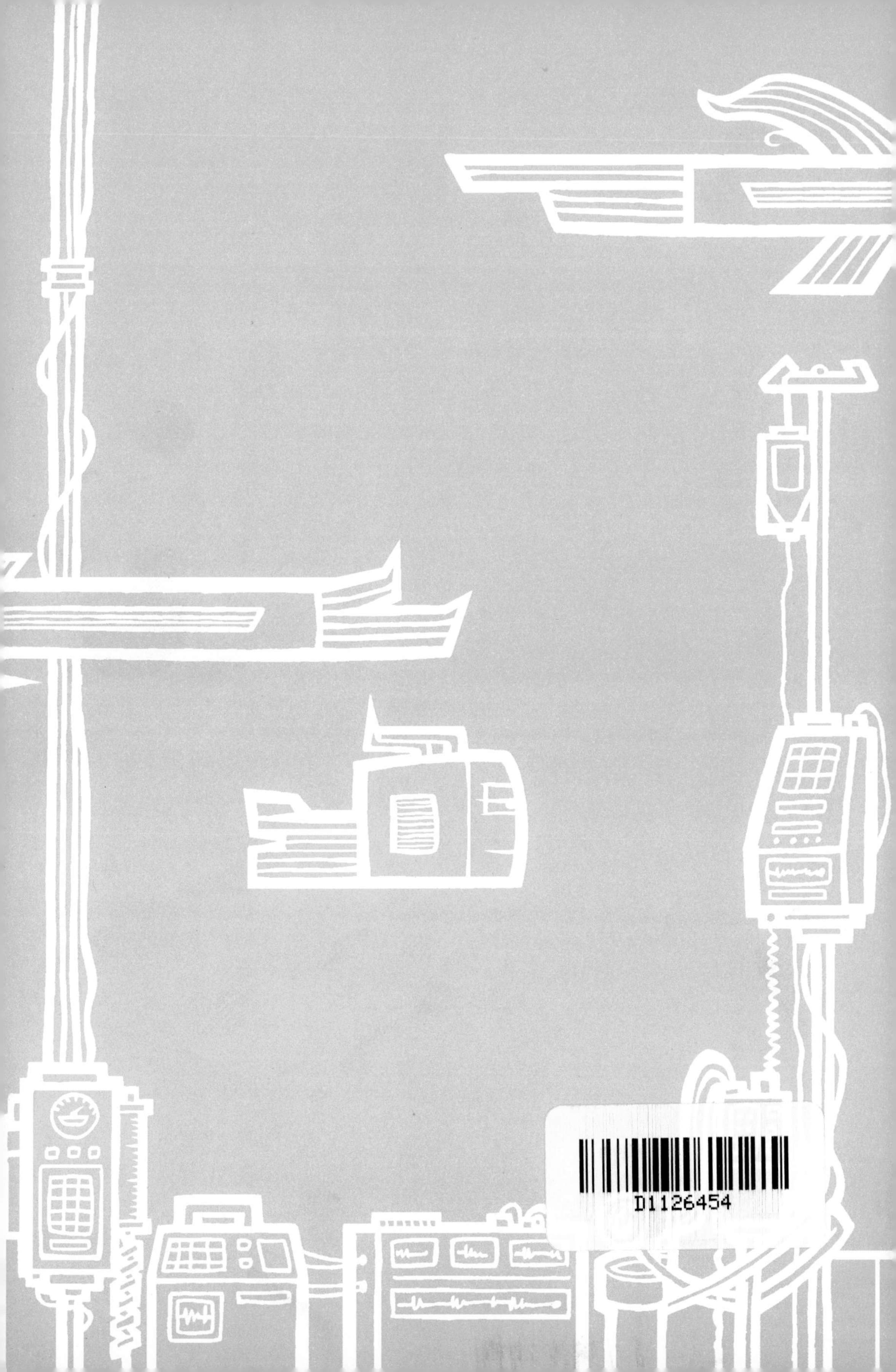

A CHANCE

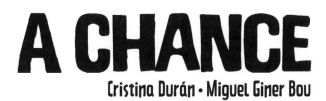

A CHANCE

Cristina Durán · Miguel Giner Bou

graphic mundi

To our parents, Elvira and Luis, Amparo and Ramón.
Especially Luis, who couldn't see this book completed.

And to Laia, of course.

To Selamawit, for accepting us at first sight.

To Tigui, Pepón, Lupe, Atnafu, and Yeneneh,
travel companions.

And to my sisters, Elvira, Encarna, and Ana,
for their kindness and constant support.

BOOK 1

ONE CHANCE IN A THOUSAND

On the pages that open chapters 1–5 in Book 1, our
translation retains the song lyrics in their original Spanish,
Catalan, and Portuguese languages. The reader will find
translations for these lyrics at the back of the book.

1.
THE ABYSS

Se aprende en la cuna,
se aprende en la cama,
se aprende en la puerta
de un hospital.

Se aprende de golpe,
se aprende de a poco
y a veces se aprende
recién al final.

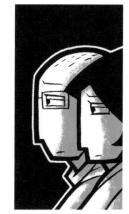

"Polvo de estrellas,"
Jorge Drexler

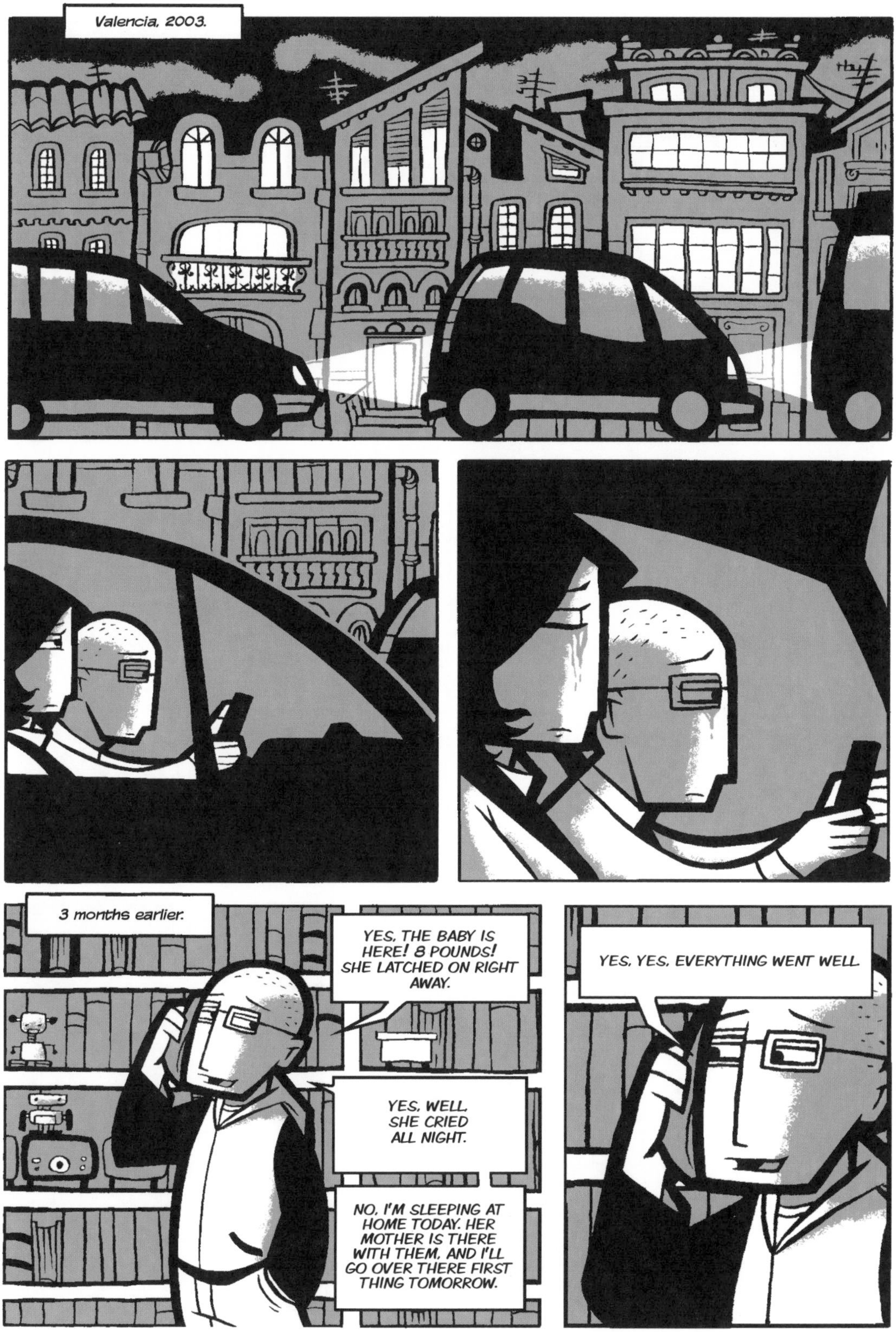
Valencia, 2003.
3 months earlier.
YES, THE BABY IS HERE! 8 POUNDS! SHE LATCHED ON RIGHT AWAY.
YES, WELL, SHE CRIED ALL NIGHT.
NO, I'M SLEEPING AT HOME TODAY. HER MOTHER IS THERE WITH THEM, AND I'LL GO OVER THERE FIRST THING TOMORROW.
YES, YES, EVERYTHING WENT WELL.

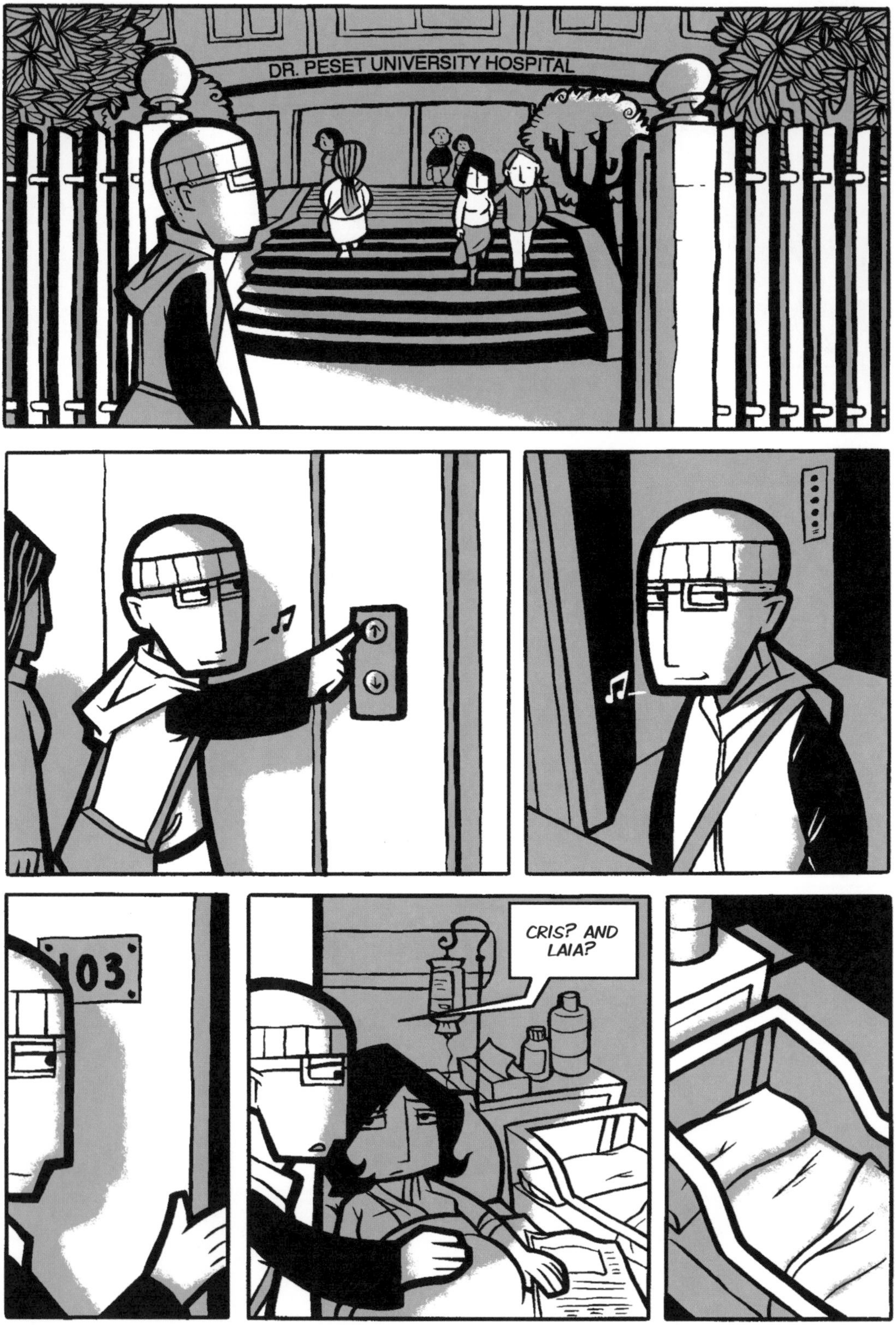
DR. PESET UNIVERSITY HOSPITAL
103
CRIS? AND LAIA?

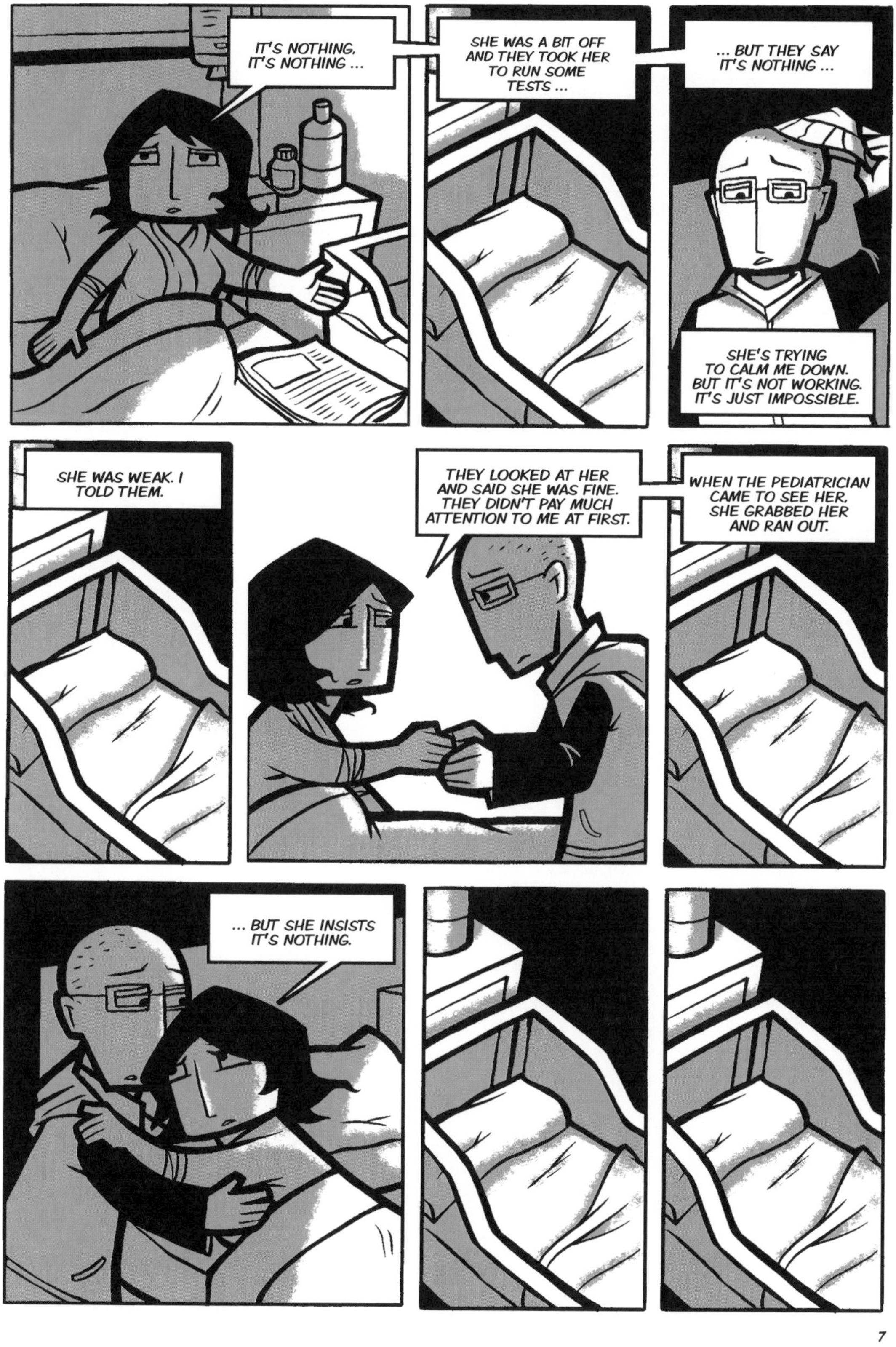
IT'S NOTHING, IT'S NOTHING ...
SHE WAS A BIT OFF AND THEY TOOK HER TO RUN SOME TESTS ...
... BUT THEY SAY IT'S NOTHING ...
SHE'S TRYING TO CALM ME DOWN. BUT IT'S NOT WORKING. IT'S JUST IMPOSSIBLE.
SHE WAS WEAK. I TOLD THEM.
THEY LOOKED AT HER AND SAID SHE WAS FINE. THEY DIDN'T PAY MUCH ATTENTION TO ME AT FIRST.
WHEN THE PEDIATRICIAN CAME TO SEE HER, SHE GRABBED HER AND RAN OUT.
... BUT SHE INSISTS IT'S NOTHING.

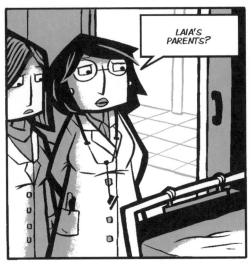

LAIA'S PARENTS?

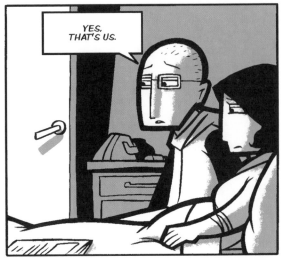

YES, THAT'S US.

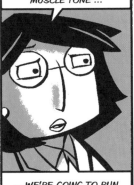

RIGHT NOW WE CAN'T TELL YOU ANYTHING, JUST THAT SHE HAS DECREASED MUSCLE TONE ...

... WE'RE GOING TO RUN ALL THE NECESSARY TESTS ...

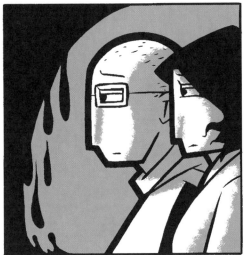

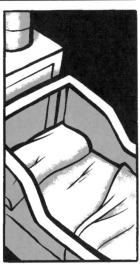

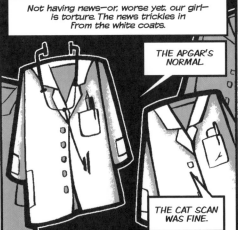

Not having news—or, worse yet, our girl—is torture. The news trickles in from the white coats.

THE APGAR'S NORMAL

THE CAT SCAN WAS FINE.

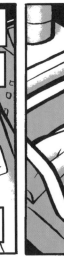

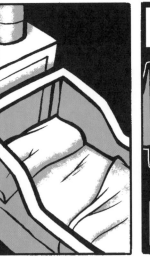

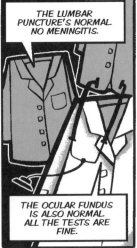

THE LUMBAR PUNCTURE'S NORMAL. NO MENINGITIS.

THE OCULAR FUNDUS IS ALSO NORMAL. ALL THE TESTS ARE FINE.

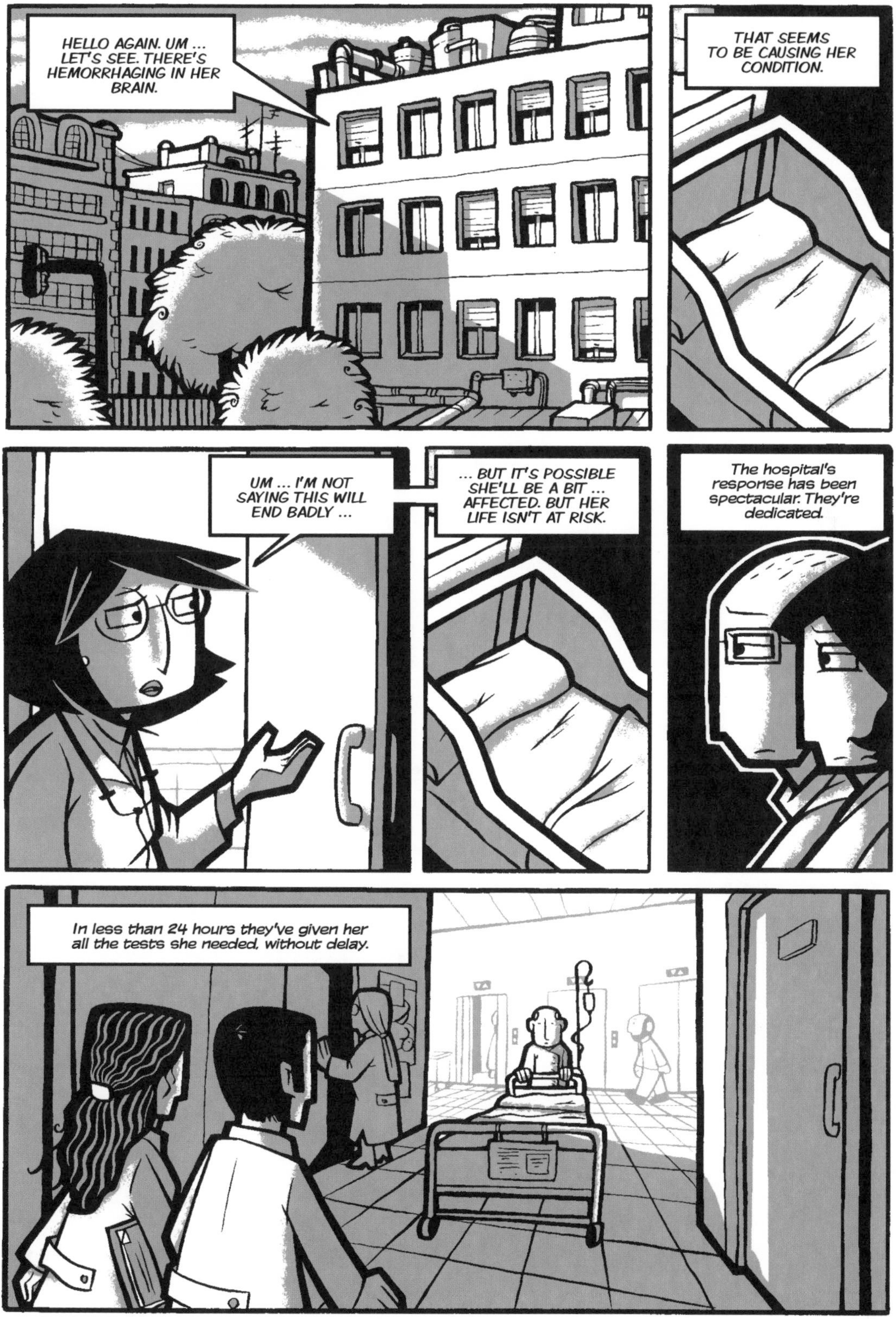
HELLO AGAIN. UM ... LET'S SEE. THERE'S HEMORRHAGING IN HER BRAIN.
THAT SEEMS TO BE CAUSING HER CONDITION.
UM ... I'M NOT SAYING THIS WILL END BADLY ...
... BUT IT'S POSSIBLE SHE'LL BE A BIT ... AFFECTED. BUT HER LIFE ISN'T AT RISK.
The hospital's response has been spectacular. They're dedicated.
In less than 24 hours they've given her all the tests she needed, without delay.

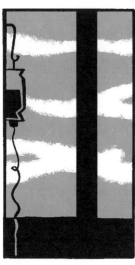

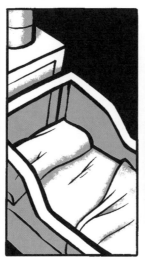

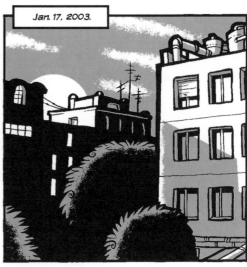
Jan. 17, 2003.

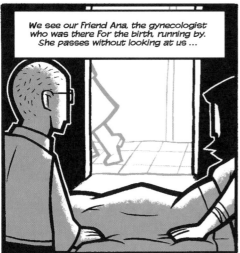
We see our friend Ana, the gynecologist who was there for the birth, running by. She passes without looking at us ...

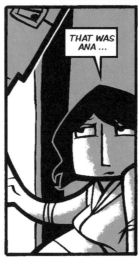
THAT WAS ANA ...

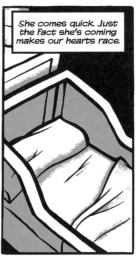
She comes quick. Just the fact she's coming makes our hearts race.

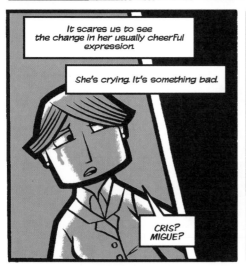
It scares us to see the change in her usually cheerful expression.

She's crying. It's something bad.

CRIS? MIGUE?

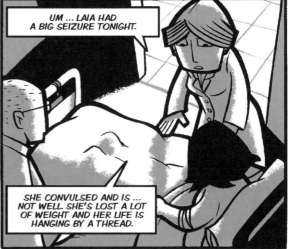
UM ... LAIA HAD A BIG SEIZURE TONIGHT.

SHE CONVULSED AND IS ... NOT WELL. SHE'S LOST A LOT OF WEIGHT AND HER LIFE IS HANGING BY A THREAD.

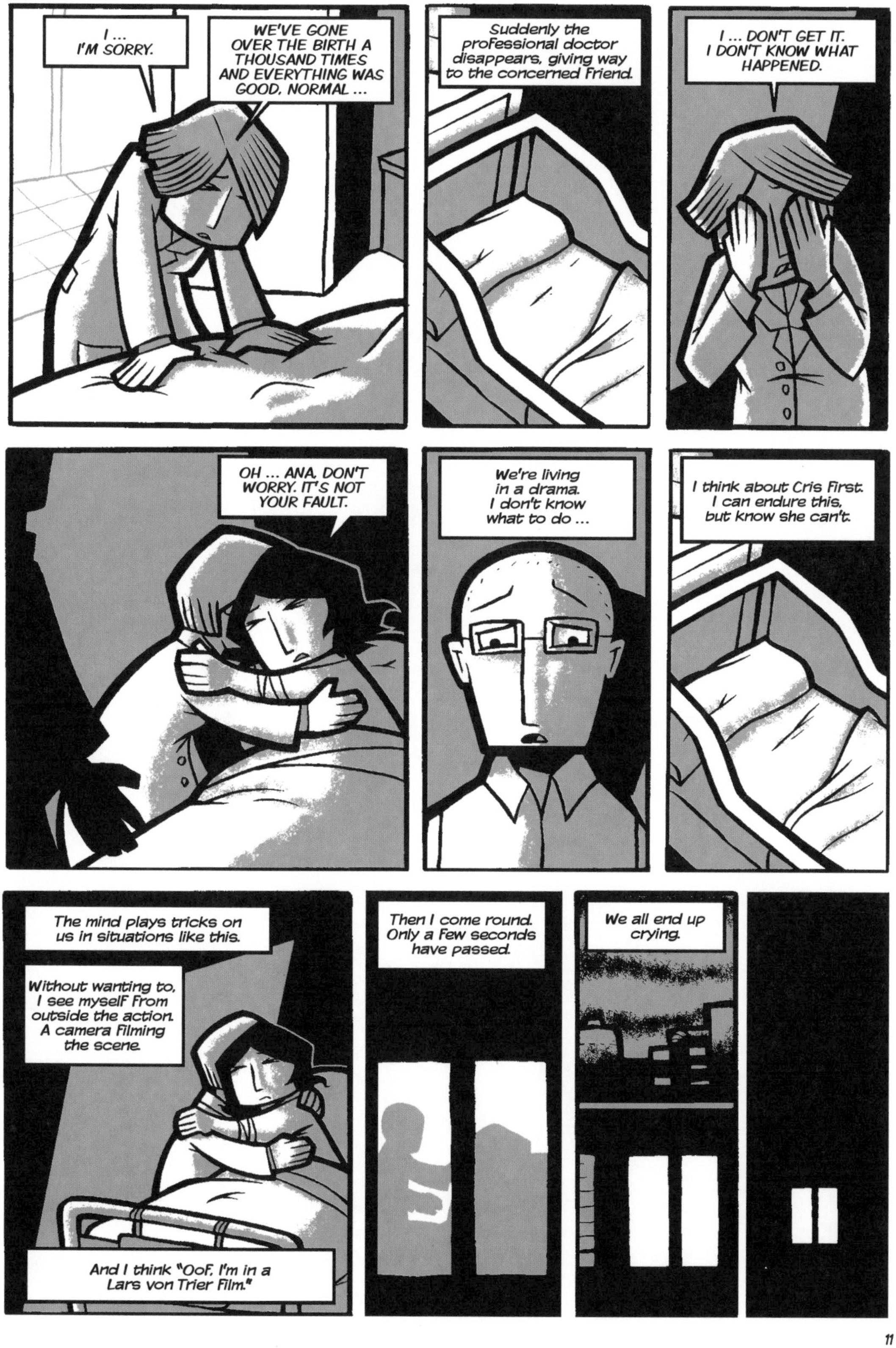
I ... I'M SORRY.
WE'VE GONE OVER THE BIRTH A THOUSAND TIMES AND EVERYTHING WAS GOOD, NORMAL ...
Suddenly the professional doctor disappears, giving way to the concerned friend.
I ... DON'T GET IT. I DON'T KNOW WHAT HAPPENED.
OH ... ANA, DON'T WORRY. IT'S NOT YOUR FAULT.
We're living in a drama. I don't know what to do ...
I think about Cris first. I can endure this, but know she can't.
The mind plays tricks on us in situations like this.
Without wanting to, I see myself from outside the action. A camera filming the scene.
And I think "Oof, I'm in a Lars von Trier film."
Then I come round. Only a few seconds have passed.
We all end up crying.

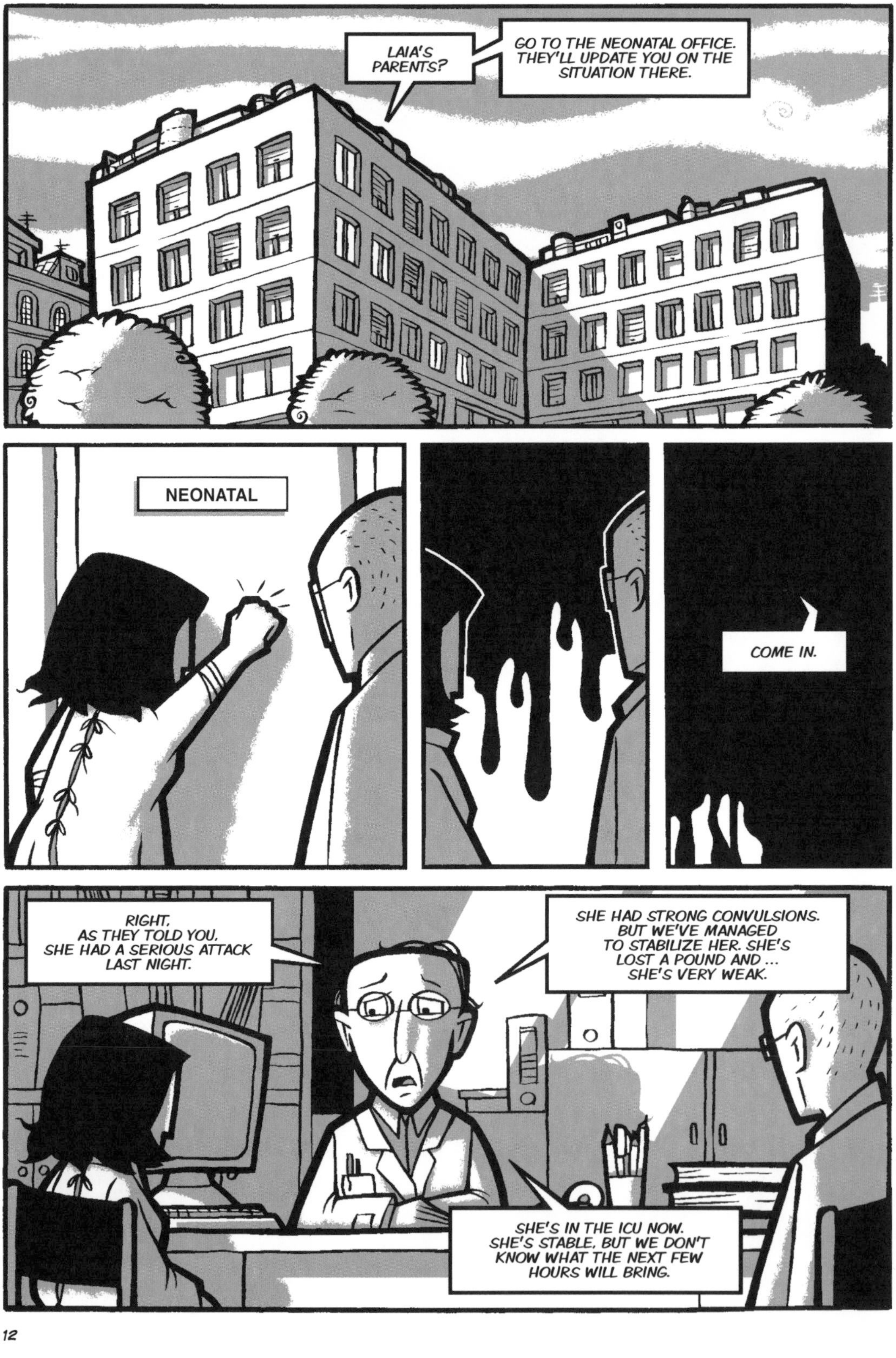
LAIA'S PARENTS?
GO TO THE NEONATAL OFFICE. THEY'LL UPDATE YOU ON THE SITUATION THERE.
NEONATAL
COME IN.
RIGHT, AS THEY TOLD YOU, SHE HAD A SERIOUS ATTACK LAST NIGHT.
SHE HAD STRONG CONVULSIONS. BUT WE'VE MANAGED TO STABILIZE HER. SHE'S LOST A POUND AND ... SHE'S VERY WEAK.
SHE'S IN THE ICU NOW. SHE'S STABLE, BUT WE DON'T KNOW WHAT THE NEXT FEW HOURS WILL BRING.

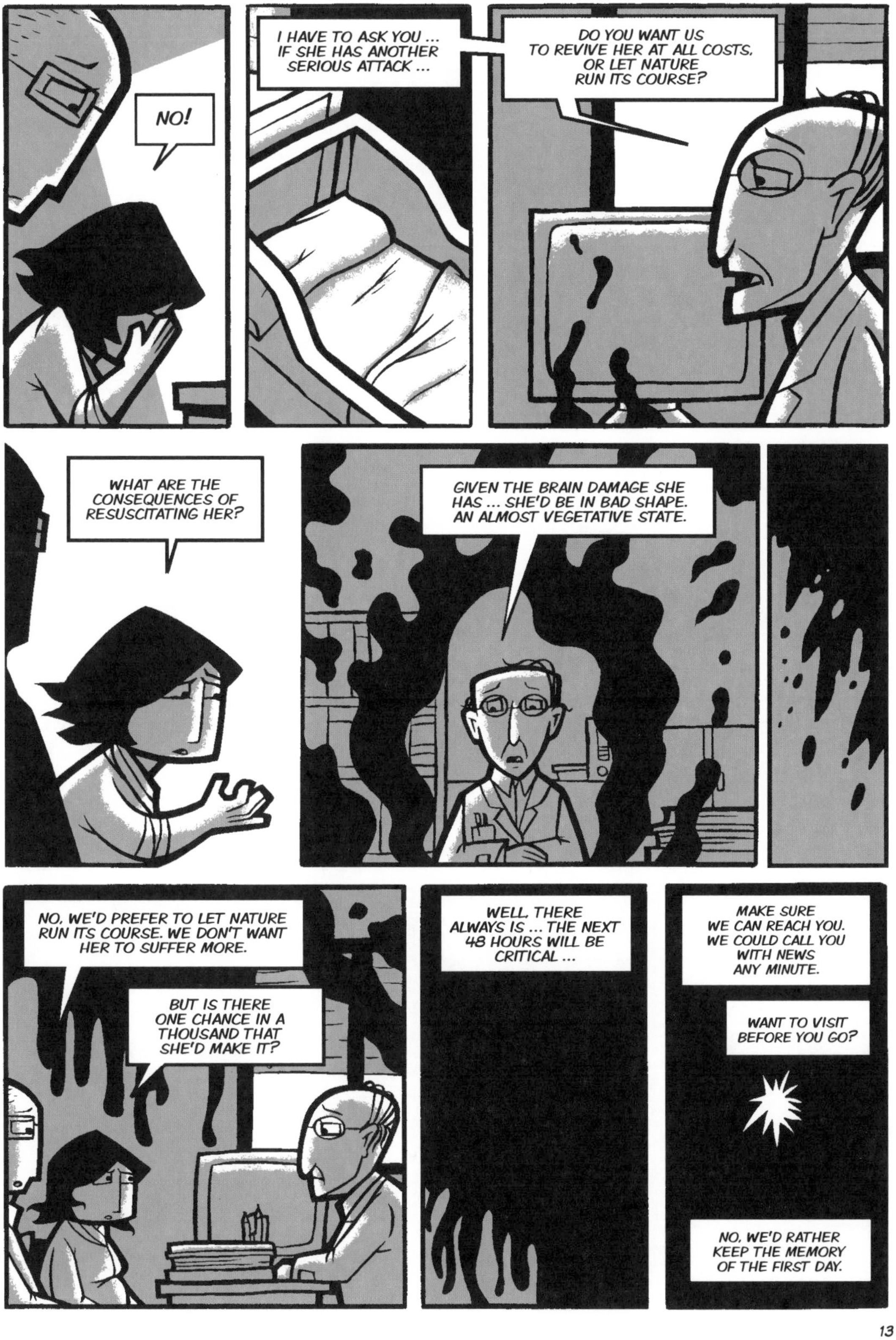
NO!
I HAVE TO ASK YOU ... IF SHE HAS ANOTHER SERIOUS ATTACK ...
DO YOU WANT US TO REVIVE HER AT ALL COSTS, OR LET NATURE RUN ITS COURSE?
WHAT ARE THE CONSEQUENCES OF RESUSCITATING HER?
GIVEN THE BRAIN DAMAGE SHE HAS ... SHE'D BE IN BAD SHAPE. AN ALMOST VEGETATIVE STATE.
NO, WE'D PREFER TO LET NATURE RUN ITS COURSE. WE DON'T WANT HER TO SUFFER MORE.
BUT IS THERE ONE CHANCE IN A THOUSAND THAT SHE'D MAKE IT?
WELL, THERE ALWAYS IS ... THE NEXT 48 HOURS WILL BE CRITICAL ...
MAKE SURE WE CAN REACH YOU. WE COULD CALL YOU WITH NEWS ANY MINUTE.
WANT TO VISIT BEFORE YOU GO?
NO, WE'D RATHER KEEP THE MEMORY OF THE FIRST DAY.

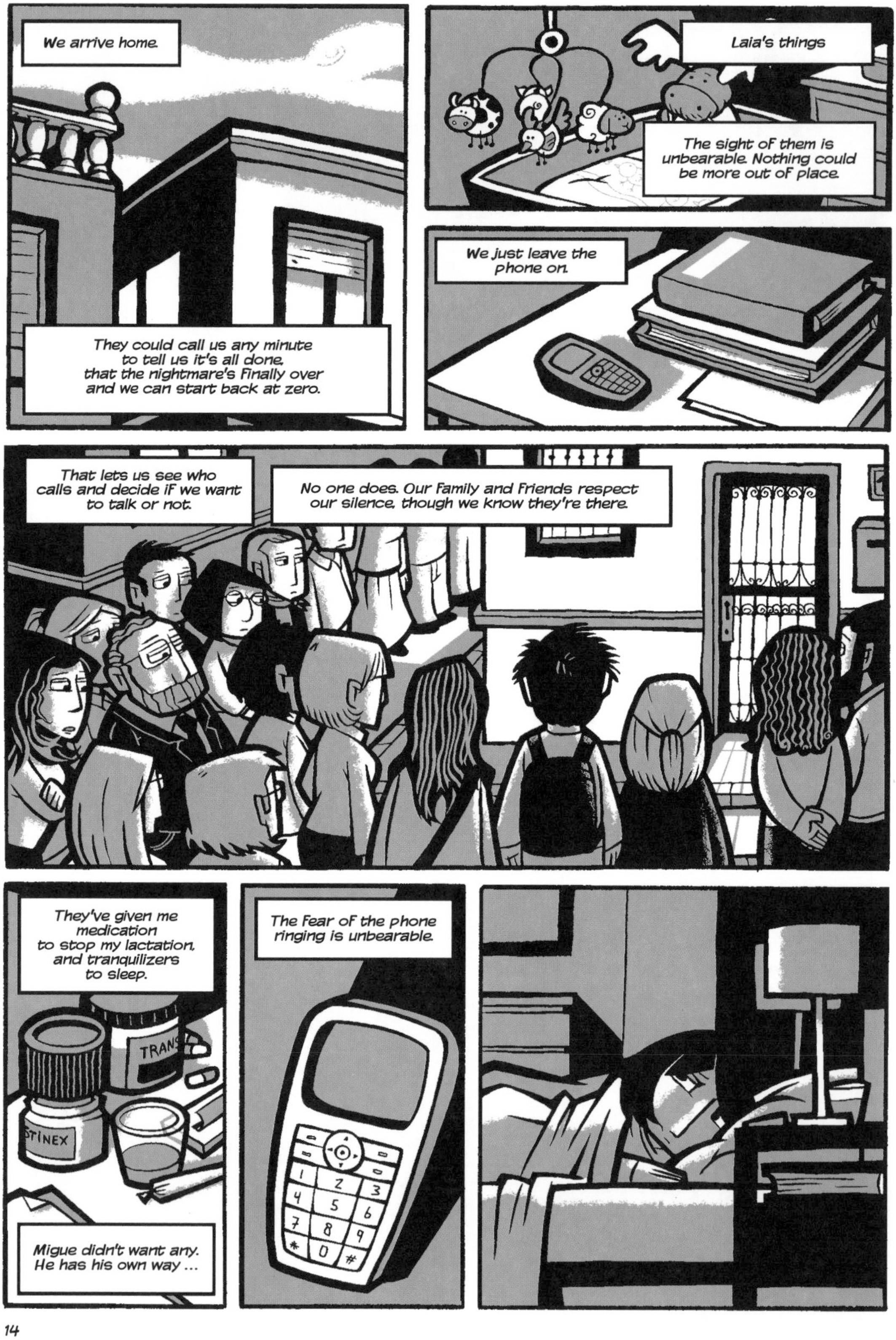
We arrive home.
They could call us any minute to tell us it's all done, that the nightmare's finally over and we can start back at zero.
Laia's things
The sight of them is unbearable. Nothing could be more out of place.
We just leave the phone on.
That lets us see who calls and decide if we want to talk or not.
No one does. Our family and friends respect our silence, though we know they're there.
They've given me medication to stop my lactation, and tranquilizers to sleep.
TRANS
STINEX
Migue didn't want any. He has his own way ...
The fear of the phone ringing is unbearable.

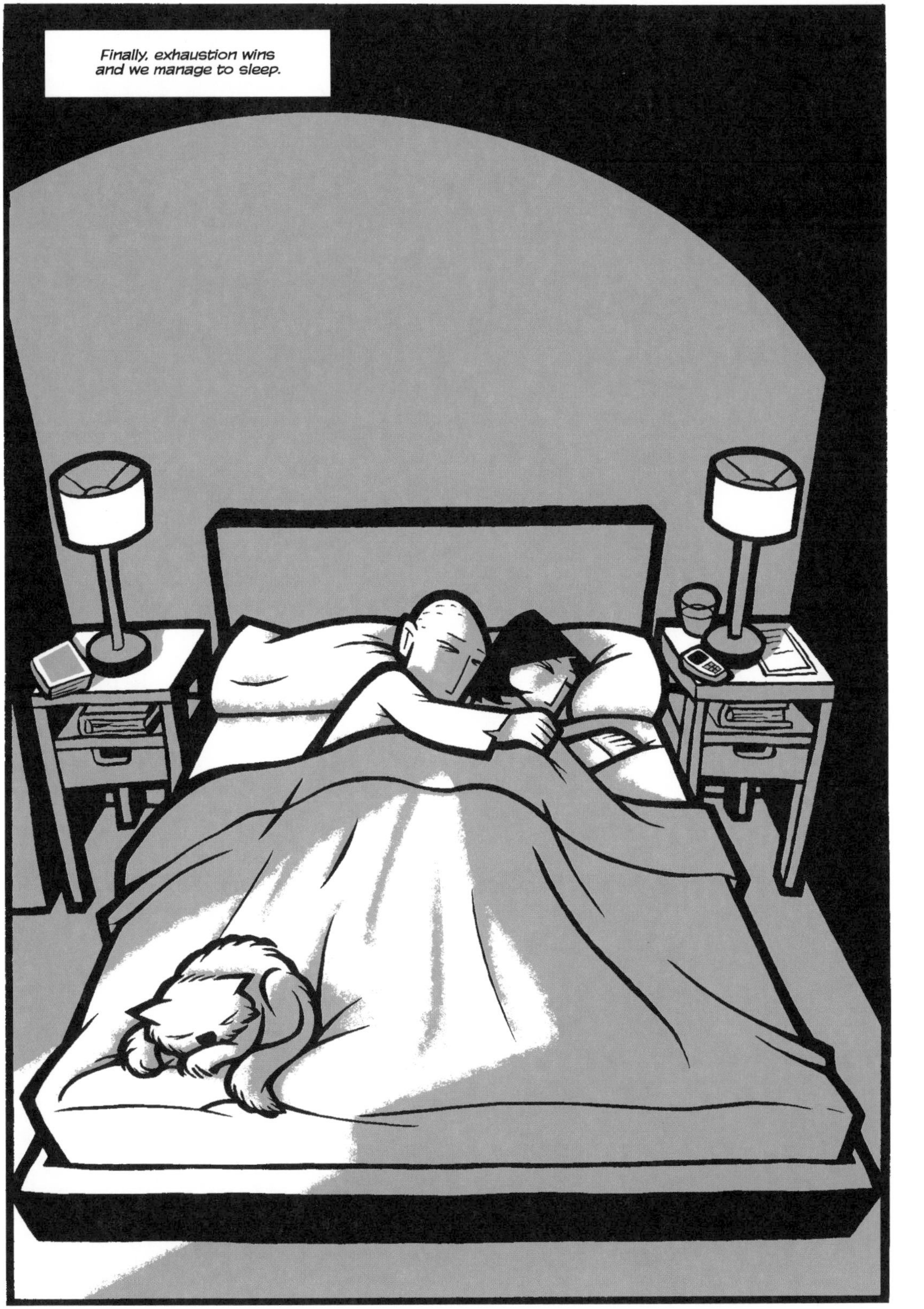
Finally, exhaustion wins
and we manage to sleep.

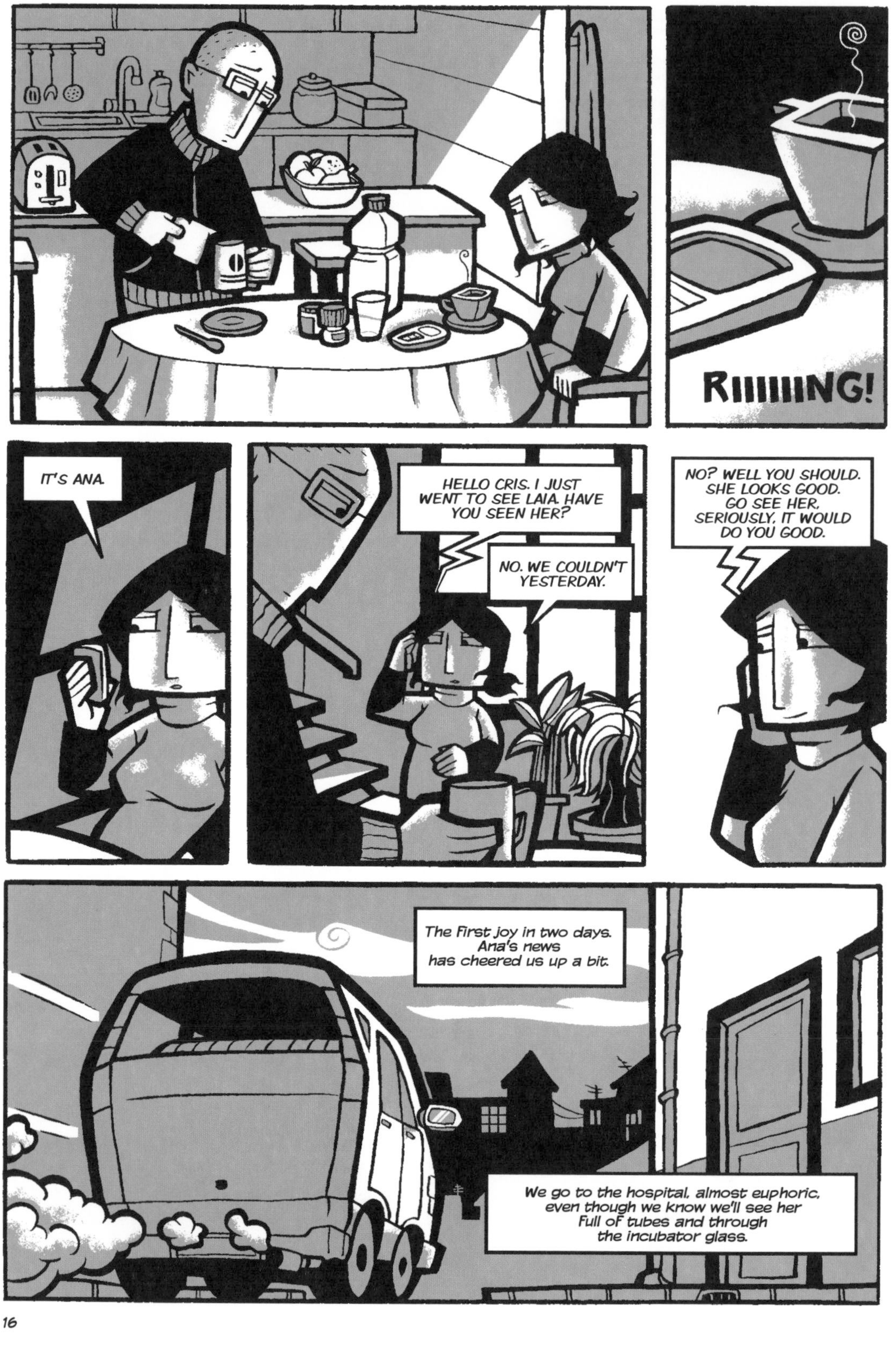
RIIIIIING!
IT'S ANA.
HELLO CRIS. I JUST WENT TO SEE LAIA. HAVE YOU SEEN HER?
NO. WE COULDN'T YESTERDAY.
NO? WELL YOU SHOULD. SHE LOOKS GOOD. GO SEE HER. SERIOUSLY, IT WOULD DO YOU GOOD.
The first joy in two days. Ana's news has cheered us up a bit.
We go to the hospital, almost euphoric, even though we know we'll see her full of tubes and through the incubator glass.

2.
The Tree

Jo tinc, per a tu, un niu
en el meu arbre
i un núvol blanc, penjat
d'alguna branca.

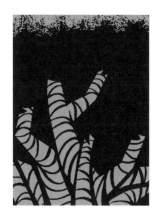

"Un núvol blanc,"
Lluís Llach

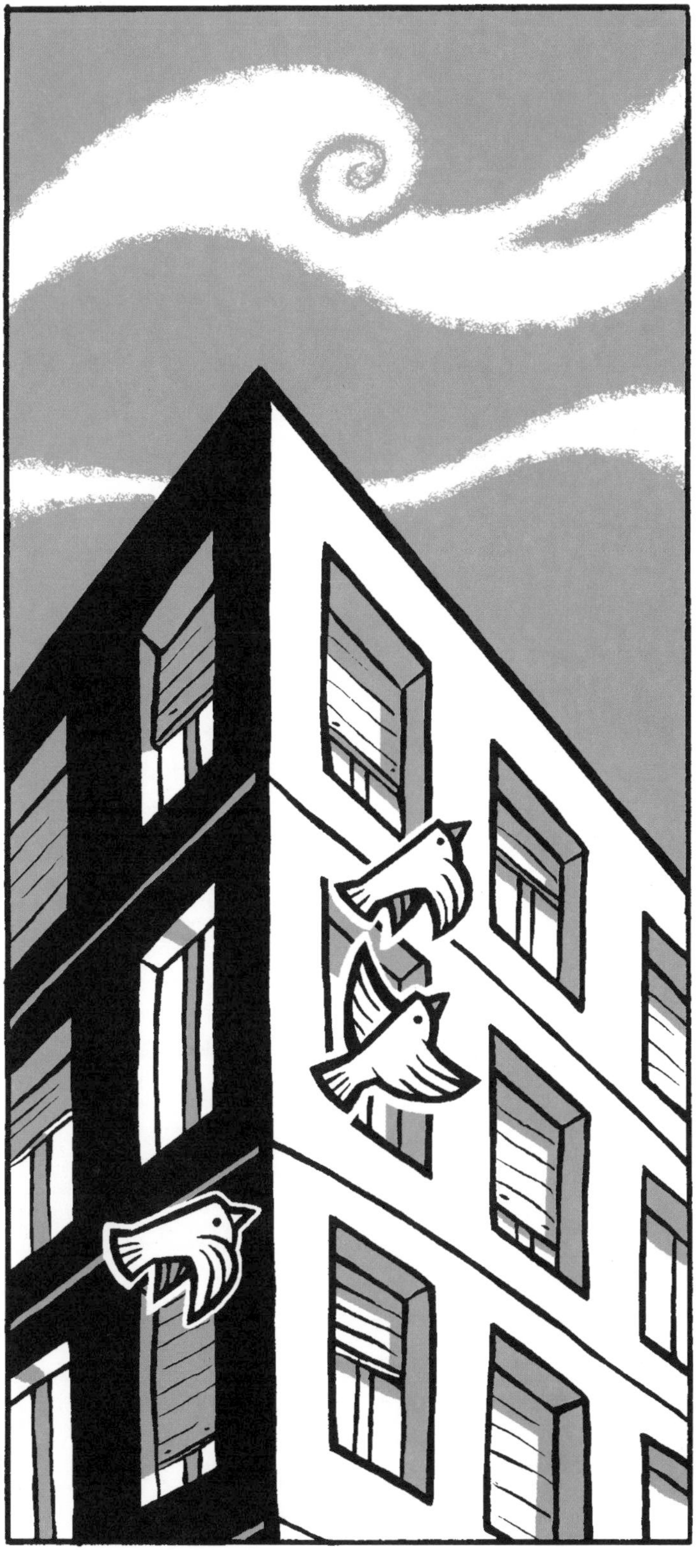

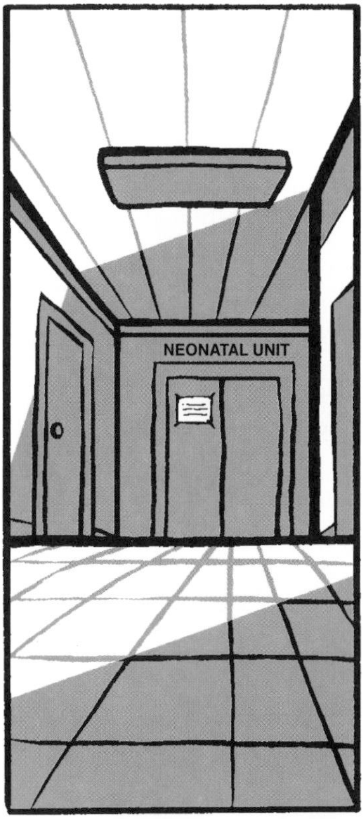
NEONATAL UNIT

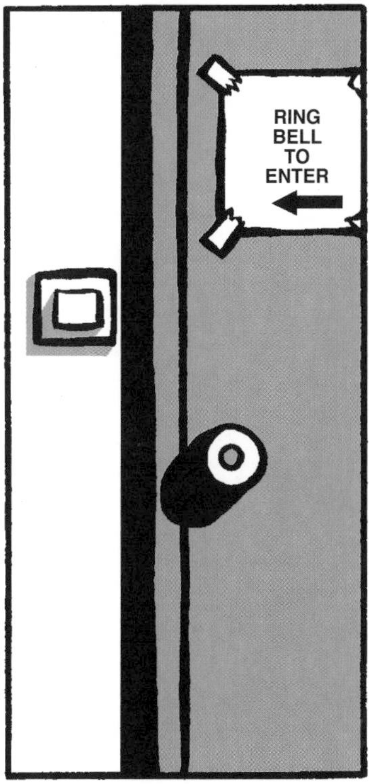
RING BELL TO ENTER

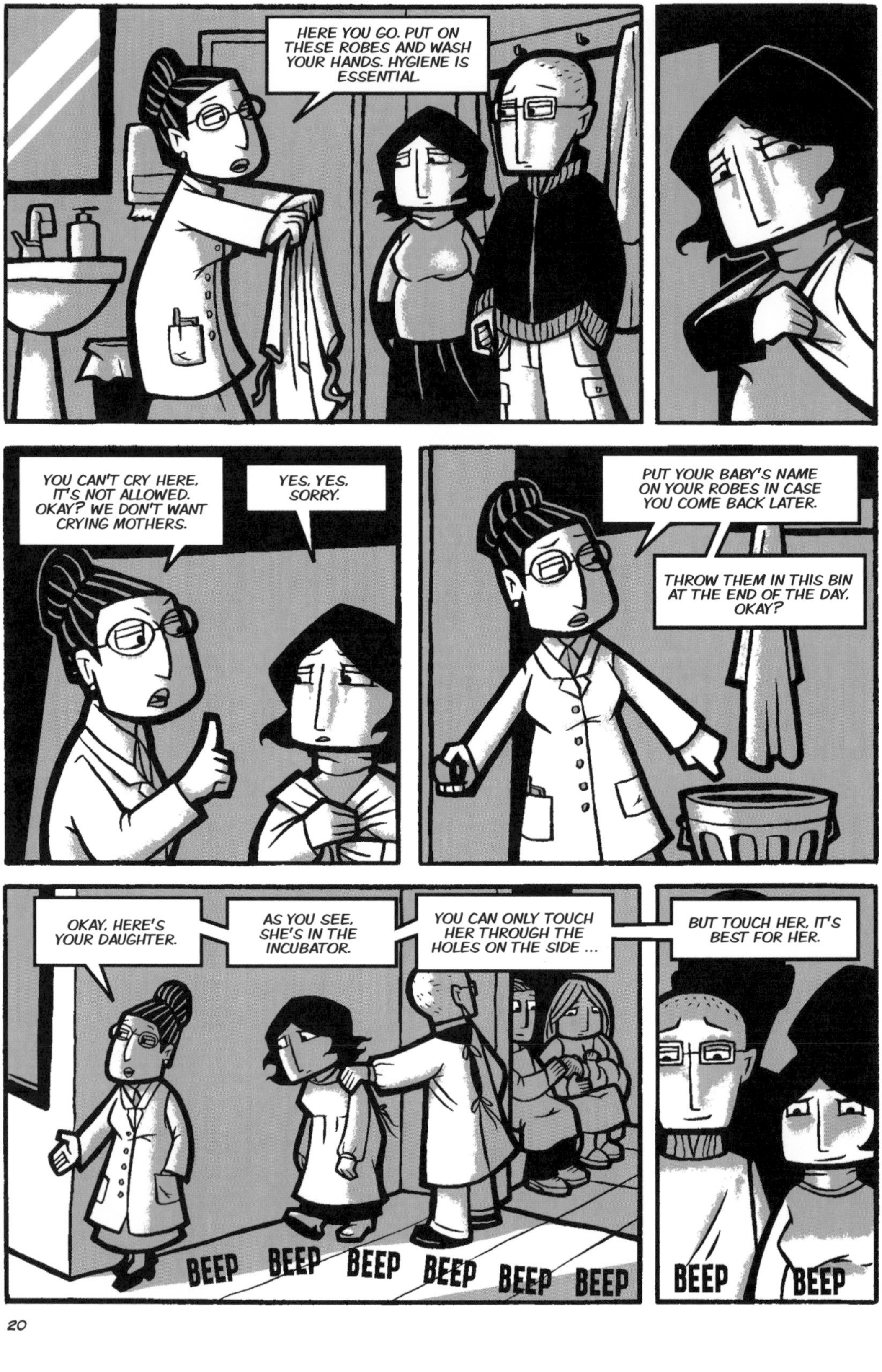
HERE YOU GO. PUT ON THESE ROBES AND WASH YOUR HANDS. HYGIENE IS ESSENTIAL.
YOU CAN'T CRY HERE. IT'S NOT ALLOWED. OKAY? WE DON'T WANT CRYING MOTHERS.
YES, YES, SORRY.
PUT YOUR BABY'S NAME ON YOUR ROBES IN CASE YOU COME BACK LATER.
THROW THEM IN THIS BIN AT THE END OF THE DAY, OKAY?
OKAY, HERE'S YOUR DAUGHTER.
AS YOU SEE, SHE'S IN THE INCUBATOR.
YOU CAN ONLY TOUCH HER THROUGH THE HOLES ON THE SIDE ...
BEEP BEEP BEEP BEEP BEEP BEEP
BUT TOUCH HER, IT'S BEST FOR HER.
BEEP BEEP

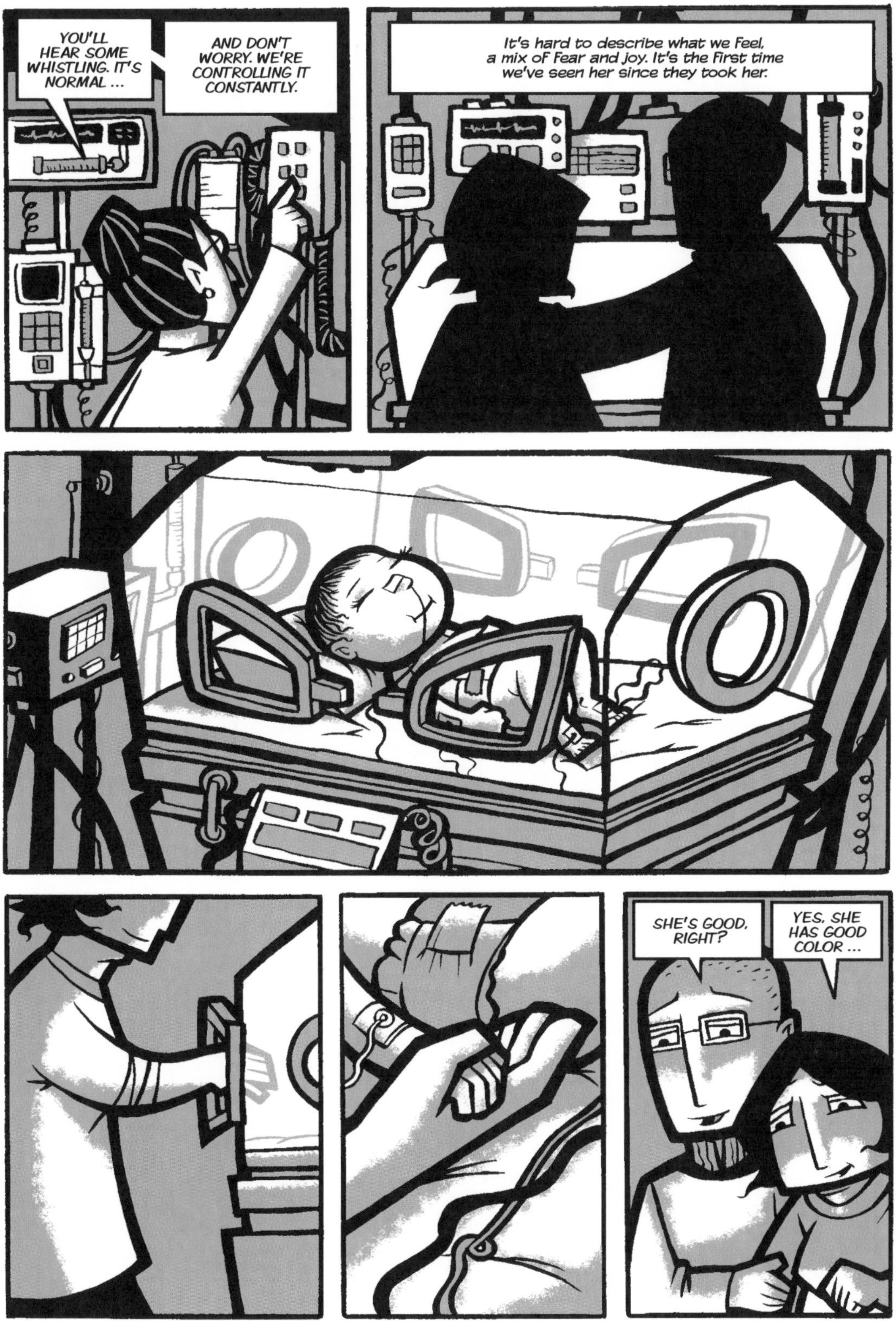
YOU'LL HEAR SOME WHISTLING. IT'S NORMAL ...
AND DON'T WORRY. WE'RE CONTROLLING IT CONSTANTLY.
It's hard to describe what we feel, a mix of fear and joy. It's the first time we've seen her since they took her.
SHE'S GOOD, RIGHT?
YES, SHE HAS GOOD COLOR ...

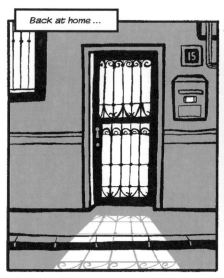

Back at home ...

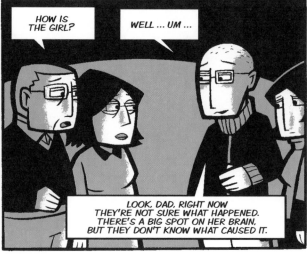

HOW IS THE GIRL?

WELL ... UM ...

LOOK, DAD, RIGHT NOW THEY'RE NOT SURE WHAT HAPPENED. THERE'S A BIG SPOT ON HER BRAIN, BUT THEY DON'T KNOW WHAT CAUSED IT.

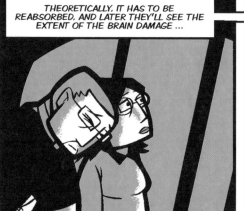

THEORETICALLY, IT HAS TO BE REABSORBED, AND LATER THEY'LL SEE THE EXTENT OF THE BRAIN DAMAGE ...

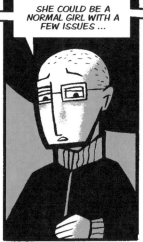

SHE COULD BE A NORMAL GIRL WITH A FEW ISSUES ...

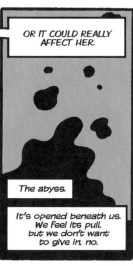

OR IT COULD REALLY AFFECT HER.

The abyss.

It's opened beneath us. We feel its pull, but we don't want to give in, no.

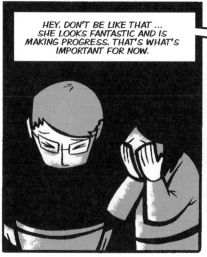

HEY, DON'T BE LIKE THAT ... SHE LOOKS FANTASTIC AND IS MAKING PROGRESS, THAT'S WHAT'S IMPORTANT FOR NOW.

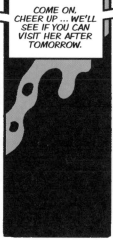

COME ON, CHEER UP ... WE'LL SEE IF YOU CAN VISIT HER AFTER TOMORROW.

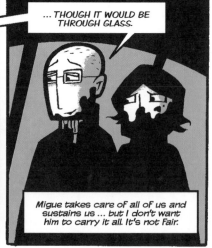

... THOUGH IT WOULD BE THROUGH GLASS.

Migue takes care of all of us and sustains us ... but I don't want him to carry it all. It's not fair.

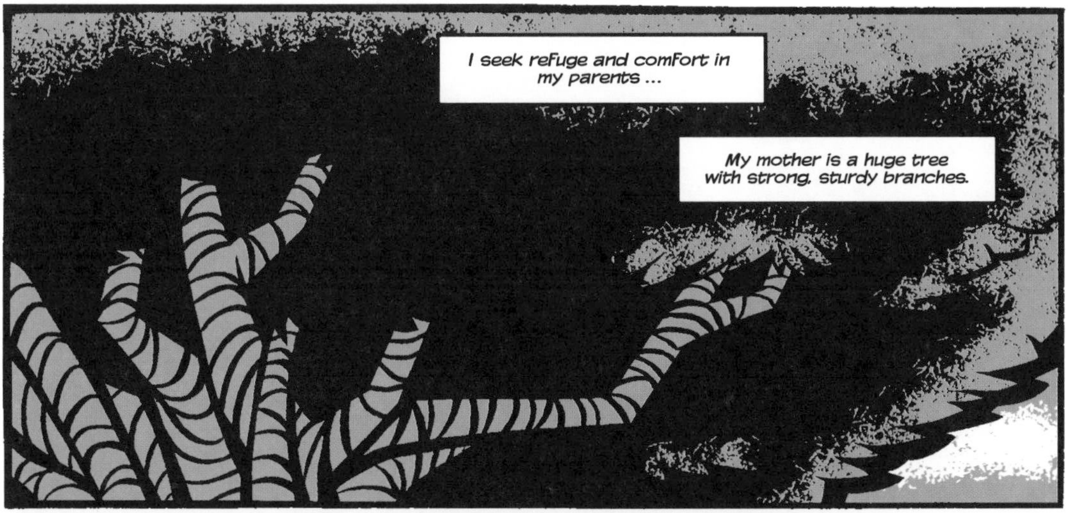
I seek refuge and comfort in my parents ...
My mother is a huge tree with strong, sturdy branches.
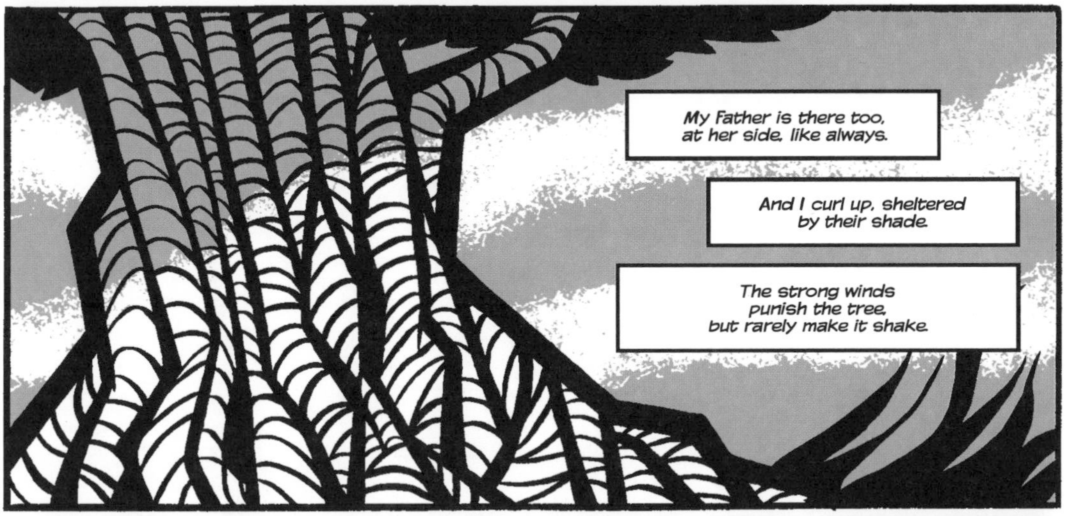
My father is there too, at her side, like always.
And I curl up, sheltered by their shade.
The strong winds punish the tree, but rarely make it shake.
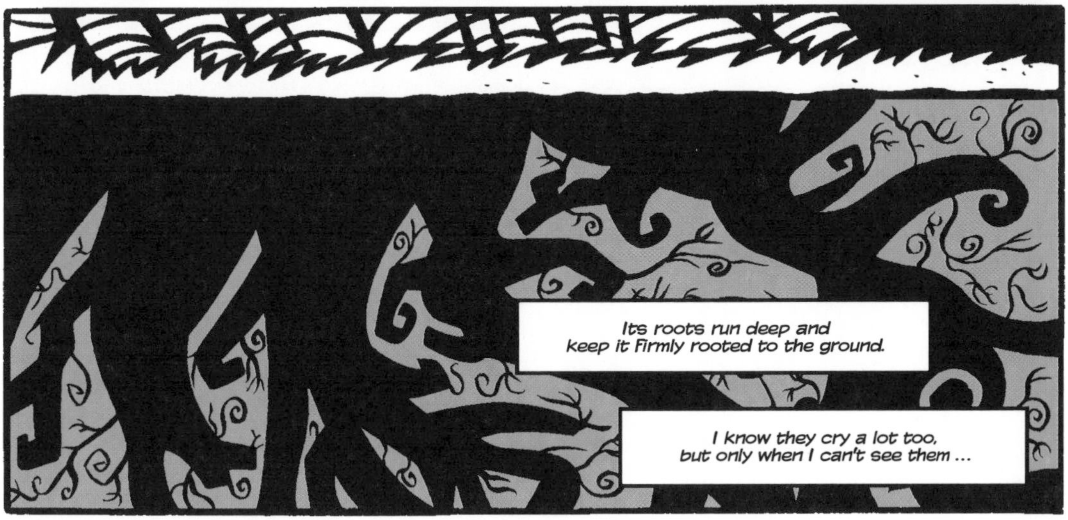
Its roots run deep and keep it firmly rooted to the ground.
I know they cry a lot too, but only when I can't see them ...

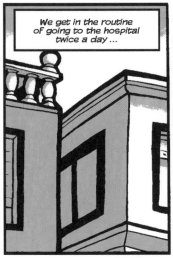

We get in the routine of going to the hospital twice a day ...

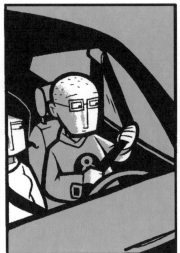

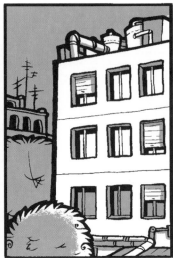

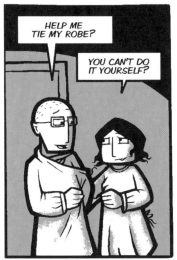

HELP ME TIE MY ROBE?

YOU CAN'T DO IT YOURSELF?

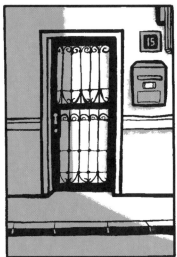

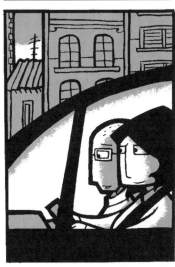

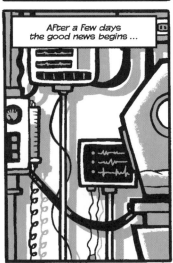

After a few days the good news begins ...

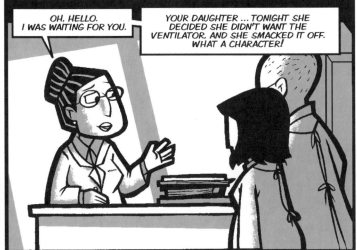

OH, HELLO. I WAS WAITING FOR YOU.

YOUR DAUGHTER ... TONIGHT SHE DECIDED SHE DIDN'T WANT THE VENTILATOR, AND SHE SMACKED IT OFF. WHAT A CHARACTER!

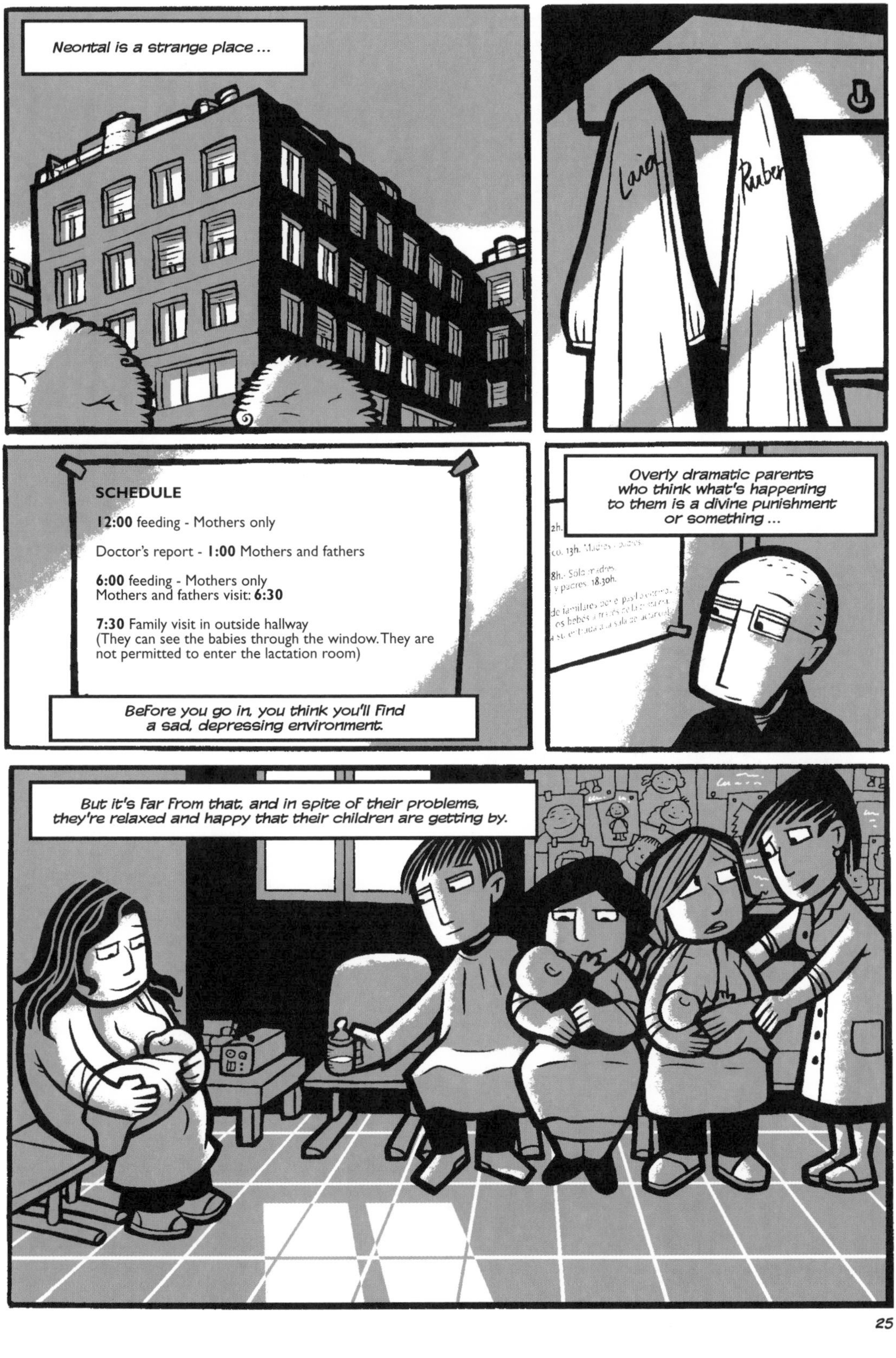
Neontal is a strange place ...
Laia
Ruben
SCHEDULE
12:00 feeding - Mothers only
Doctor's report - 1:00 Mothers and fathers
6:00 feeding - Mothers only
Mothers and fathers visit: 6:30
7:30 Family visit in outside hallway
(They can see the babies through the window. They are not permitted to enter the lactation room)
Before you go in, you think you'll find a sad, depressing environment.
Overly dramatic parents who think what's happening to them is a divine punishment or something ...
But it's far from that, and in spite of their problems, they're relaxed and happy that their children are getting by.

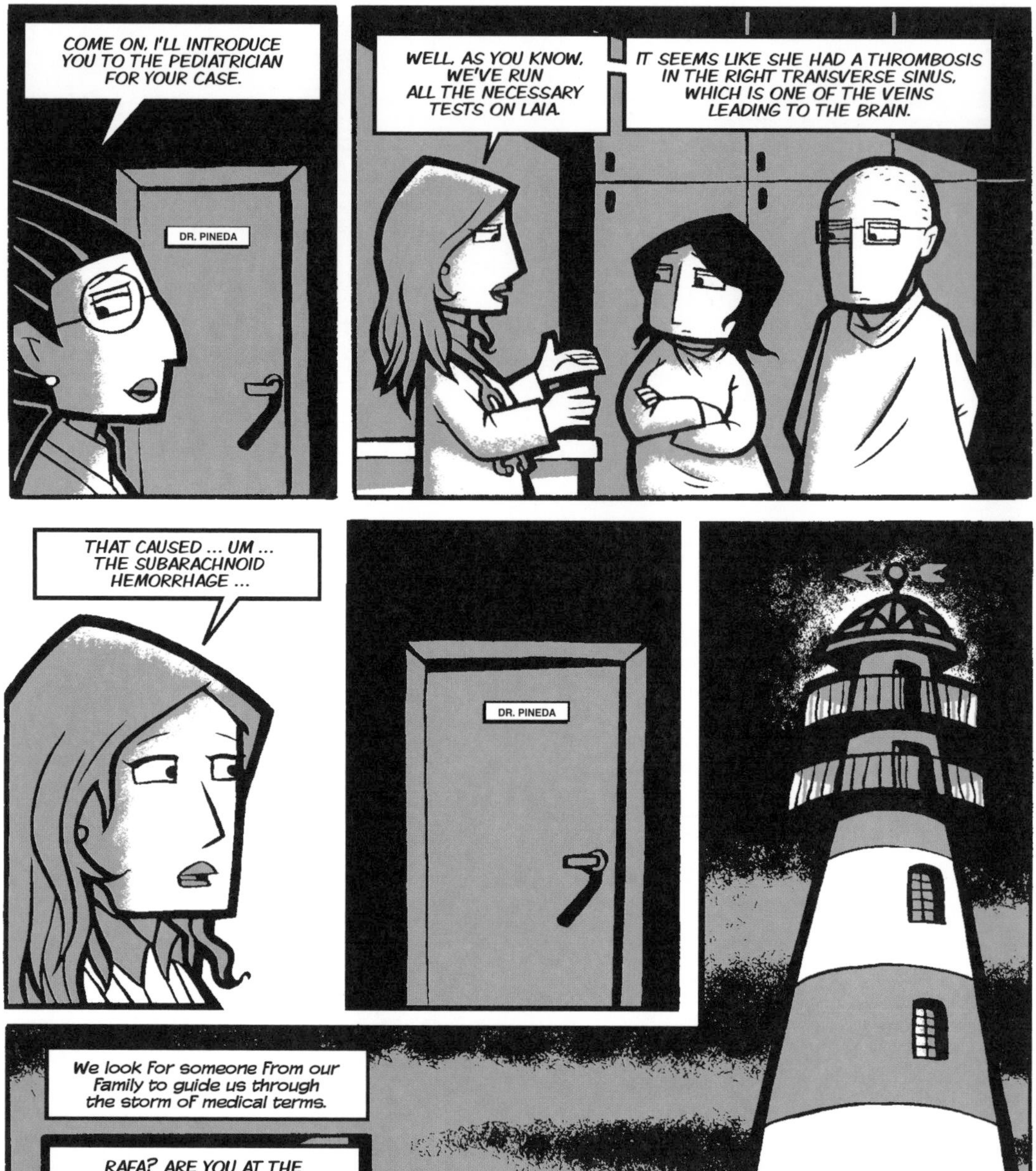
COME ON, I'LL INTRODUCE YOU TO THE PEDIATRICIAN FOR YOUR CASE.
DR. PINEDA
WELL, AS YOU KNOW, WE'VE RUN ALL THE NECESSARY TESTS ON LAIA.
IT SEEMS LIKE SHE HAD A THROMBOSIS IN THE RIGHT TRANSVERSE SINUS, WHICH IS ONE OF THE VEINS LEADING TO THE BRAIN.
THAT CAUSED ... UM ... THE SUBARACHNOID HEMORRHAGE ...
DR. PINEDA
We look for someone from our family to guide us through the storm of medical terms.
RAFA? ARE YOU AT THE HOSPITAL? CAN YOU TALK NOW?
His calm voice and the way he explains things calmly help us understand everything.
A SUBARACHNOID HEMORRHAGE IS ... IMAGINE A FIELD FULL OF WATER, AND THE WATER IS SLOWLY REABSORBED ...

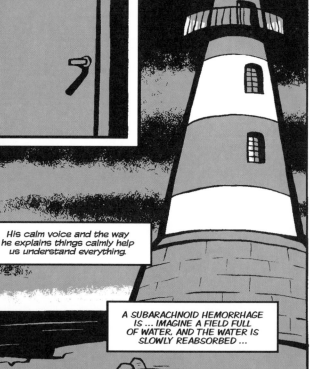

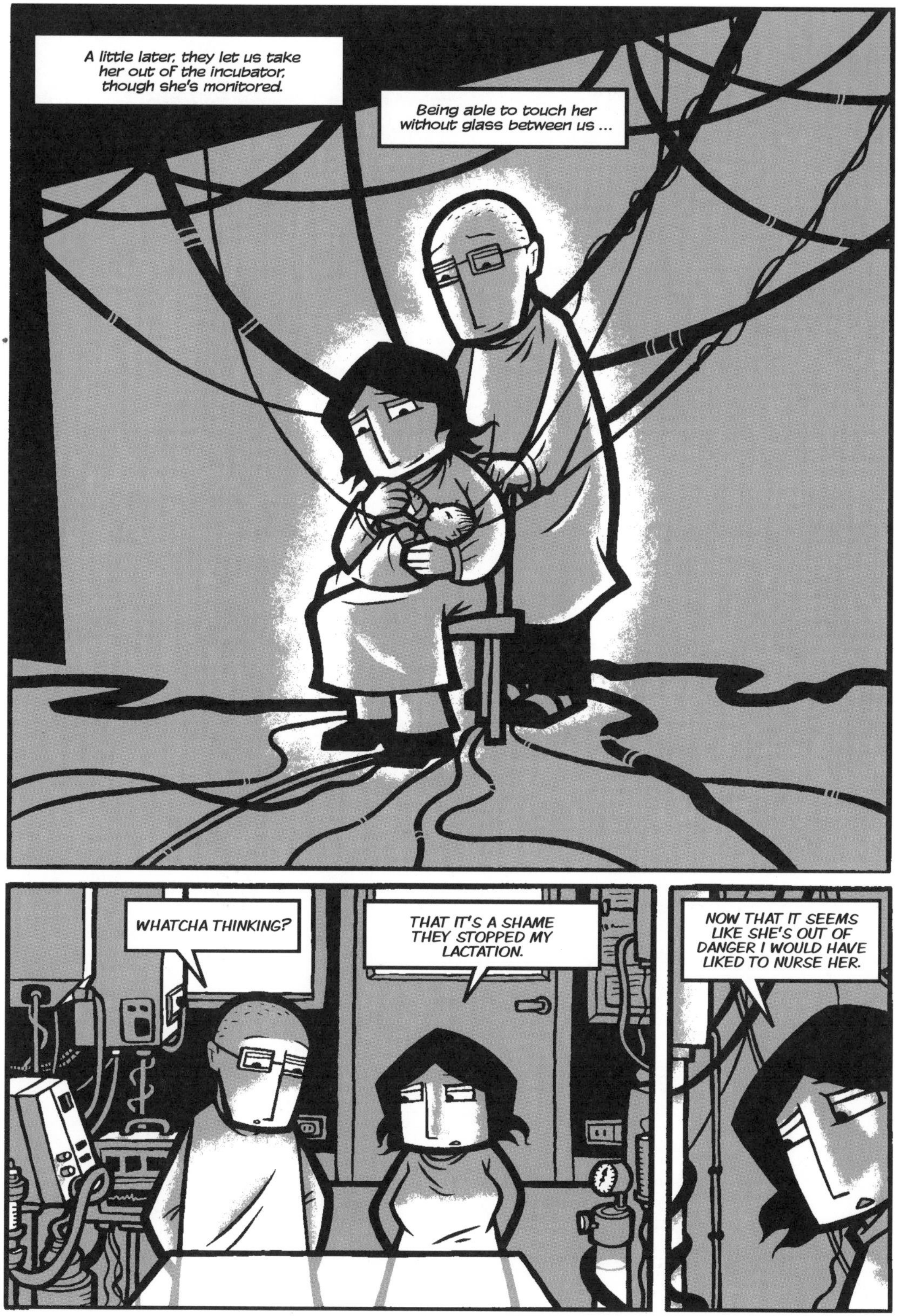
A little later, they let us take her out of the incubator, though she's monitored.
Being able to touch her without glass between us ...
WHATCHA THINKING?
THAT IT'S A SHAME THEY STOPPED MY LACTATION.
NOW THAT IT SEEMS LIKE SHE'S OUT OF DANGER I WOULD HAVE LIKED TO NURSE HER.

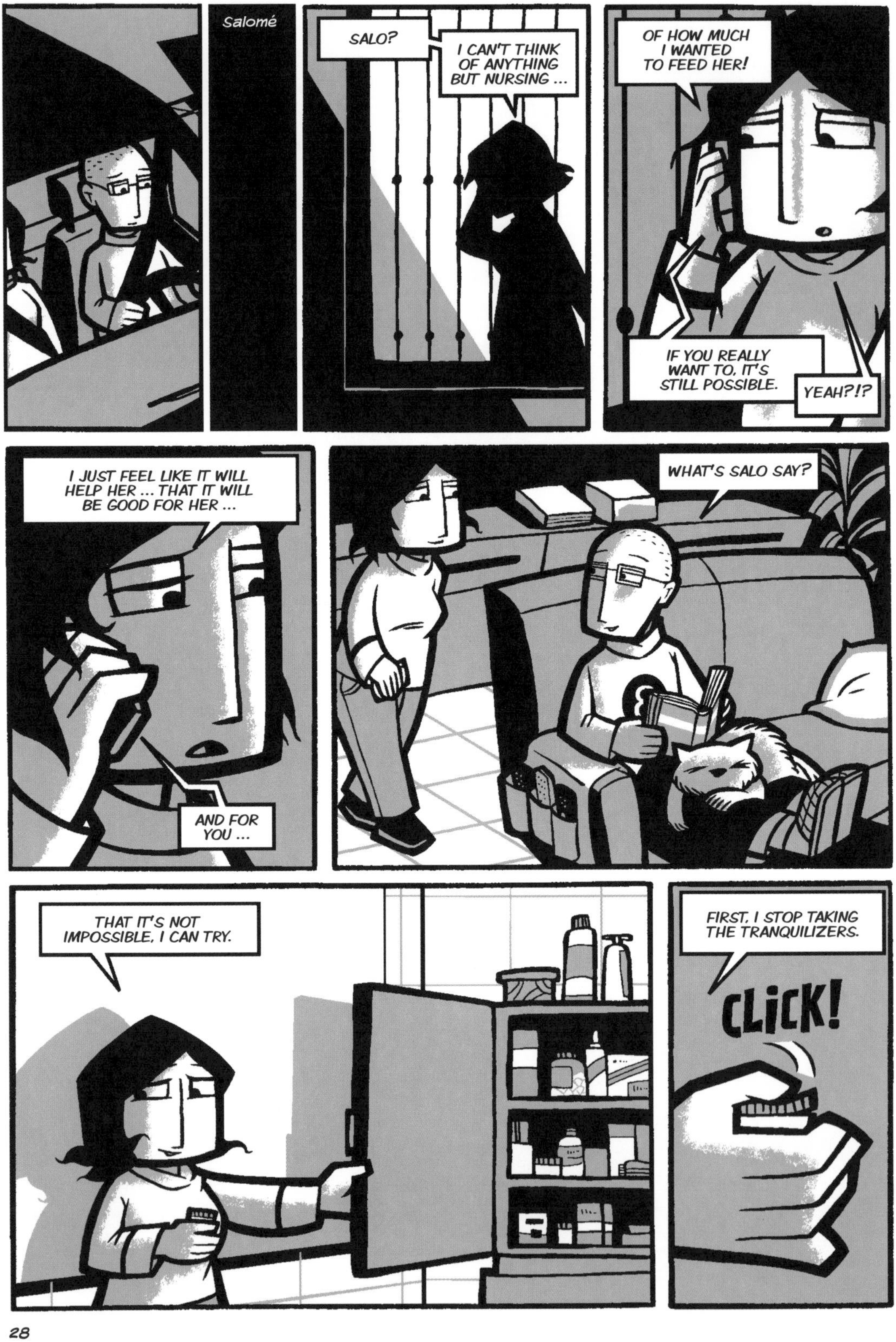
Salomé
SALO?
I CAN'T THINK OF ANYTHING BUT NURSING ...
OF HOW MUCH I WANTED TO FEED HER!
IF YOU REALLY WANT TO, IT'S STILL POSSIBLE.
YEAH?!?
I JUST FEEL LIKE IT WILL HELP HER ... THAT IT WILL BE GOOD FOR HER ...
AND FOR YOU ...
WHAT'S SALO SAY?
THAT IT'S NOT IMPOSSIBLE, I CAN TRY.
FIRST, I STOP TAKING THE TRANQUILIZERS.
CLICK!

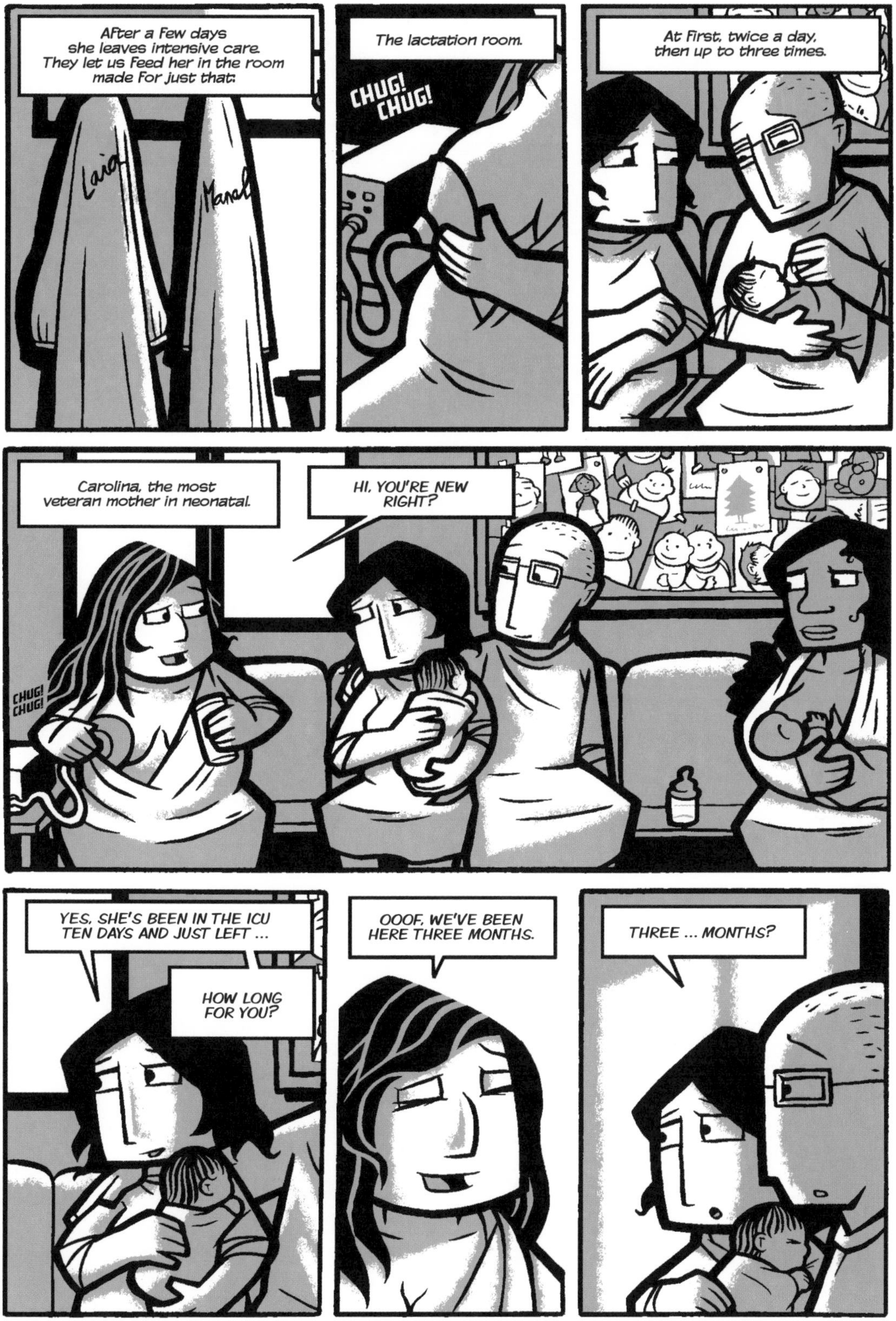
After a Few days she leaves intensive care. They let us Feed her in the room made For just that:
Laia
Manal
The lactation room.
CHUG! CHUG!
At First, twice a day, then up to three times.
Carolina, the most veteran mother in neonatal.
HI, YOU'RE NEW RIGHT?
CHUG! CHUG!
YES, SHE'S BEEN IN THE ICU TEN DAYS AND JUST LEFT ...
HOW LONG FOR YOU?
OOOF, WE'VE BEEN HERE THREE MONTHS.
THREE ... MONTHS?

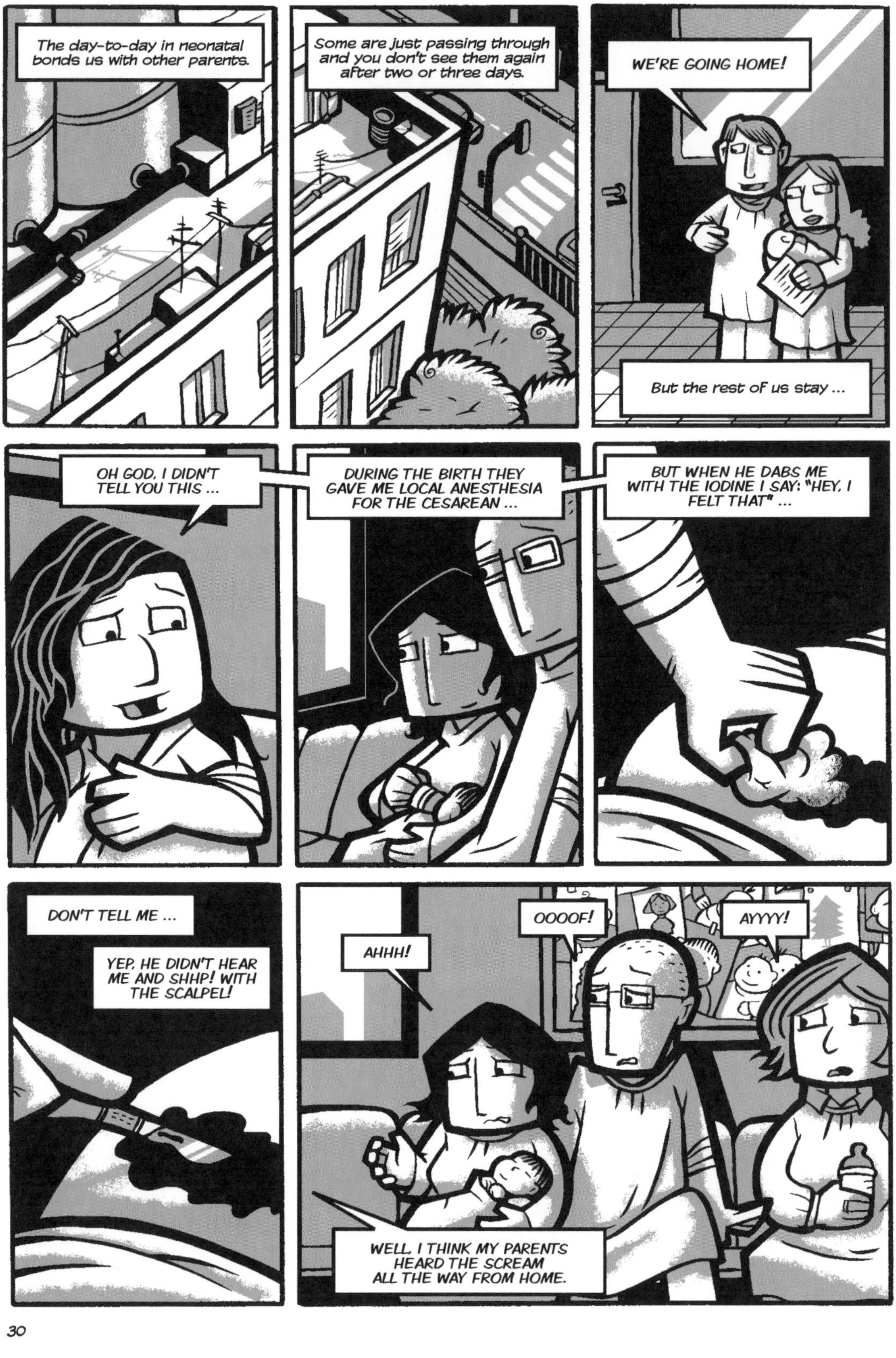
The day-to-day in neonatal bonds us with other parents.
Some are just passing through and you don't see them again after two or three days.
WE'RE GOING HOME!
But the rest of us stay ...
OH GOD, I DIDN'T TELL YOU THIS ...
DURING THE BIRTH THEY GAVE ME LOCAL ANESTHESIA FOR THE CESAREAN ...
BUT WHEN HE DABS ME WITH THE IODINE I SAY: "HEY, I FELT THAT" ...
DON'T TELL ME ...
YEP, HE DIDN'T HEAR ME AND SHHP! WITH THE SCALPEL!
AHHH!
OOOOF!
AYYYY!
WELL, I THINK MY PARENTS HEARD THE SCREAM ALL THE WAY FROM HOME.

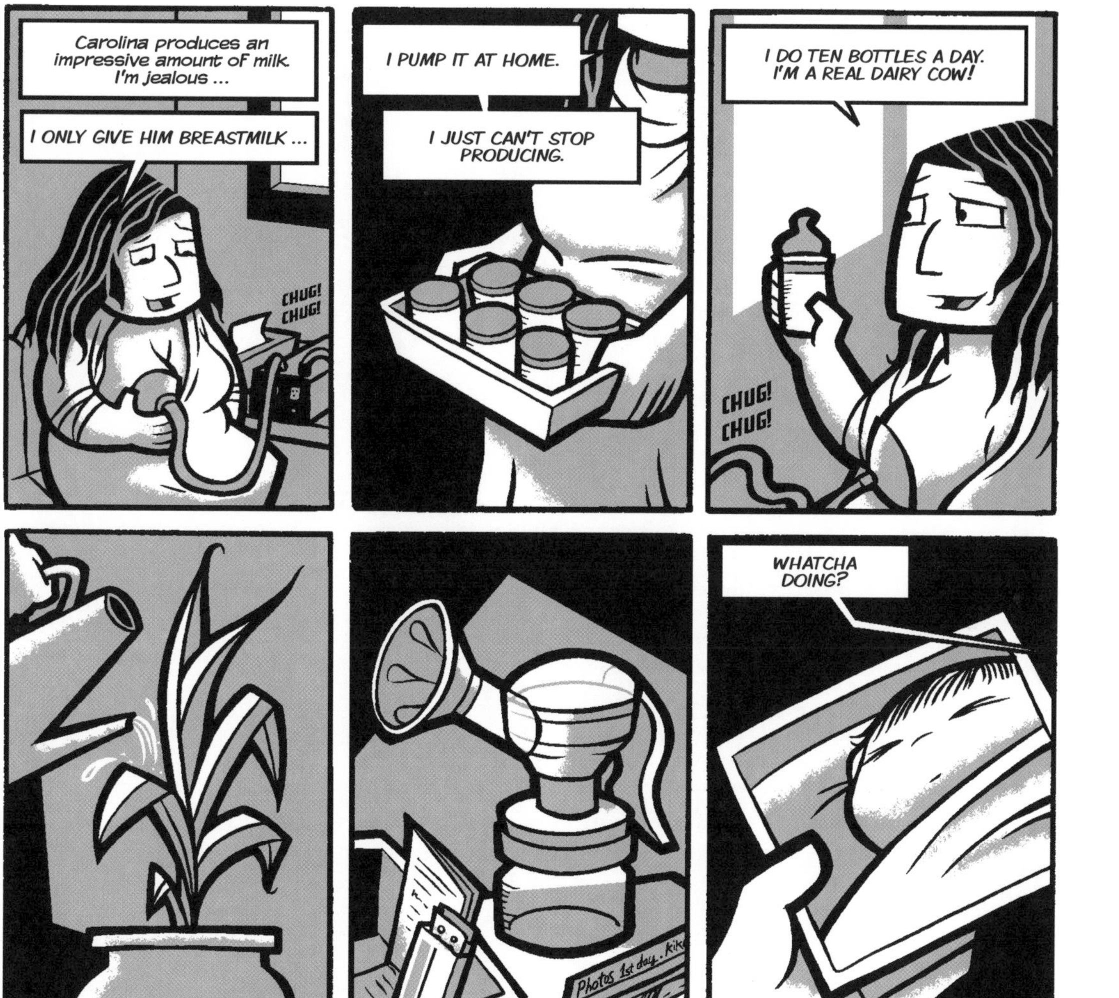
Carolina produces an impressive amount of milk. I'm jealous ...
I ONLY GIVE HIM BREASTMILK ...
CHUG! CHUG!
I PUMP IT AT HOME.
I JUST CAN'T STOP PRODUCING.
I DO TEN BOTTLES A DAY. I'M A REAL DAIRY COW!
CHUG! CHUG!
Photos 1st day
WHATCHA DOING?
LACTATION IS PARTLY EMOTIONAL. I'M LOOKING AT A PHOTO OF HER AND THINKING OF HER ...
THE STIMULATION OF PROLACTIN IS MENTAL MORE THAN ANYTHING.
THOUGH, OF COURSE, IDEALLY I COULD TOUCH HER. SMELL HER ... KISS HER.

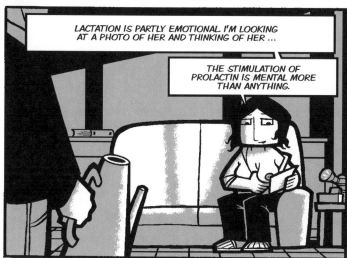

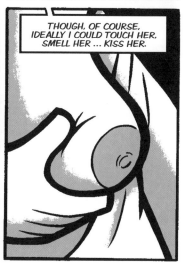

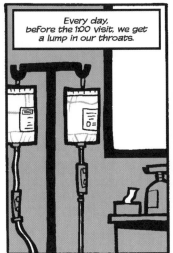

Every day, before the 1:00 visit, we get a lump in our throats.

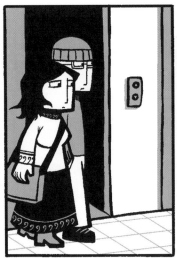

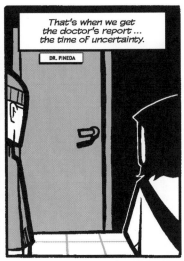

That's when we get the doctor's report ... the time of uncertainty.

DR. PINEDA

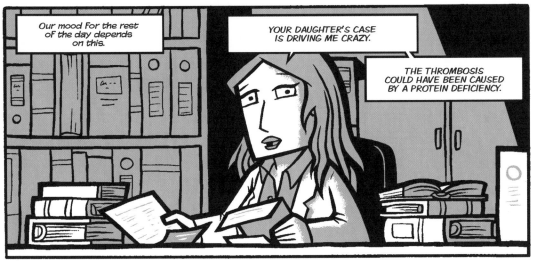

Our mood for the rest of the day depends on this.

YOUR DAUGHTER'S CASE IS DRIVING ME CRAZY.

THE THROMBOSIS COULD HAVE BEEN CAUSED BY A PROTEIN DEFICIENCY.

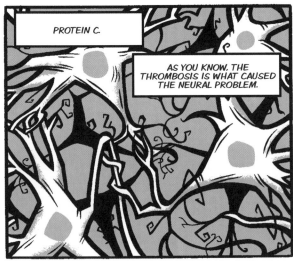

PROTEIN C.

AS YOU KNOW, THE THROMBOSIS IS WHAT CAUSED THE NEURAL PROBLEM.

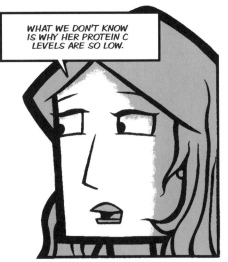

WHAT WE DON'T KNOW IS WHY HER PROTEIN C LEVELS ARE SO LOW.

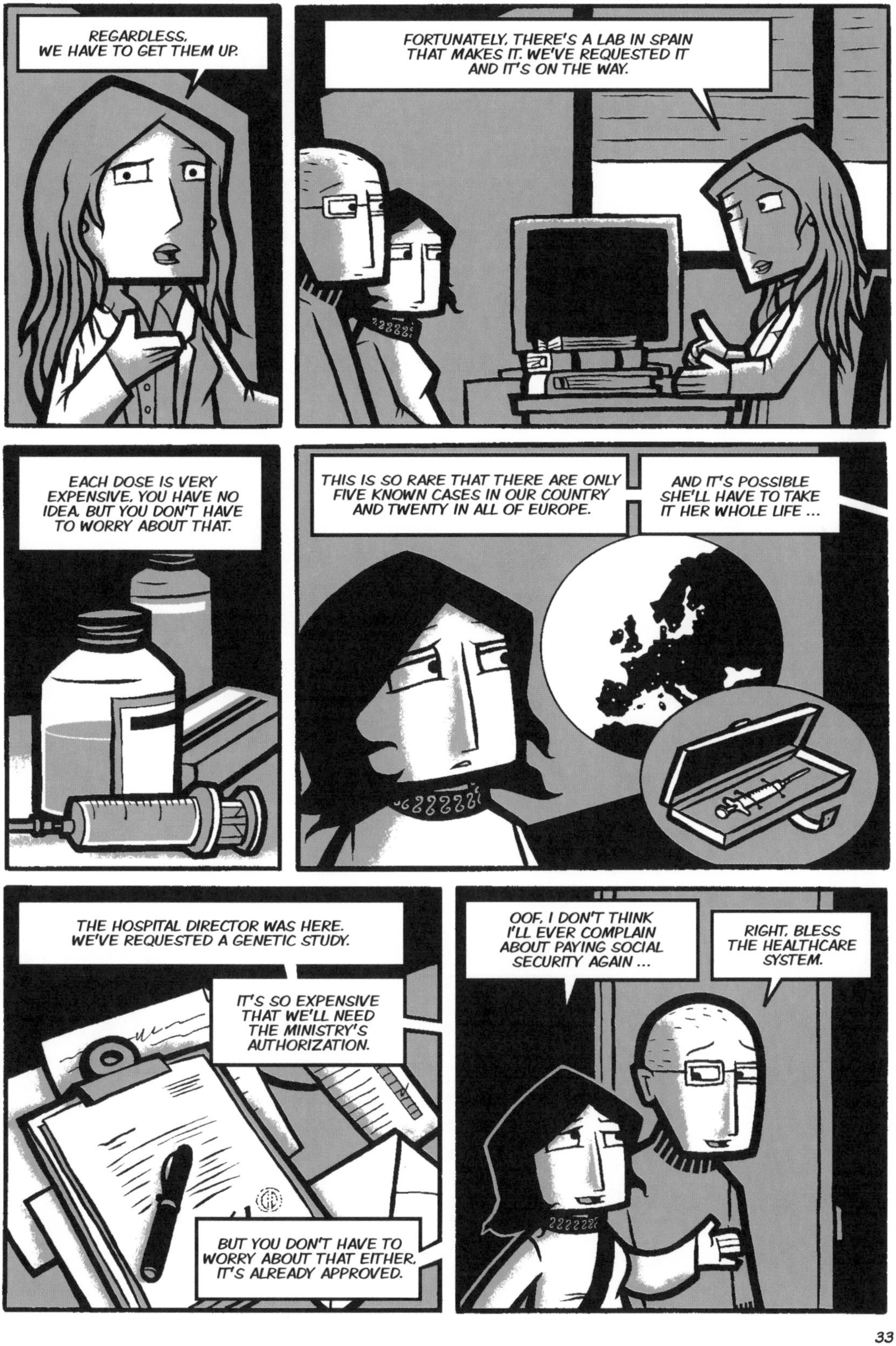
REGARDLESS, WE HAVE TO GET THEM UP.
FORTUNATELY, THERE'S A LAB IN SPAIN THAT MAKES IT. WE'VE REQUESTED IT AND IT'S ON THE WAY.
EACH DOSE IS VERY EXPENSIVE, YOU HAVE NO IDEA, BUT YOU DON'T HAVE TO WORRY ABOUT THAT.
THIS IS SO RARE THAT THERE ARE ONLY FIVE KNOWN CASES IN OUR COUNTRY AND TWENTY IN ALL OF EUROPE.
AND IT'S POSSIBLE SHE'LL HAVE TO TAKE IT HER WHOLE LIFE ...
THE HOSPITAL DIRECTOR WAS HERE. WE'VE REQUESTED A GENETIC STUDY.
IT'S SO EXPENSIVE THAT WE'LL NEED THE MINISTRY'S AUTHORIZATION.
BUT YOU DON'T HAVE TO WORRY ABOUT THAT EITHER. IT'S ALREADY APPROVED.
OOF, I DON'T THINK I'LL EVER COMPLAIN ABOUT PAYING SOCIAL SECURITY AGAIN ...
RIGHT, BLESS THE HEALTHCARE SYSTEM.

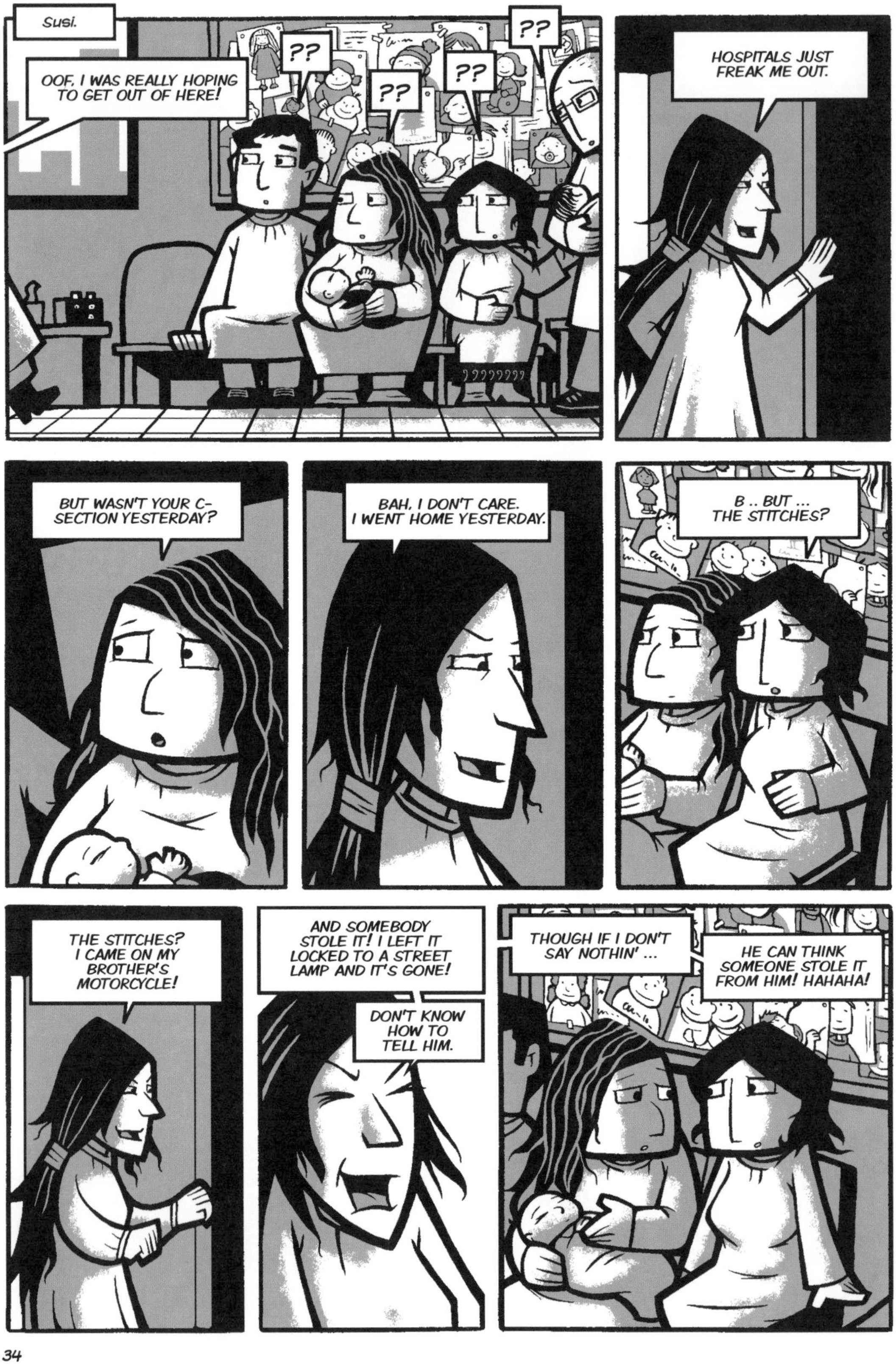

Susi.
OOF, I WAS REALLY HOPING TO GET OUT OF HERE!
??
??
??
??
HOSPITALS JUST FREAK ME OUT.
BUT WASN'T YOUR C-SECTION YESTERDAY?
BAH, I DON'T CARE. I WENT HOME YESTERDAY.
B .. BUT ... THE STITCHES?
THE STITCHES? I CAME ON MY BROTHER'S MOTORCYCLE!
AND SOMEBODY STOLE IT! I LEFT IT LOCKED TO A STREET LAMP AND IT'S GONE!
DON'T KNOW HOW TO TELL HIM.
THOUGH IF I DON'T SAY NOTHIN' ...
HE CAN THINK SOMEONE STOLE IT FROM HIM! HAHAHA!

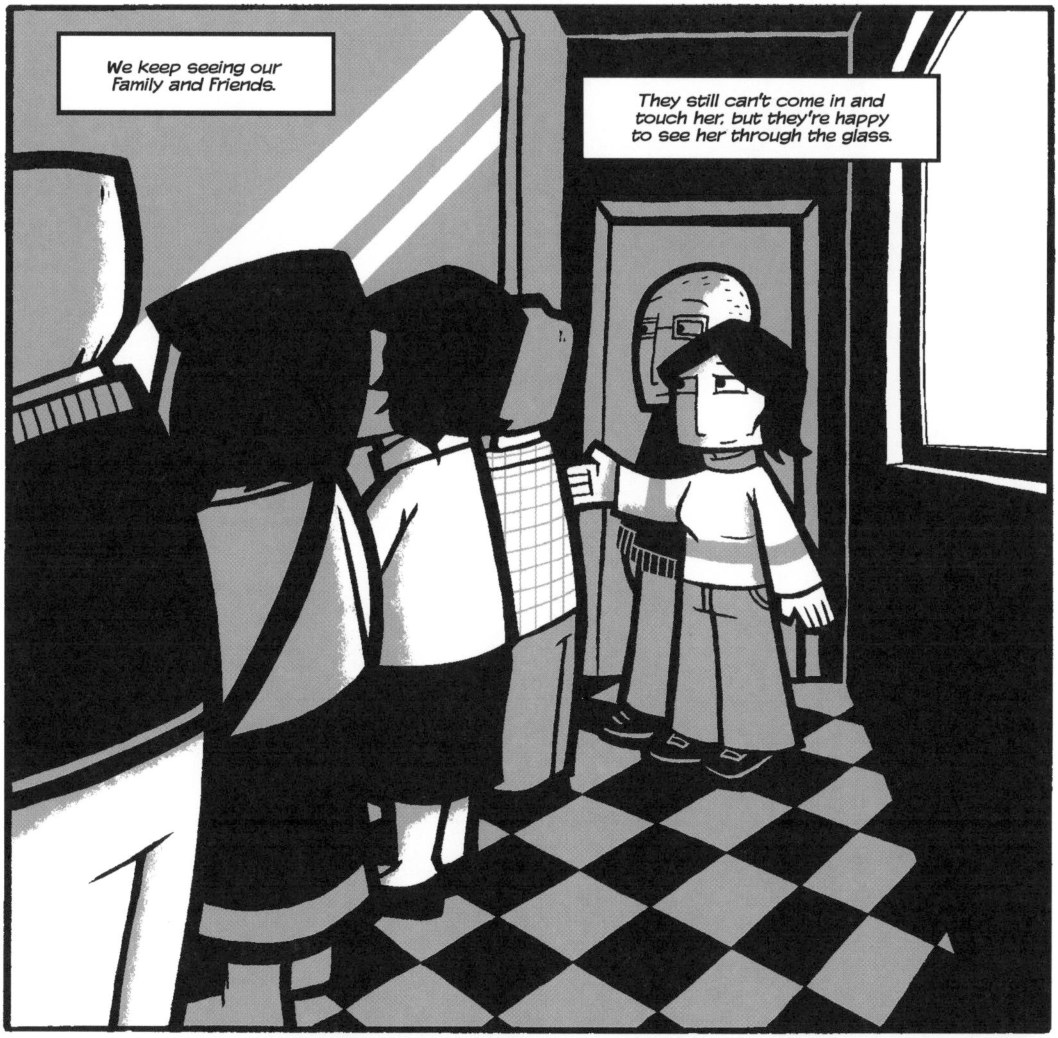
We keep seeing our Family and Friends.
They still can't come in and touch her, but they're happy to see her through the glass.

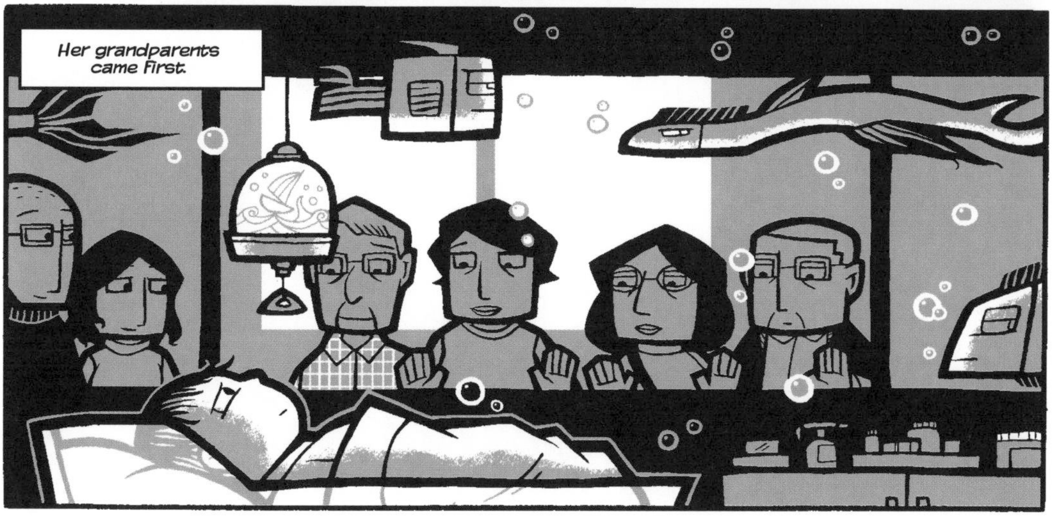
Her grandparents came First.

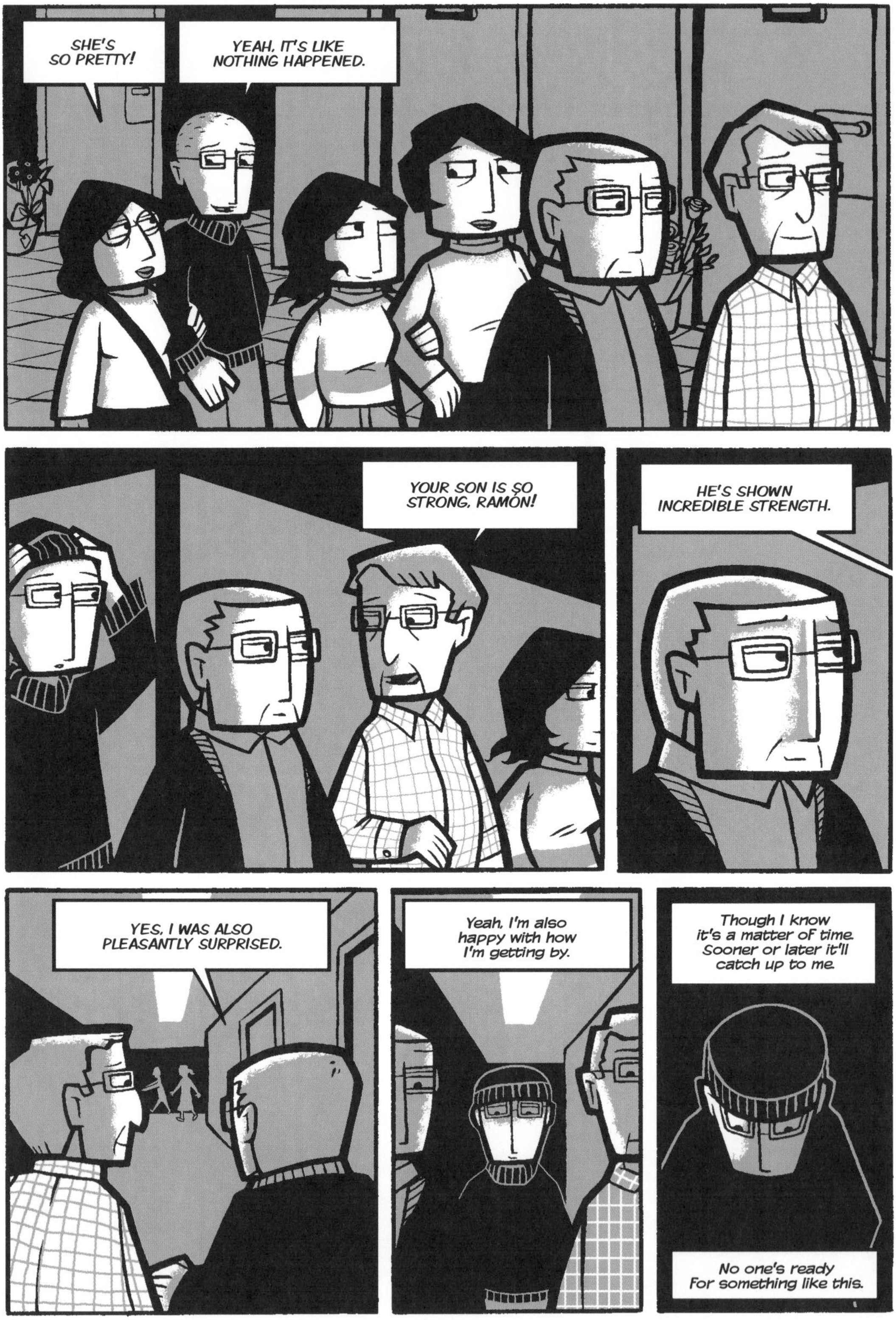
SHE'S SO PRETTY!
YEAH, IT'S LIKE NOTHING HAPPENED.
YOUR SON IS SO STRONG, RAMÓN!
HE'S SHOWN INCREDIBLE STRENGTH.
YES, I WAS ALSO PLEASANTLY SURPRISED.
Yeah, I'm also happy with how I'm getting by.
Though I know it's a matter of time. Sooner or later it'll catch up to me.
No one's ready for something like this.

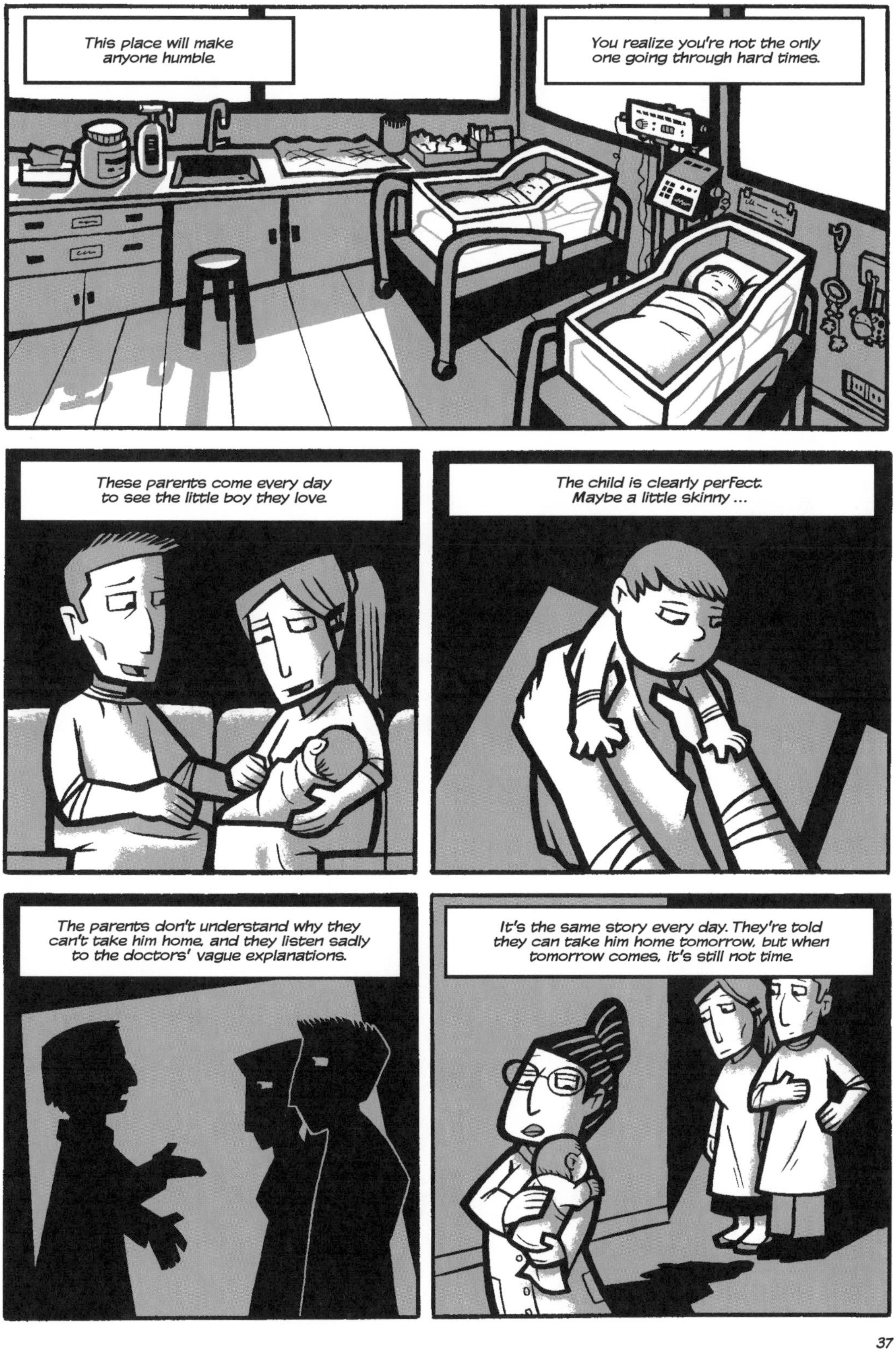
This place will make anyone humble.
You realize you're not the only one going through hard times.
These parents come every day to see the little boy they love.
The child is clearly perfect. Maybe a little skinny ...
The parents don't understand why they can't take him home, and they listen sadly to the doctors' vague explanations.
It's the same story every day. They're told they can take him home tomorrow, but when tomorrow comes, it's still not time.

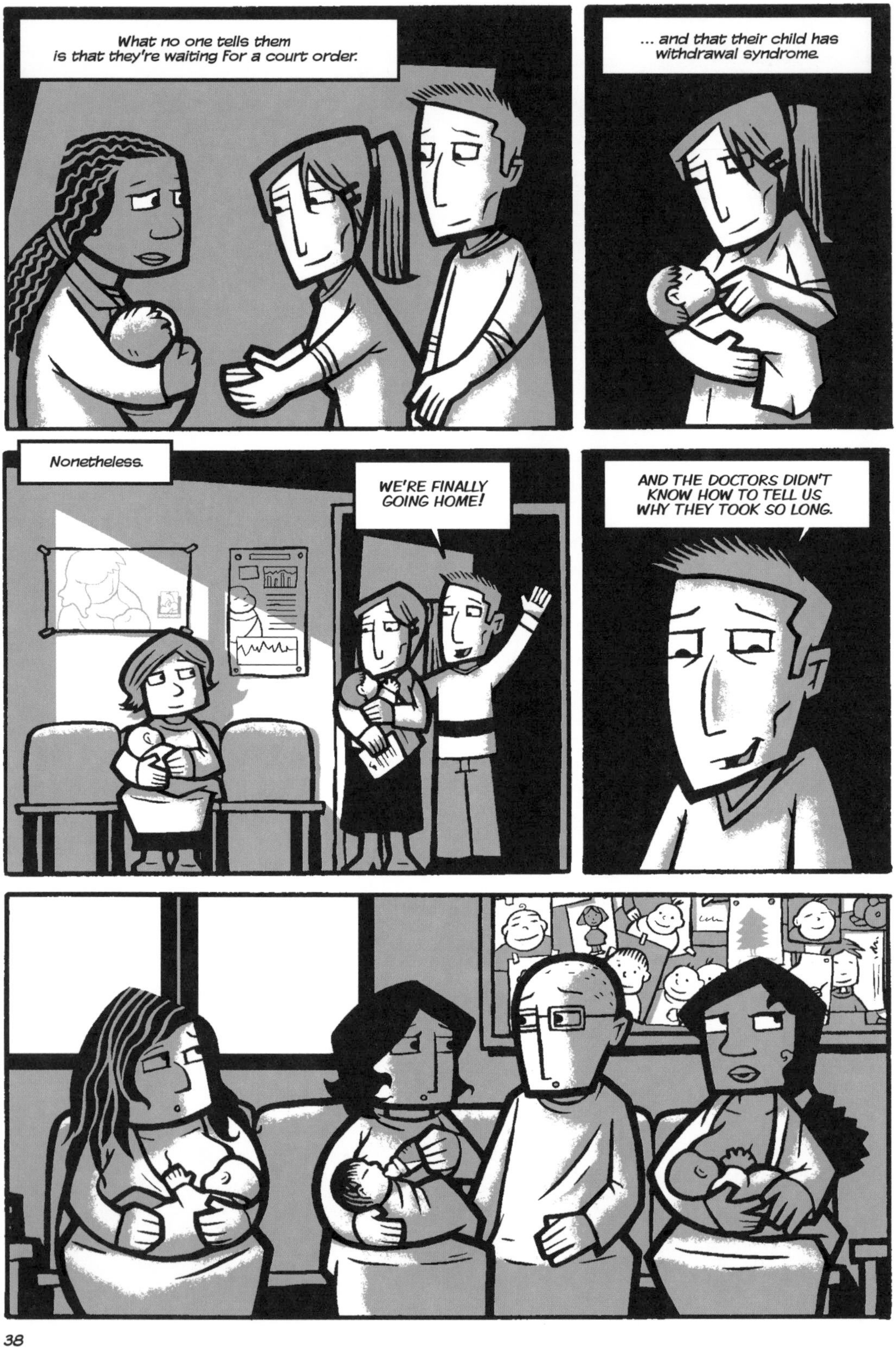
What no one tells them is that they're waiting for a court order.
... and that their child has withdrawal syndrome.
Nonetheless.
WE'RE FINALLY GOING HOME!
AND THE DOCTORS DIDN'T KNOW HOW TO TELL US WHY THEY TOOK SO LONG.

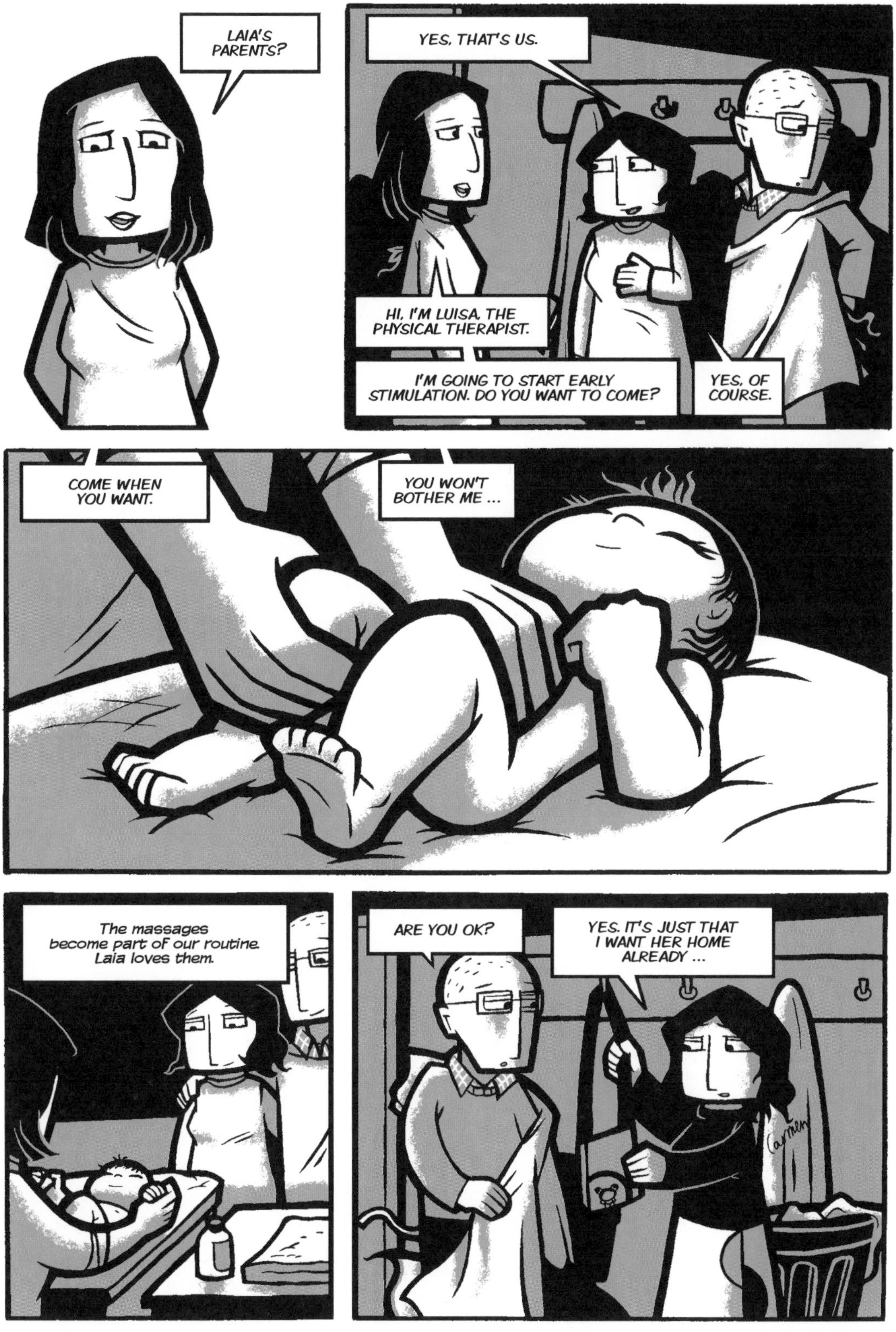
LAIA'S PARENTS?
YES, THAT'S US.
HI, I'M LUISA, THE PHYSICAL THERAPIST.
I'M GOING TO START EARLY STIMULATION. DO YOU WANT TO COME?
YES, OF COURSE.
COME WHEN YOU WANT.
YOU WON'T BOTHER ME ...
The massages become part of our routine. Laia loves them.
ARE YOU OK?
YES. IT'S JUST THAT I WANT HER HOME ALREADY ...

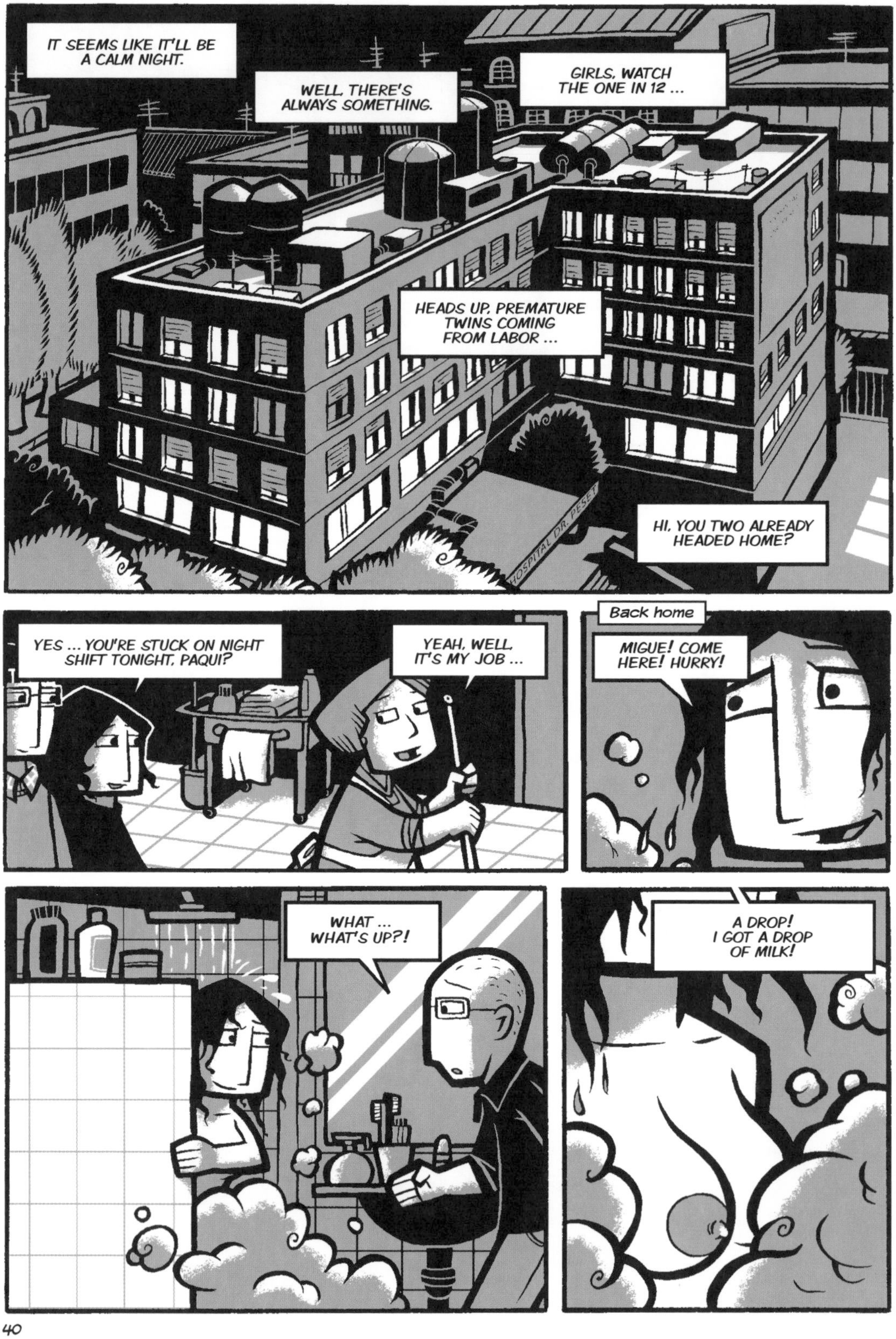
IT SEEMS LIKE IT'LL BE A CALM NIGHT.
WELL, THERE'S ALWAYS SOMETHING.
GIRLS, WATCH THE ONE IN 12 ...
HEADS UP, PREMATURE TWINS COMING FROM LABOR ...
HOSPITAL DR. PESET
HI, YOU TWO ALREADY HEADED HOME?
YES ... YOU'RE STUCK ON NIGHT SHIFT TONIGHT, PAQUI?
YEAH, WELL, IT'S MY JOB ...
Back home
MIGUE! COME HERE! HURRY!
WHAT ... WHAT'S UP?!
A DROP! I GOT A DROP OF MILK!

3.
EARTH

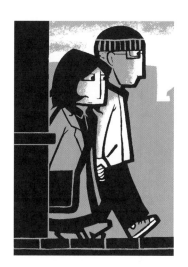

Terra para o pé, firmeza
Terra para a mâo, carícia

"Terra,"
Caetano Veloso

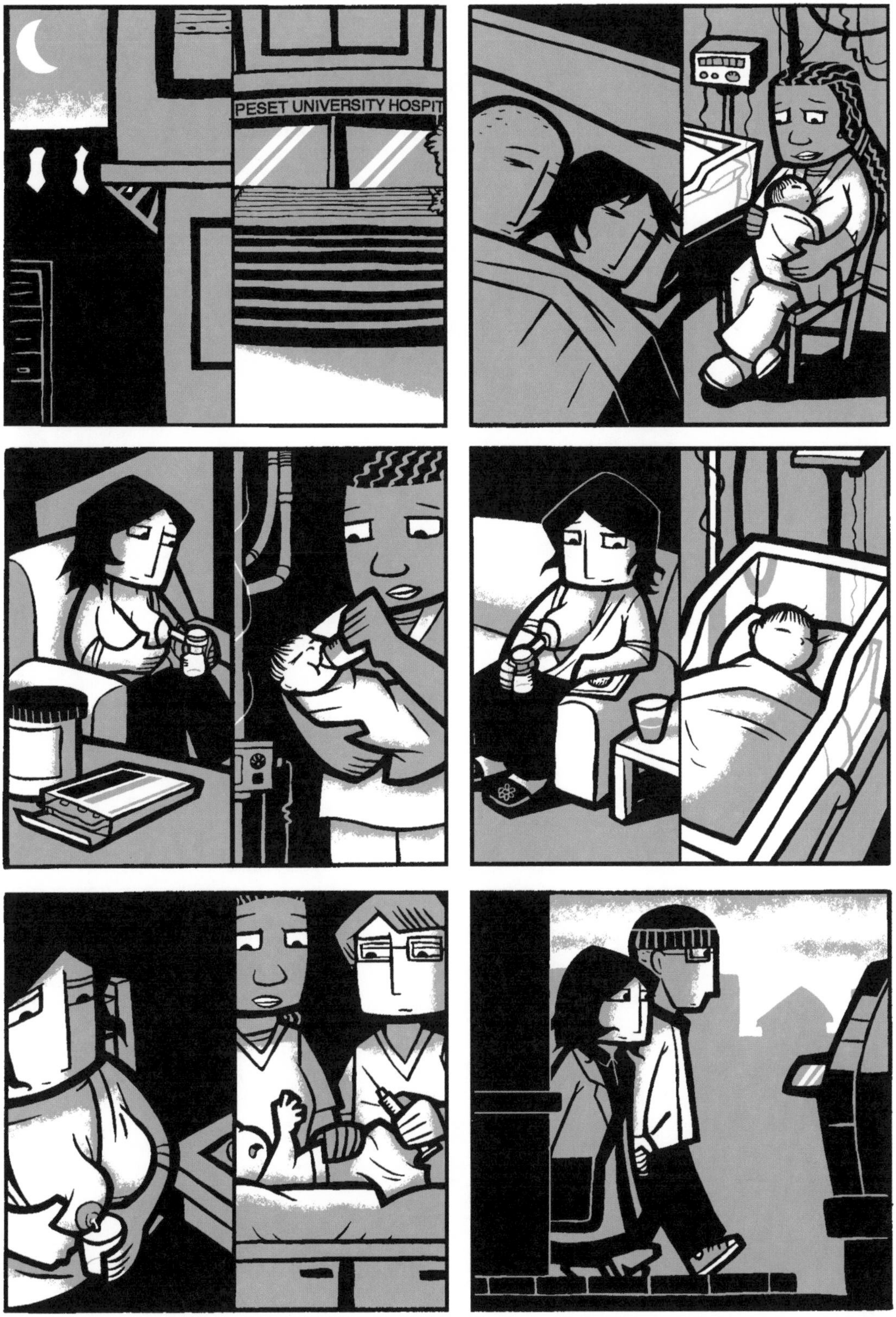
PESET UNIVERSITY HOSPIT

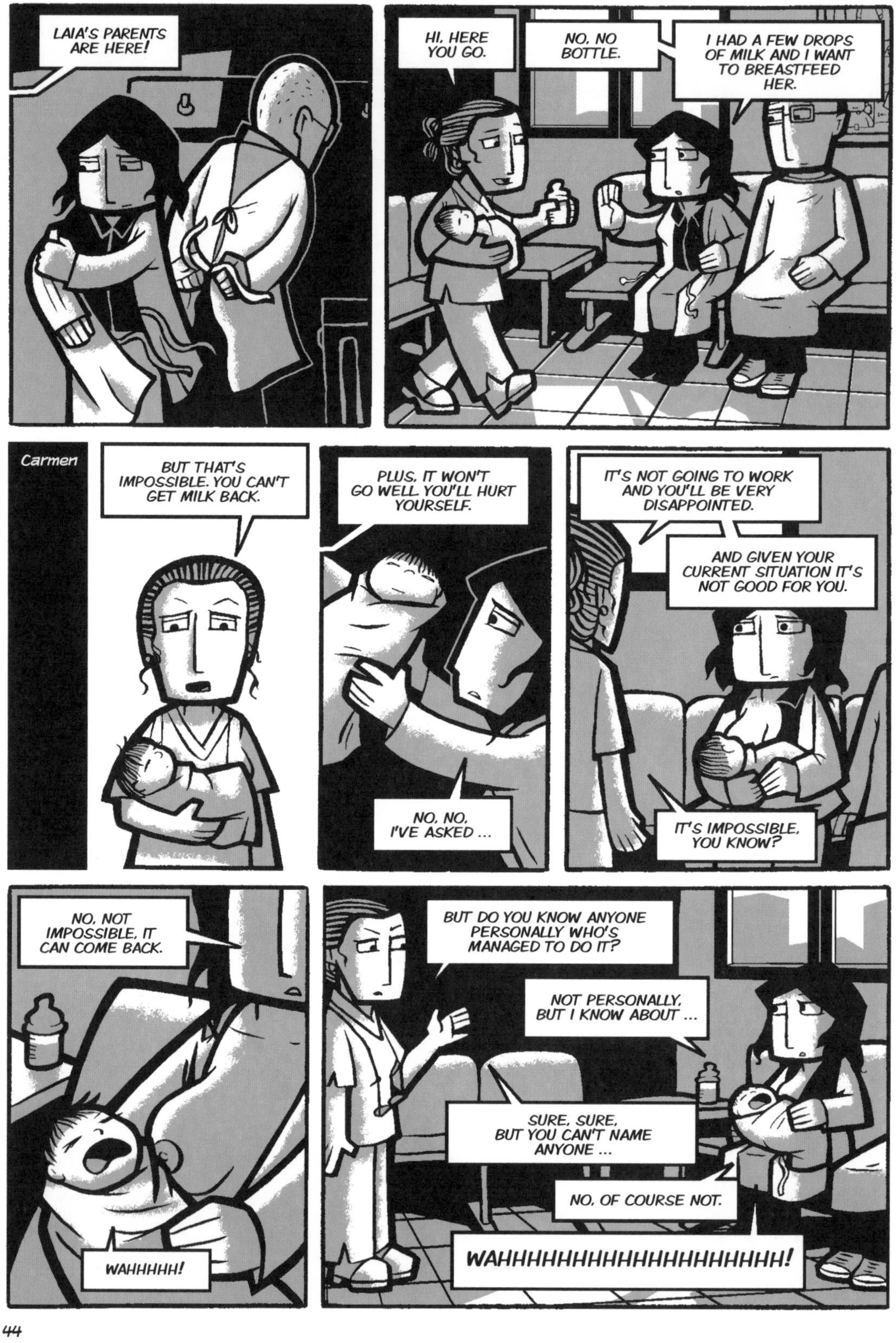
LAIA'S PARENTS ARE HERE!
HI, HERE YOU GO.
NO, NO BOTTLE.
I HAD A FEW DROPS OF MILK AND I WANT TO BREASTFEED HER.
Carmen
BUT THAT'S IMPOSSIBLE. YOU CAN'T GET MILK BACK.
PLUS, IT WON'T GO WELL. YOU'LL HURT YOURSELF.
NO, NO, I'VE ASKED ...
IT'S NOT GOING TO WORK AND YOU'LL BE VERY DISAPPOINTED.
AND GIVEN YOUR CURRENT SITUATION IT'S NOT GOOD FOR YOU.
IT'S IMPOSSIBLE, YOU KNOW?
NO, NOT IMPOSSIBLE, IT CAN COME BACK.
WAHHHHH!
BUT DO YOU KNOW ANYONE PERSONALLY WHO'S MANAGED TO DO IT?
NOT PERSONALLY, BUT I KNOW ABOUT ...
SURE, SURE, BUT YOU CAN'T NAME ANYONE ...
NO, OF COURSE NOT.
WAHHHHHHHHHHHHHHHHHHHH!

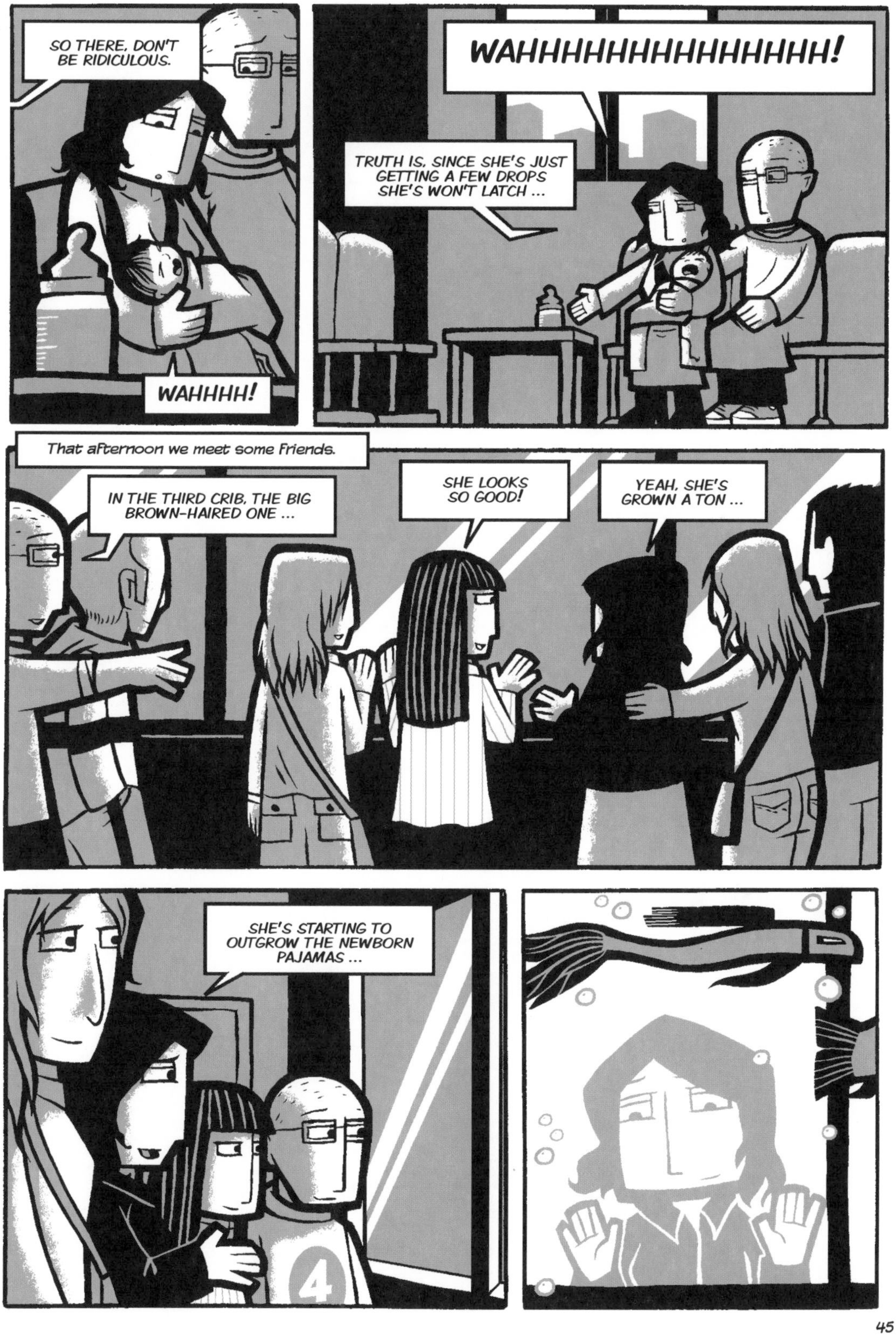
SO THERE, DON'T BE RIDICULOUS.
WAHHHH!
WAHHHHHHHHHHHHHH!
TRUTH IS, SINCE SHE'S JUST GETTING A FEW DROPS SHE'S WON'T LATCH ...
That afternoon we meet some friends.
IN THE THIRD CRIB, THE BIG BROWN-HAIRED ONE ...
SHE LOOKS SO GOOD!
YEAH, SHE'S GROWN A TON ...
SHE'S STARTING TO OUTGROW THE NEWBORN PAJAMAS ...
4

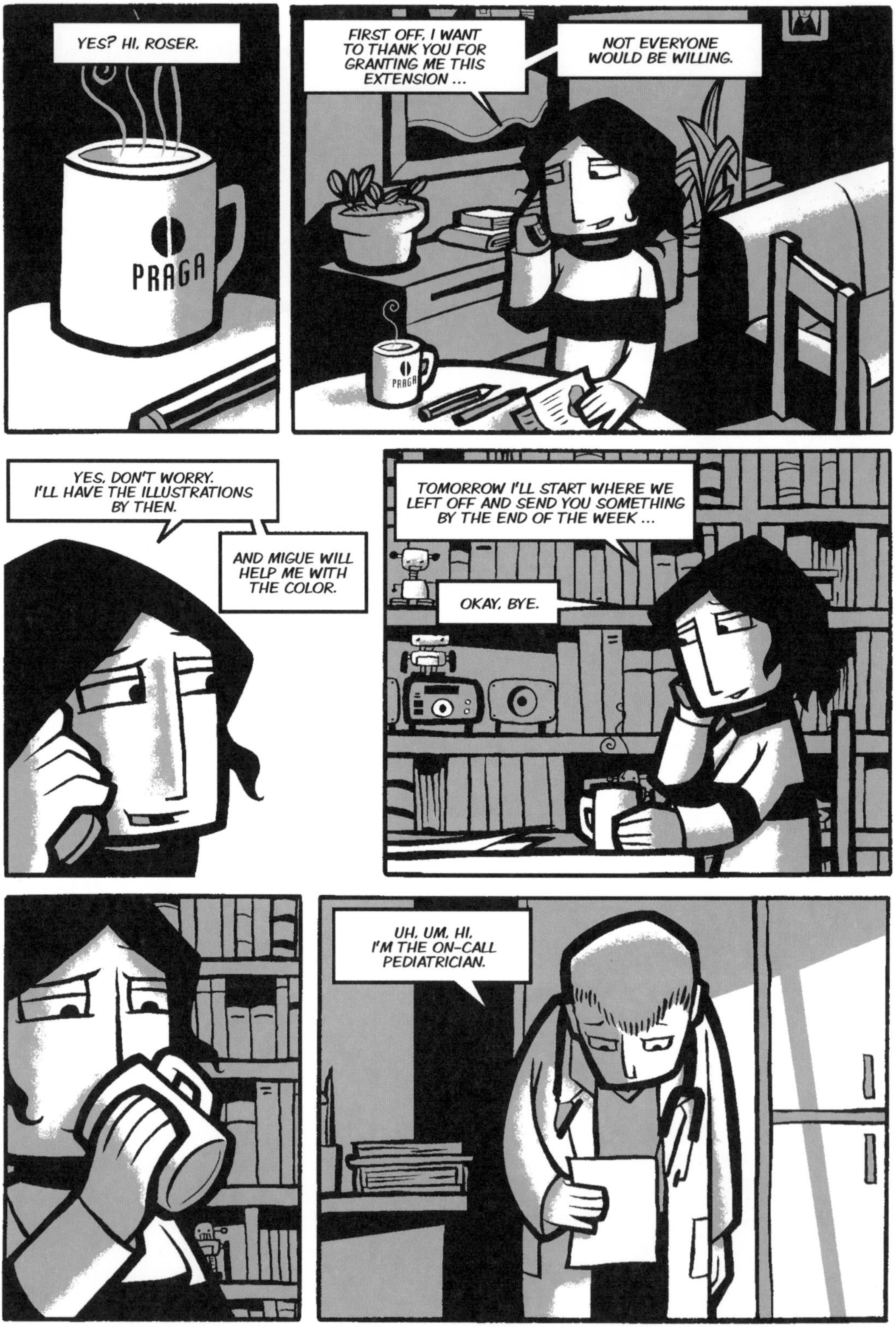
YES? HI, ROSER.
PRAGA
FIRST OFF, I WANT TO THANK YOU FOR GRANTING ME THIS EXTENSION ...
NOT EVERYONE WOULD BE WILLING.
PRAGA
YES, DON'T WORRY. I'LL HAVE THE ILLUSTRATIONS BY THEN.
AND MIGUE WILL HELP ME WITH THE COLOR.
TOMORROW I'LL START WHERE WE LEFT OFF AND SEND YOU SOMETHING BY THE END OF THE WEEK ...
OKAY, BYE.
UH, UM, HI, I'M THE ON-CALL PEDIATRICIAN.

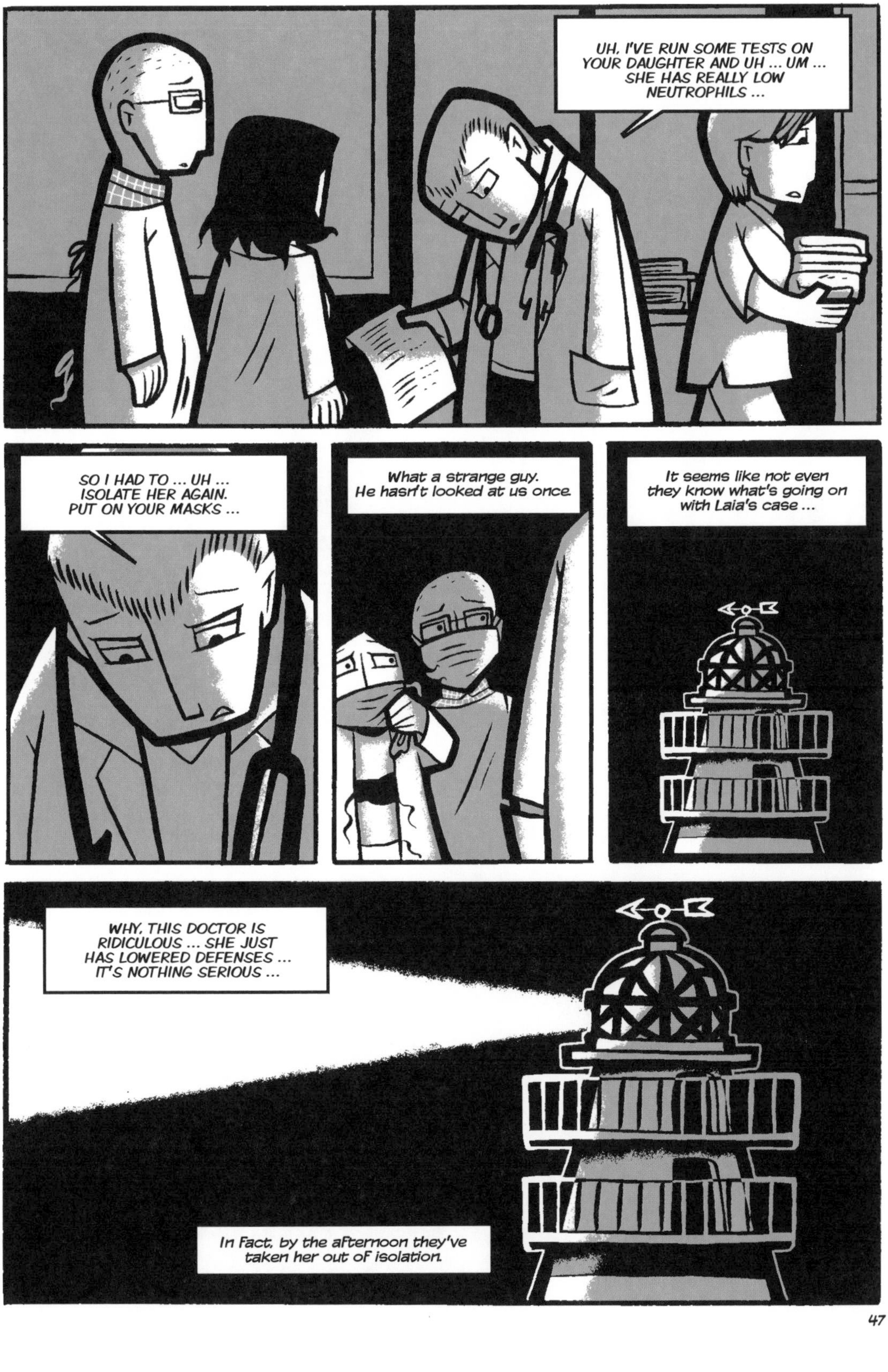
UH, I'VE RUN SOME TESTS ON YOUR DAUGHTER AND UH ... UM ... SHE HAS REALLY LOW NEUTROPHILS ...
SO I HAD TO ... UH ... ISOLATE HER AGAIN. PUT ON YOUR MASKS ...
What a strange guy. He hasn't looked at us once.
It seems like not even they know what's going on with Laia's case ...
WHY, THIS DOCTOR IS RIDICULOUS ... SHE JUST HAS LOWERED DEFENSES ... IT'S NOTHING SERIOUS ...
In Fact, by the afternoon they've taken her out of isolation.

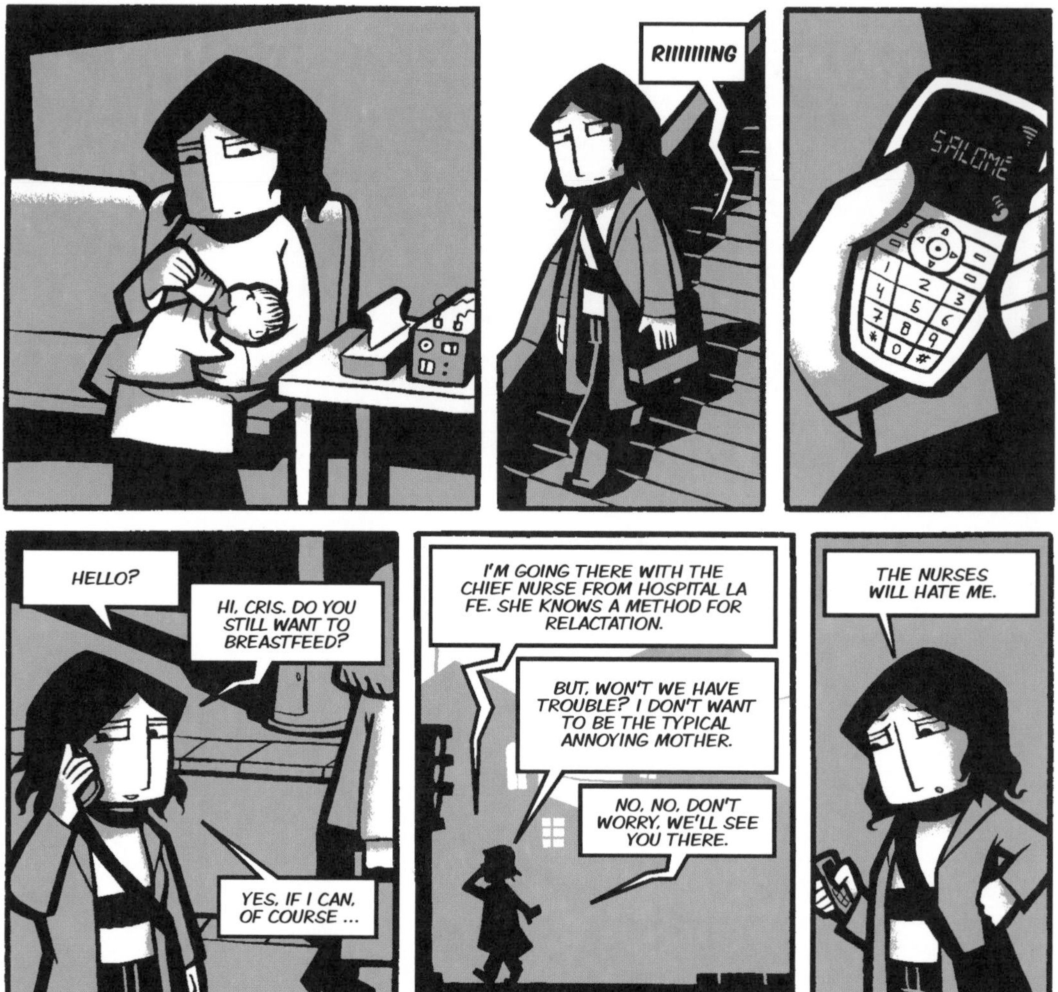
RIIIIIING
SALOMÉ
HELLO?
HI, CRIS. DO YOU STILL WANT TO BREASTFEED?
YES, IF I CAN, OF COURSE ...
I'M GOING THERE WITH THE CHIEF NURSE FROM HOSPITAL LA FE. SHE KNOWS A METHOD FOR RELACTATION.
BUT, WON'T WE HAVE TROUBLE? I DON'T WANT TO BE THE TYPICAL ANNOYING MOTHER.
NO, NO, DON'T WORRY, WE'LL SEE YOU THERE.
THE NURSES WILL HATE ME.
Ah, Carmen's here. They're going make her mad. We're invading her territory with outsiders ...
Salomé Laredo. President of Amamanta.*
Lola Bernabeu, Neonatal Supervisor of Hospital La Fe.
I don't know if it was a good idea. They'll turn against me ... but I can't stop it now.

*Amamanta: Association of breastfeeding mothers.

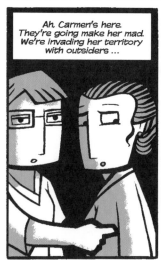

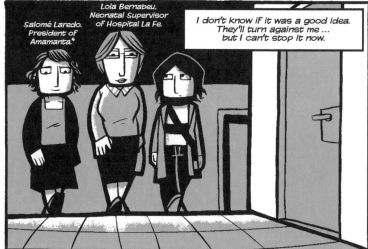

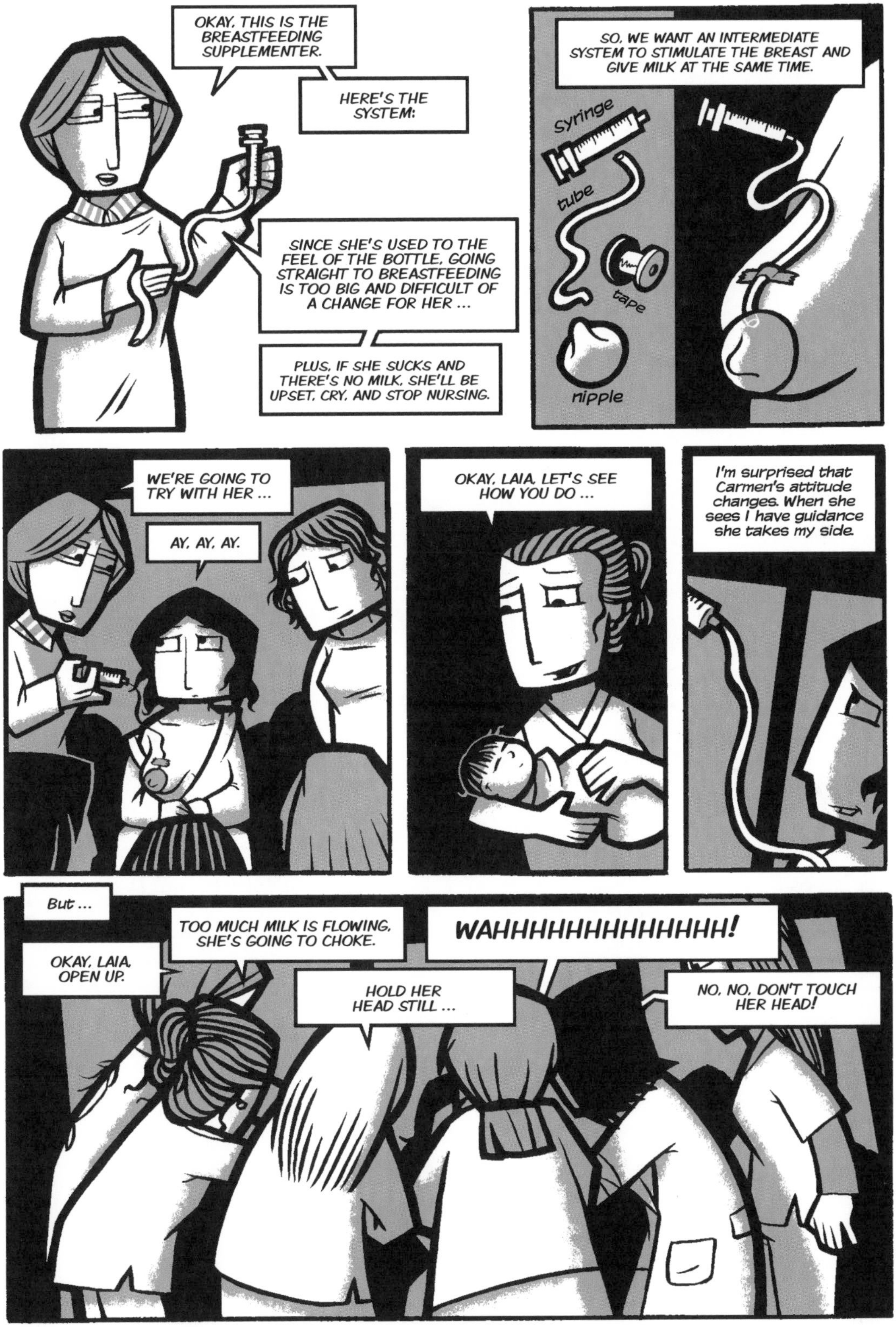
OKAY, THIS IS THE BREASTFEEDING SUPPLEMENTER.
HERE'S THE SYSTEM:
SINCE SHE'S USED TO THE FEEL OF THE BOTTLE, GOING STRAIGHT TO BREASTFEEDING IS TOO BIG AND DIFFICULT OF A CHANGE FOR HER ...
PLUS, IF SHE SUCKS AND THERE'S NO MILK, SHE'LL BE UPSET, CRY, AND STOP NURSING.
SO, WE WANT AN INTERMEDIATE SYSTEM TO STIMULATE THE BREAST AND GIVE MILK AT THE SAME TIME.
syringe
tube
tape
nipple
WE'RE GOING TO TRY WITH HER ...
AY, AY, AY.
OKAY, LAIA, LET'S SEE HOW YOU DO ...
I'm surprised that Carmen's attitude changes. When she sees I have guidance she takes my side.
But ...
OKAY, LAIA, OPEN UP.
TOO MUCH MILK IS FLOWING, SHE'S GOING TO CHOKE.
HOLD HER HEAD STILL ...
WAHHHHHHHHHHHHHH!
NO, NO, DON'T TOUCH HER HEAD!

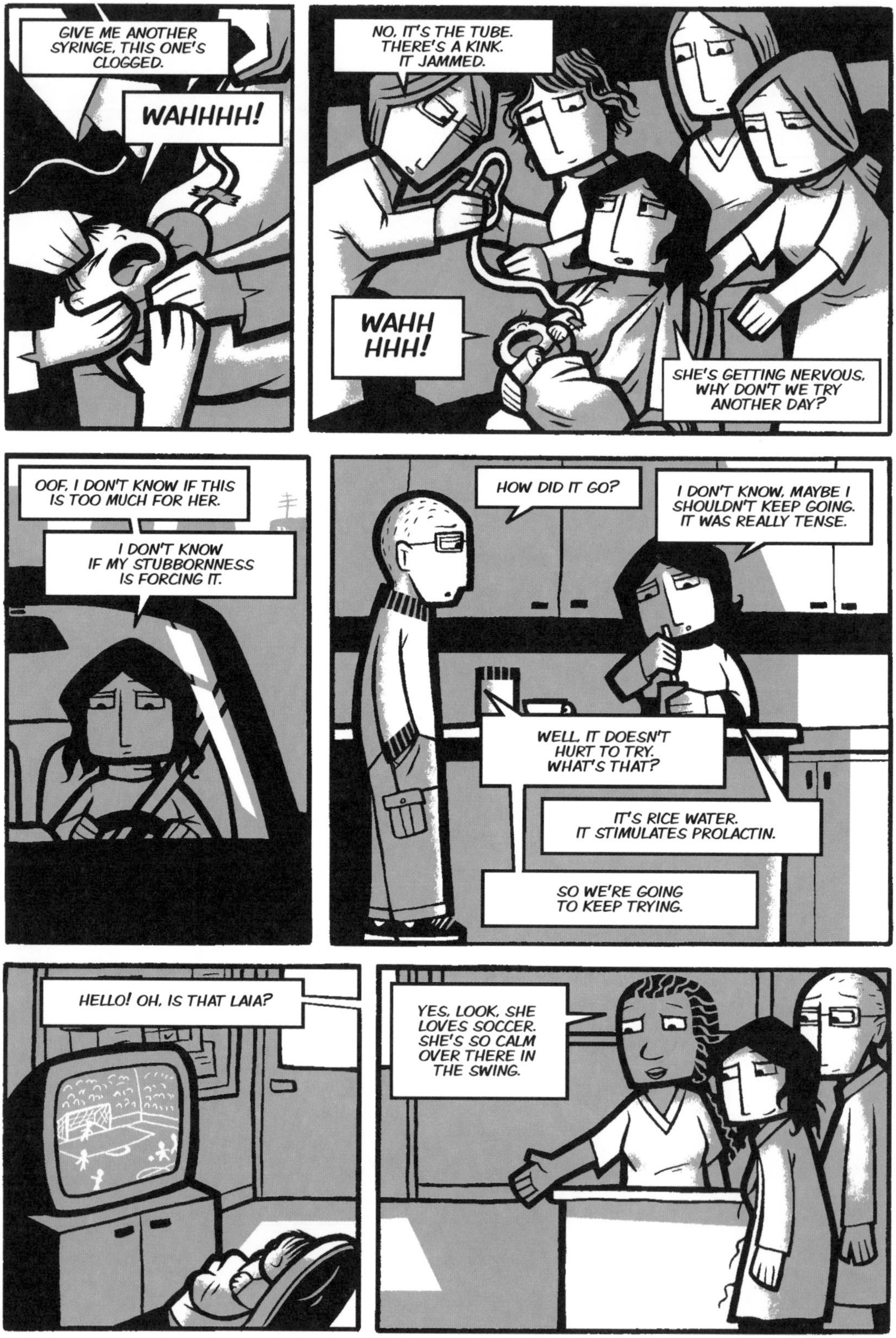
GIVE ME ANOTHER SYRINGE, THIS ONE'S CLOGGED.
WAHHHH!
NO, IT'S THE TUBE. THERE'S A KINK. IT JAMMED.
WAHH HHH!
SHE'S GETTING NERVOUS. WHY DON'T WE TRY ANOTHER DAY?
OOF, I DON'T KNOW IF THIS IS TOO MUCH FOR HER.
I DON'T KNOW IF MY STUBBORNNESS IS FORCING IT.
HOW DID IT GO?
I DON'T KNOW. MAYBE I SHOULDN'T KEEP GOING. IT WAS REALLY TENSE.
WELL, IT DOESN'T HURT TO TRY. WHAT'S THAT?
IT'S RICE WATER. IT STIMULATES PROLACTIN.
SO WE'RE GOING TO KEEP TRYING.
HELLO! OH, IS THAT LAIA?
YES, LOOK, SHE LOVES SOCCER. SHE'S SO CALM OVER THERE IN THE SWING.

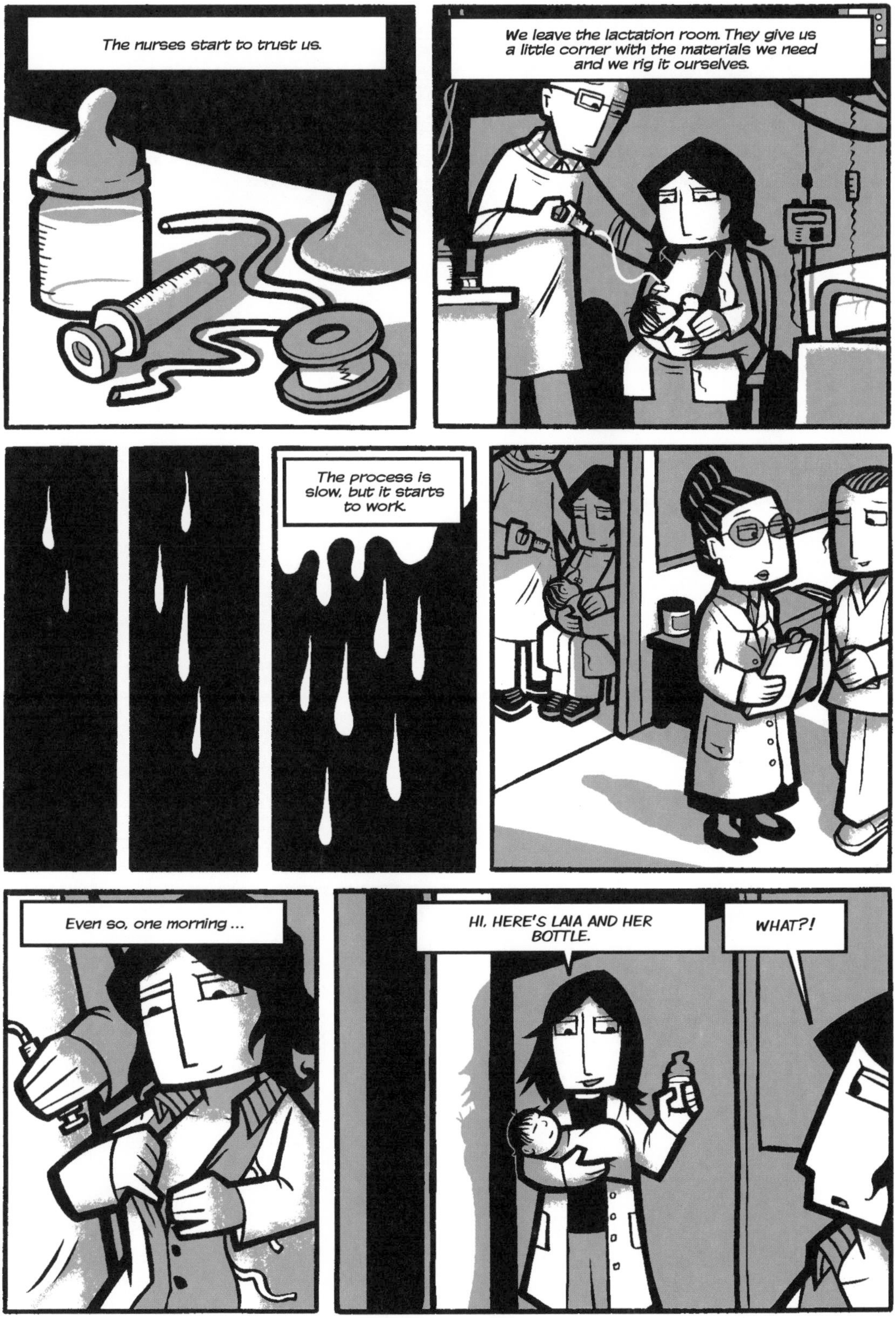
The nurses start to trust us.
We leave the lactation room. They give us a little corner with the materials we need and we rig it ourselves.
The process is slow, but it starts to work.
Even so, one morning ...
HI, HERE'S LAIA AND HER BOTTLE.
WHAT?!

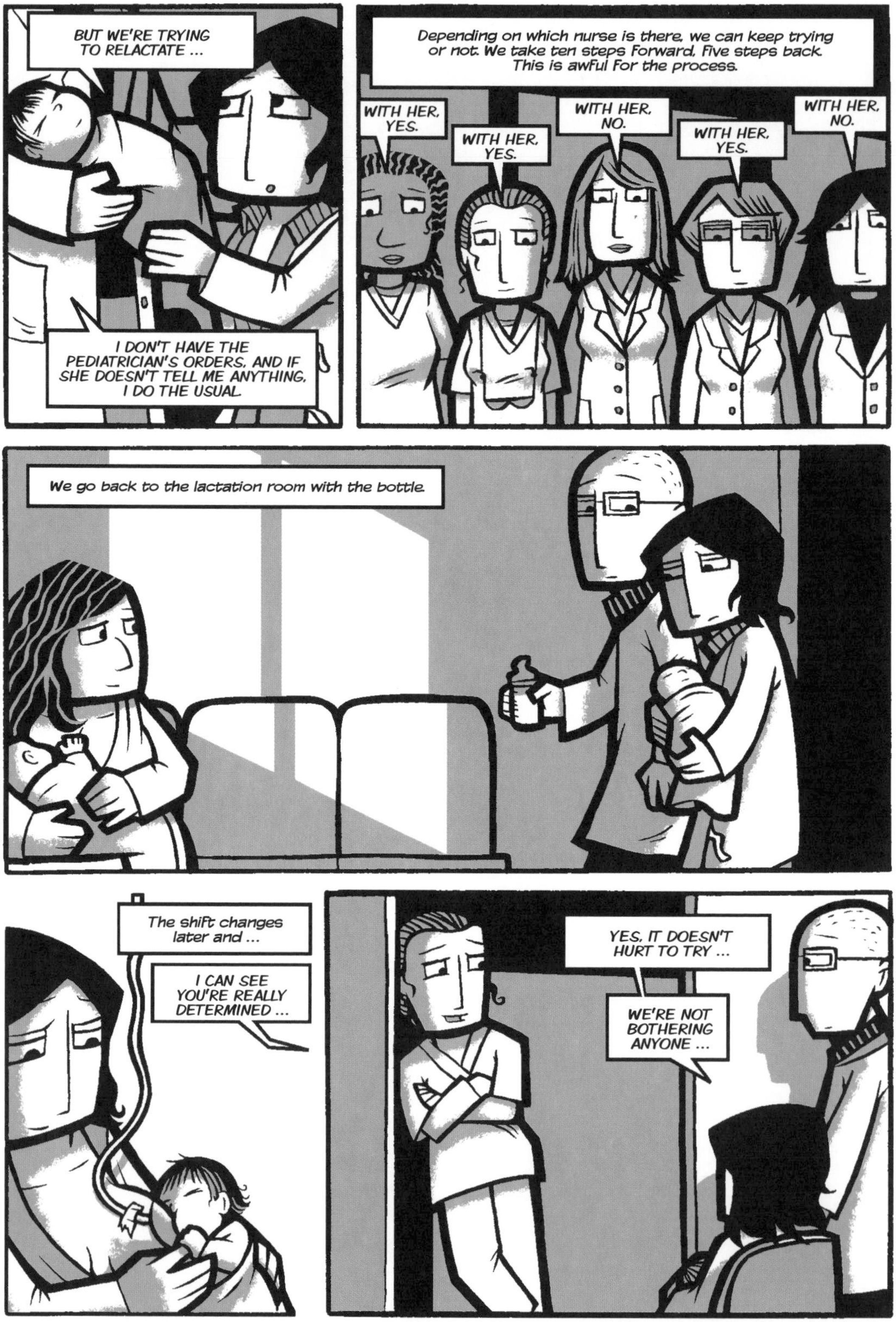
BUT WE'RE TRYING TO RELACTATE ...
I DON'T HAVE THE PEDIATRICIAN'S ORDERS, AND IF SHE DOESN'T TELL ME ANYTHING, I DO THE USUAL.
Depending on which nurse is there, we can keep trying or not. We take ten steps forward, five steps back. This is awful for the process.
WITH HER, YES.
WITH HER, YES.
WITH HER, NO.
WITH HER, YES.
WITH HER, NO.
We go back to the lactation room with the bottle.
The shift changes later and ...
I CAN SEE YOU'RE REALLY DETERMINED ...
YES, IT DOESN'T HURT TO TRY ...
WE'RE NOT BOTHERING ANYONE ...

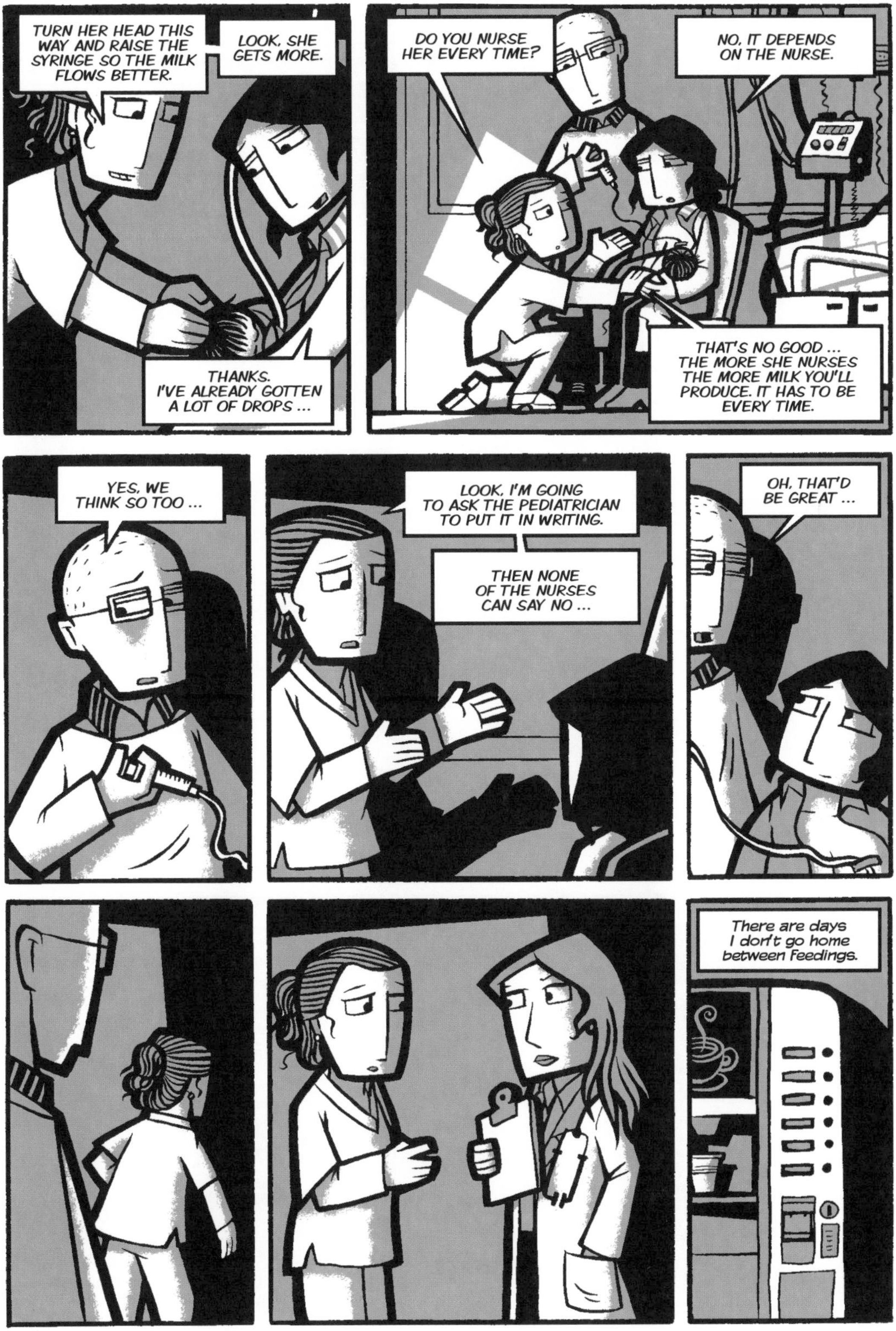
TURN HER HEAD THIS WAY AND RAISE THE SYRINGE SO THE MILK FLOWS BETTER.
LOOK, SHE GETS MORE.
THANKS. I'VE ALREADY GOTTEN A LOT OF DROPS ...
DO YOU NURSE HER EVERY TIME?
NO, IT DEPENDS ON THE NURSE.
THAT'S NO GOOD ... THE MORE SHE NURSES THE MORE MILK YOU'LL PRODUCE. IT HAS TO BE EVERY TIME.
YES, WE THINK SO TOO ...
LOOK, I'M GOING TO ASK THE PEDIATRICIAN TO PUT IT IN WRITING.
THEN NONE OF THE NURSES CAN SAY NO ...
OH, THAT'D BE GREAT ...
There are days I don't go home between feedings.

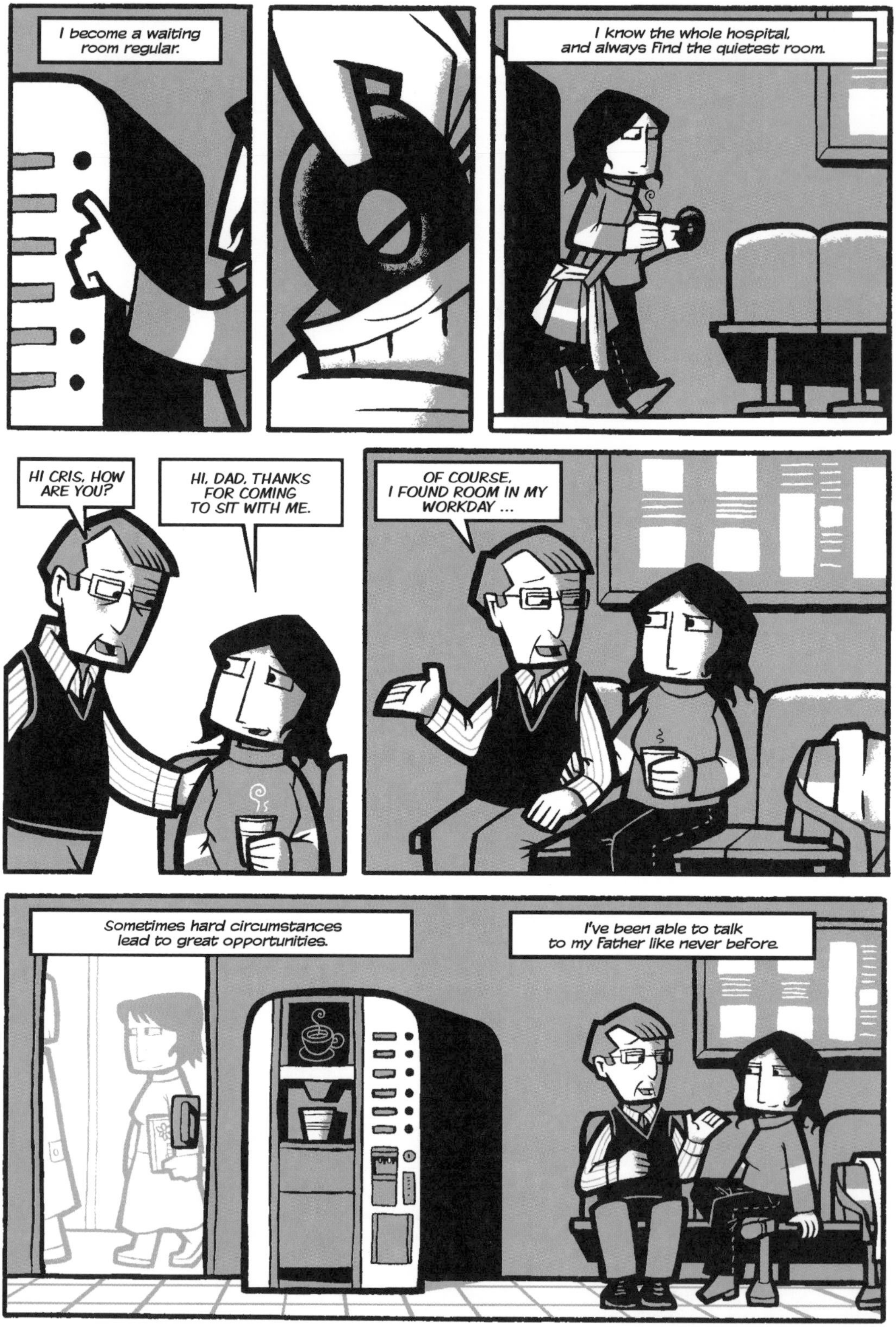
I become a waiting room regular.
I know the whole hospital, and always find the quietest room.
HI CRIS, HOW ARE YOU?
HI, DAD, THANKS FOR COMING TO SIT WITH ME.
OF COURSE, I FOUND ROOM IN MY WORKDAY ...
Sometimes hard circumstances lead to great opportunities.
I've been able to talk to my father like never before.

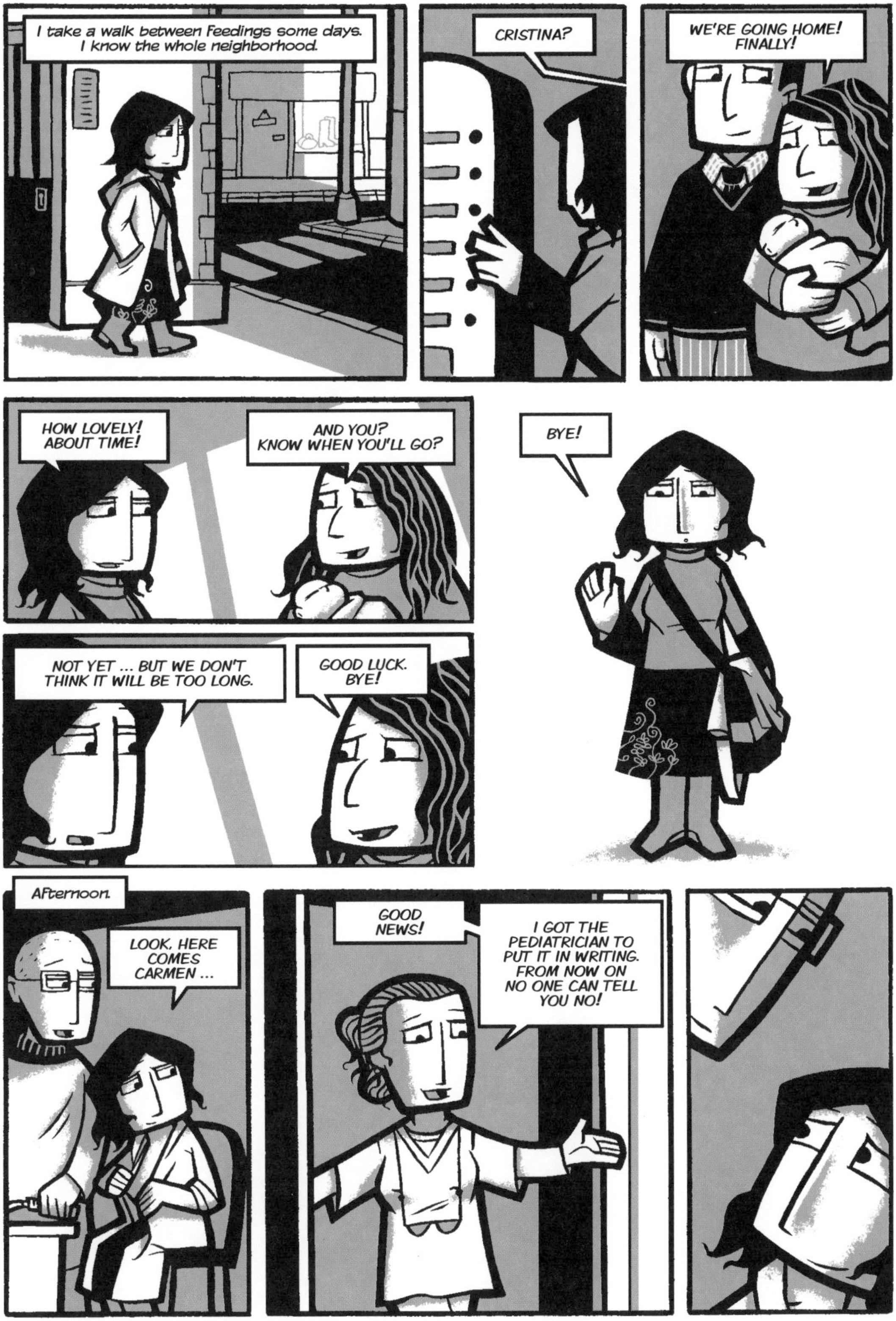
I take a walk between Feedings some days. I know the whole neighborhood.
CRISTINA?
WE'RE GOING HOME! FINALLY!
HOW LOVELY! ABOUT TIME!
AND YOU? KNOW WHEN YOU'LL GO?
BYE!
NOT YET ... BUT WE DON'T THINK IT WILL BE TOO LONG.
GOOD LUCK. BYE!
Afternoon.
LOOK, HERE COMES CARMEN ...
GOOD NEWS!
I GOT THE PEDIATRICIAN TO PUT IT IN WRITING. FROM NOW ON NO ONE CAN TELL YOU NO!

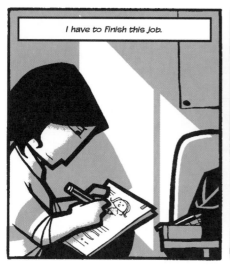

I have to finish this job.

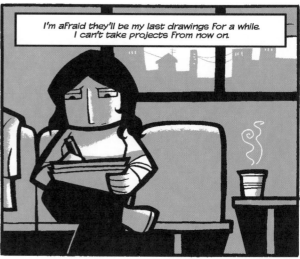

I'm afraid they'll be my last drawings for a while. I can't take projects from now on.

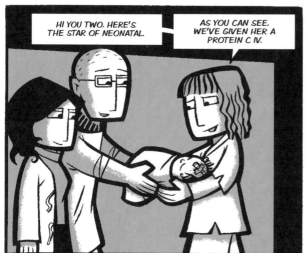

HI YOU TWO. HERE'S THE STAR OF NEONATAL.

AS YOU CAN SEE, WE'VE GIVEN HER A PROTEIN C IV.

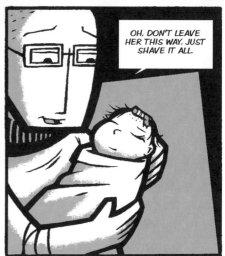

OH, DON'T LEAVE HER THIS WAY. JUST SHAVE IT ALL.

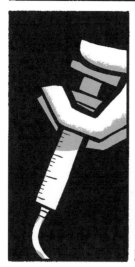

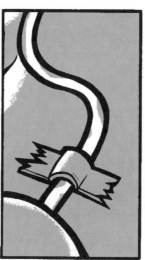

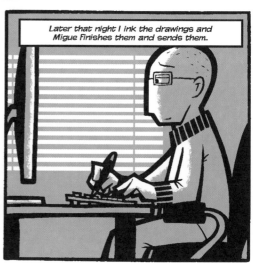

Later that night I ink the drawings and Migue finishes them and sends them.

56

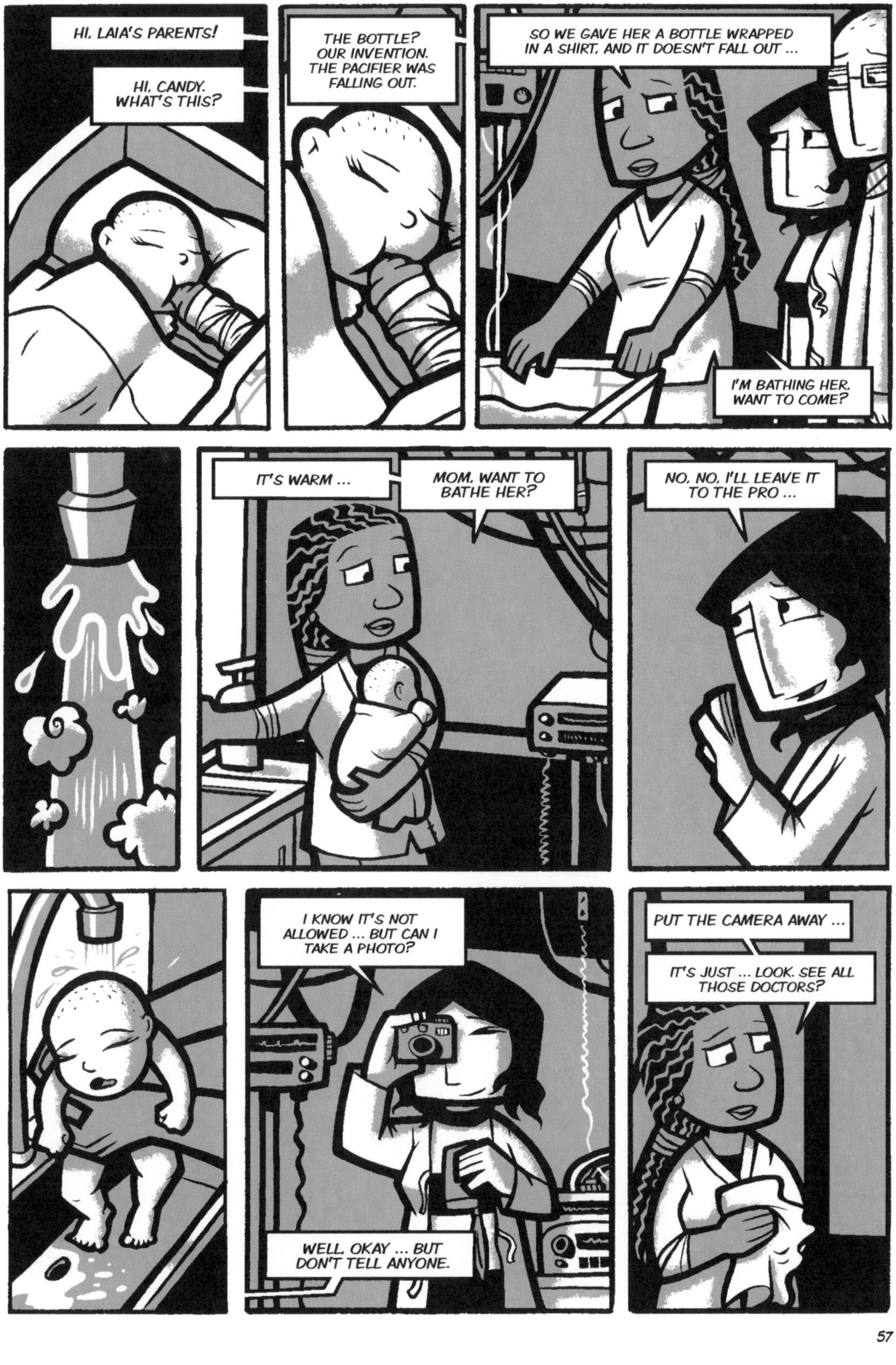
HI, LAIA'S PARENTS!
HI, CANDY. WHAT'S THIS?
THE BOTTLE? OUR INVENTION. THE PACIFIER WAS FALLING OUT.
SO WE GAVE HER A BOTTLE WRAPPED IN A SHIRT, AND IT DOESN'T FALL OUT ...
I'M BATHING HER. WANT TO COME?
IT'S WARM ...
MOM, WANT TO BATHE HER?
NO, NO, I'LL LEAVE IT TO THE PRO ...
I KNOW IT'S NOT ALLOWED ... BUT CAN I TAKE A PHOTO?
WELL, OKAY ... BUT DON'T TELL ANYONE.
PUT THE CAMERA AWAY ...
IT'S JUST ... LOOK. SEE ALL THOSE DOCTORS?

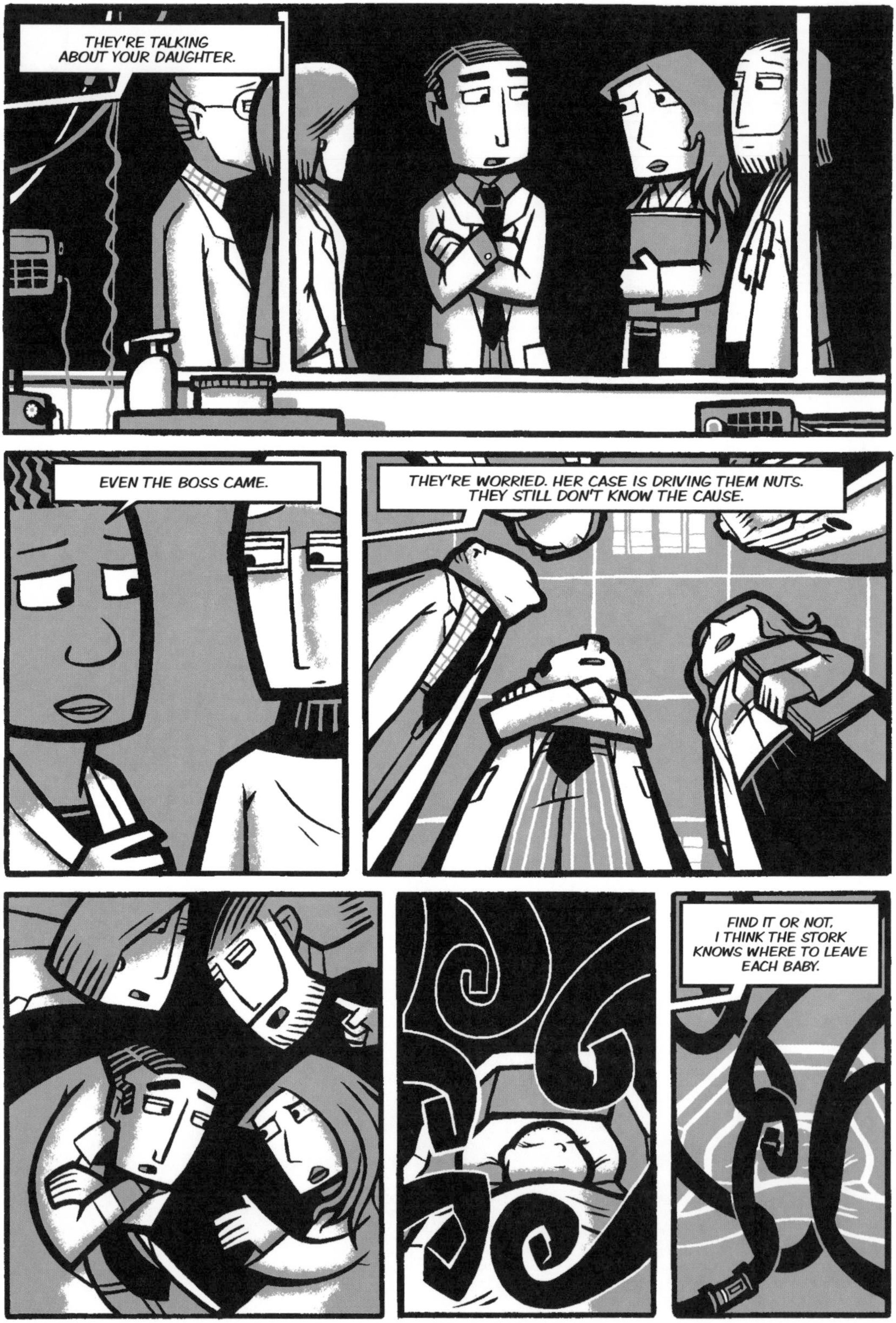
THEY'RE TALKING ABOUT YOUR DAUGHTER.
EVEN THE BOSS CAME.
THEY'RE WORRIED. HER CASE IS DRIVING THEM NUTS. THEY STILL DON'T KNOW THE CAUSE.
FIND IT OR NOT, I THINK THE STORK KNOWS WHERE TO LEAVE EACH BABY.

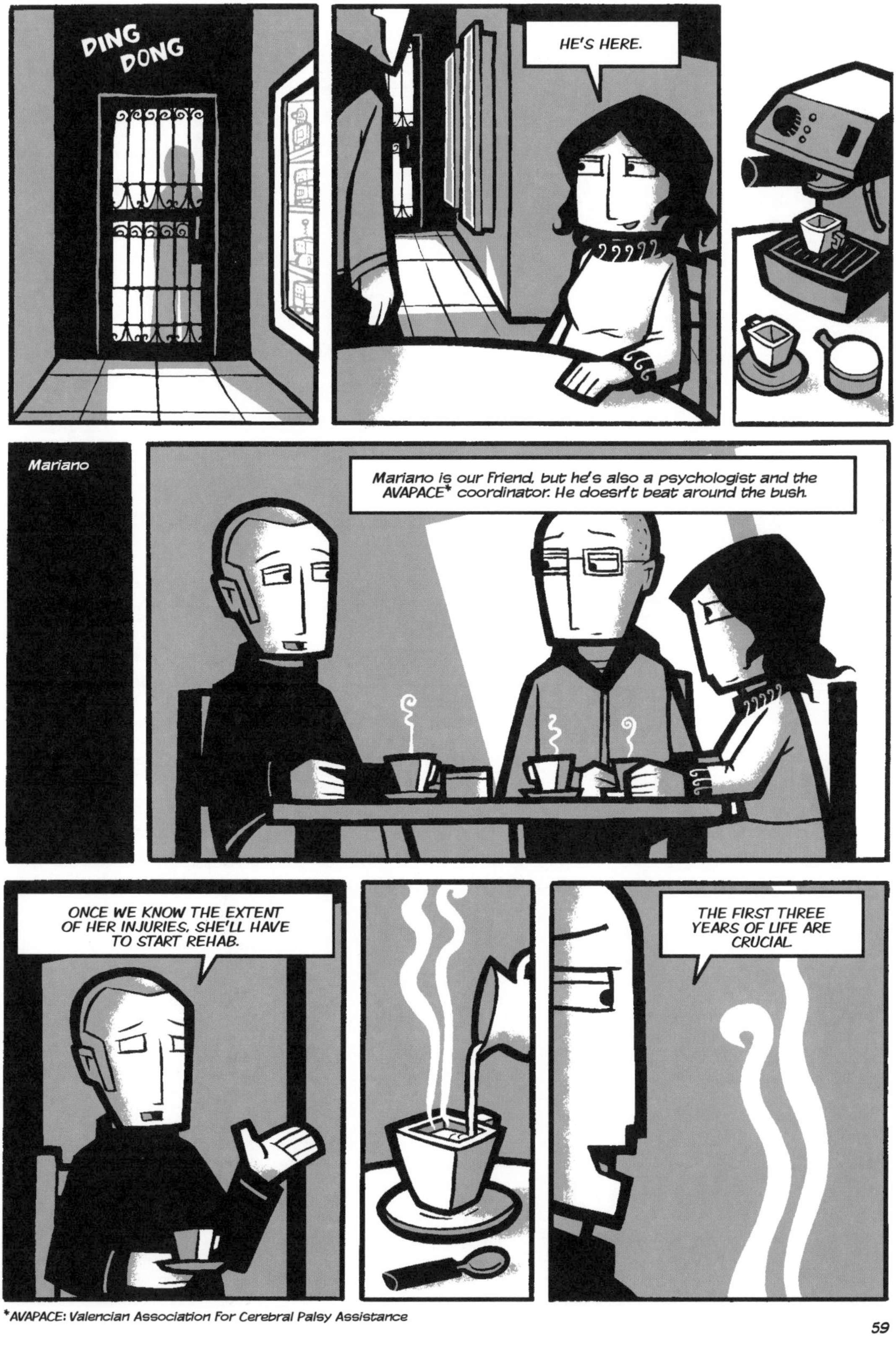
DING DONG
HE'S HERE.
Mariano
Mariano is our friend, but he's also a psychologist and the AVAPACE* coordinator. He doesn't beat around the bush.
ONCE WE KNOW THE EXTENT OF HER INJURIES, SHE'LL HAVE TO START REHAB.
THE FIRST THREE YEARS OF LIFE ARE CRUCIAL.

*AVAPACE: Valencian Association For Cerebral Palsy Assistance

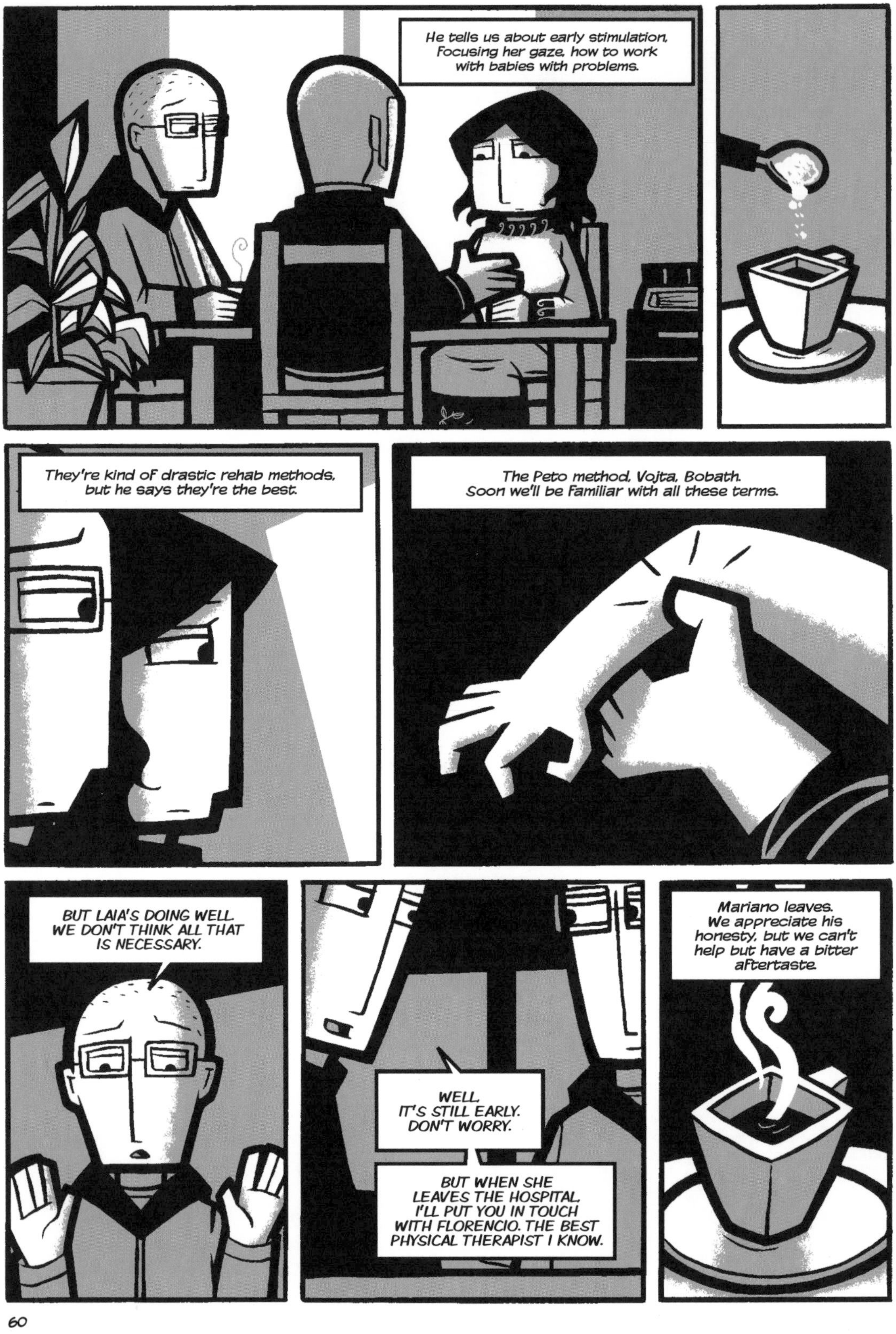
He tells us about early stimulation, focusing her gaze, how to work with babies with problems.
They're kind of drastic rehab methods, but he says they're the best.
The Peto method, Vojta, Bobath. Soon we'll be familiar with all these terms.
BUT LAIA'S DOING WELL. WE DON'T THINK ALL THAT IS NECESSARY.
WELL, IT'S STILL EARLY. DON'T WORRY.
BUT WHEN SHE LEAVES THE HOSPITAL, I'LL PUT YOU IN TOUCH WITH FLORENCIO. THE BEST PHYSICAL THERAPIST I KNOW.
Mariano leaves. We appreciate his honesty, but we can't help but have a bitter aftertaste.

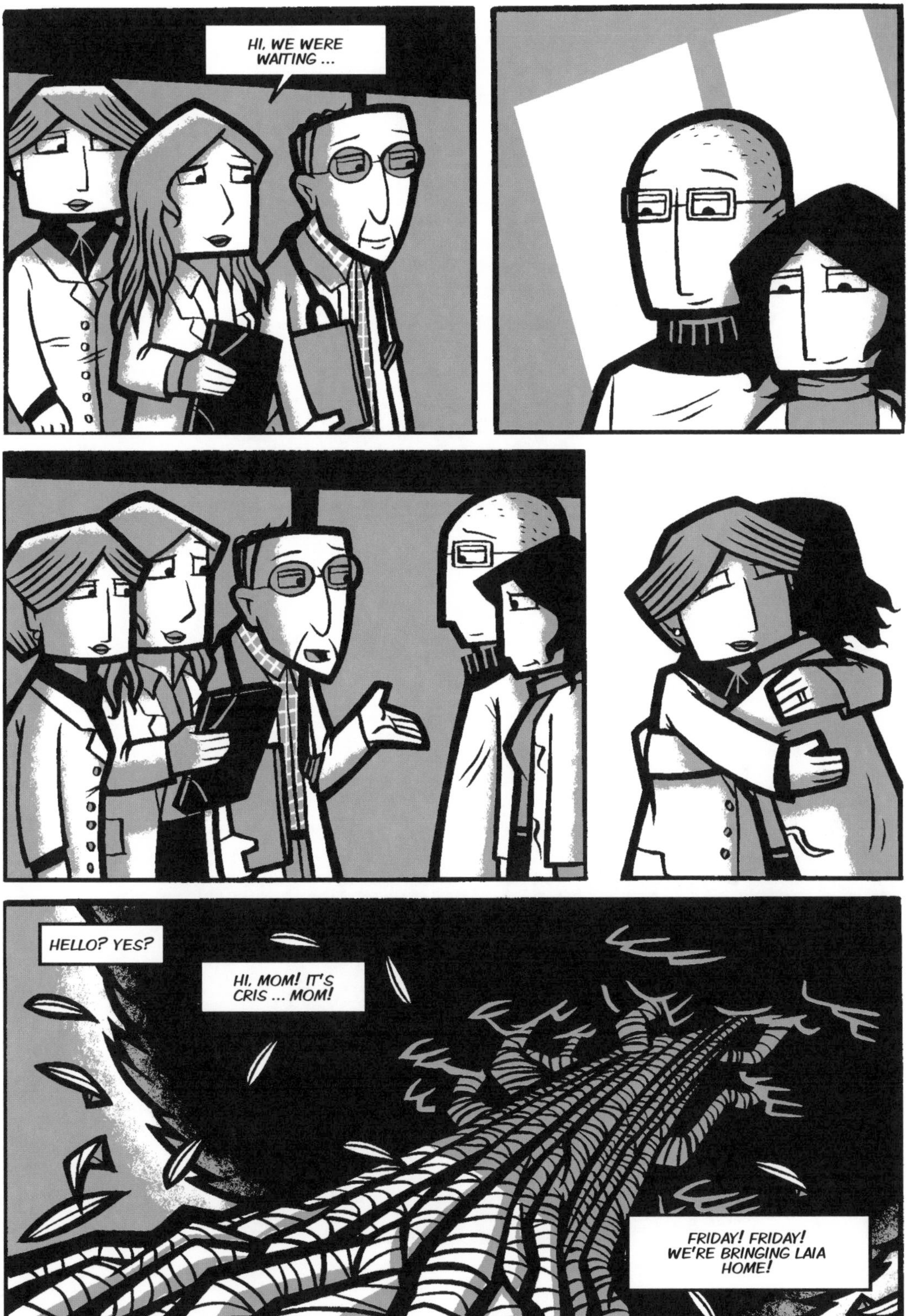
HI, WE WERE WAITING ...
HELLO? YES?
HI, MOM! IT'S CRIS ... MOM!
FRIDAY! FRIDAY! WE'RE BRINGING LAIA HOME!

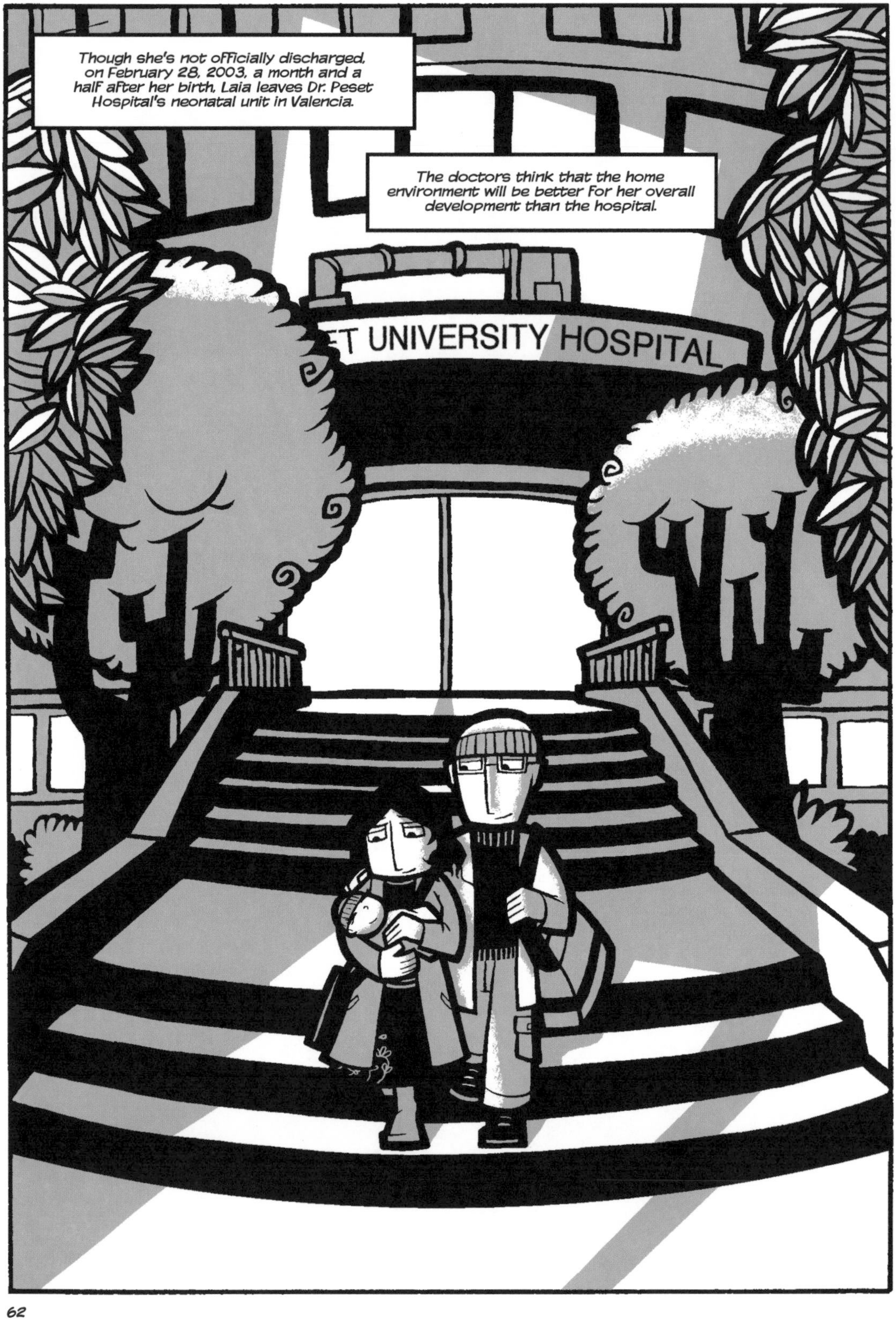
Though she's not officially discharged, on February 28, 2003, a month and a half after her birth, Laia leaves Dr. Peset Hospital's neonatal unit in Valencia.
The doctors think that the home environment will be better for her overall development than the hospital.
ET UNIVERSITY HOSPITAL

4.
MUD

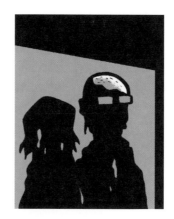

Lo más terrible se aprende enseguida y lo hermoso nos cuesta la vida.

"Canción del elegido,"
Silvio Rodríguez

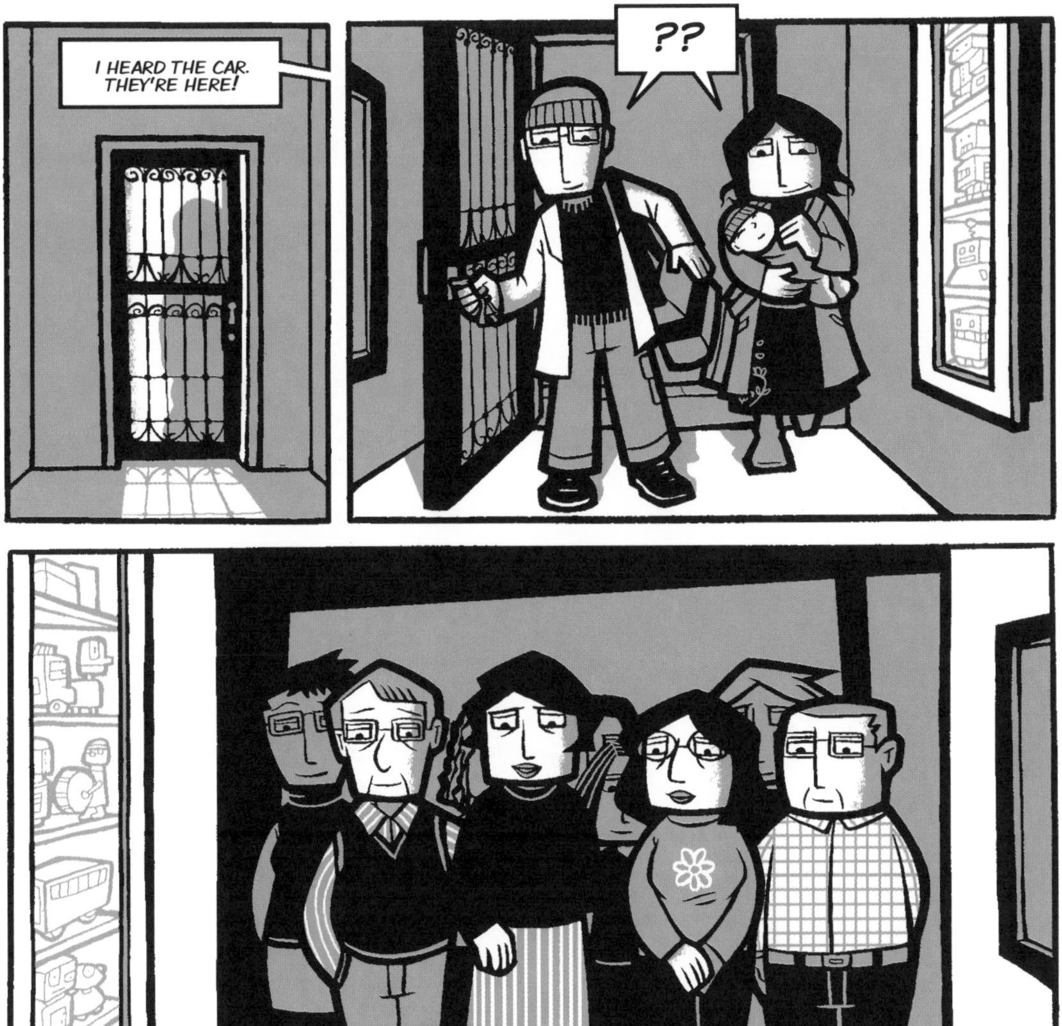
I HEARD THE CAR.
THEY'RE HERE!
??
SHE'S SO PRETTY!
WOW ... THE FIRST BABY
I'VE EVER HELD!
HAHA RAMÓN,
YOU CAN TELL
15

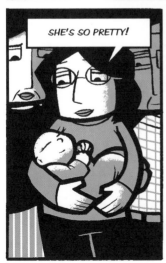

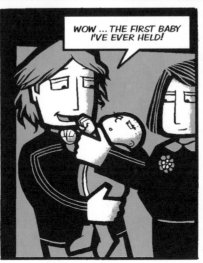

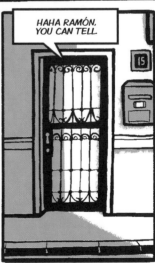

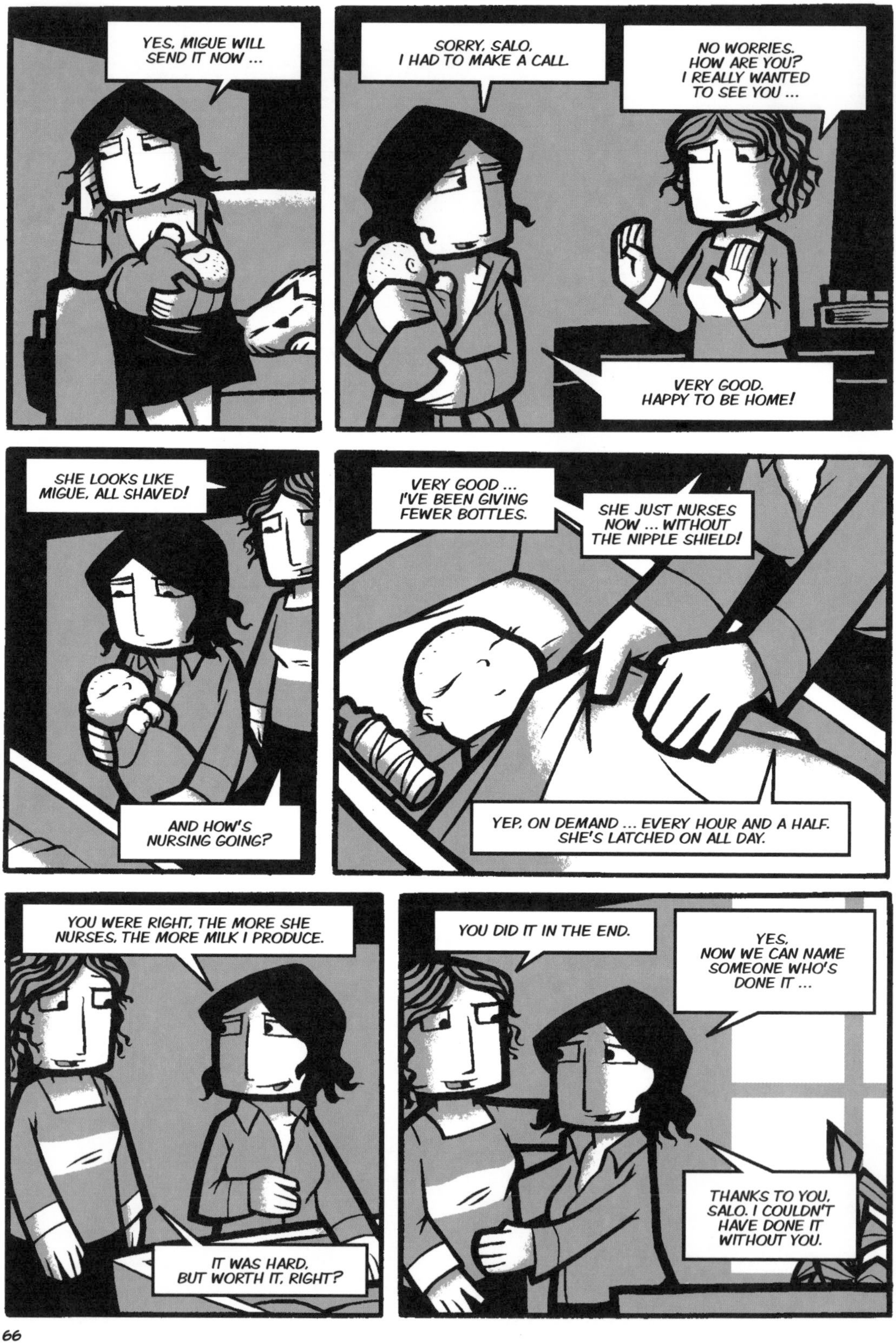
YES, MIGUE WILL SEND IT NOW ...
SORRY, SALO, I HAD TO MAKE A CALL.
NO WORRIES. HOW ARE YOU? I REALLY WANTED TO SEE YOU ...
VERY GOOD. HAPPY TO BE HOME!
SHE LOOKS LIKE MIGUE, ALL SHAVED!
AND HOW'S NURSING GOING?
VERY GOOD ... I'VE BEEN GIVING FEWER BOTTLES.
SHE JUST NURSES NOW ... WITHOUT THE NIPPLE SHIELD!
YEP, ON DEMAND ... EVERY HOUR AND A HALF. SHE'S LATCHED ON ALL DAY.
YOU WERE RIGHT, THE MORE SHE NURSES, THE MORE MILK I PRODUCE.
IT WAS HARD, BUT WORTH IT, RIGHT?
YOU DID IT IN THE END.
YES, NOW WE CAN NAME SOMEONE WHO'S DONE IT ...
THANKS TO YOU, SALO. I COULDN'T HAVE DONE IT WITHOUT YOU.

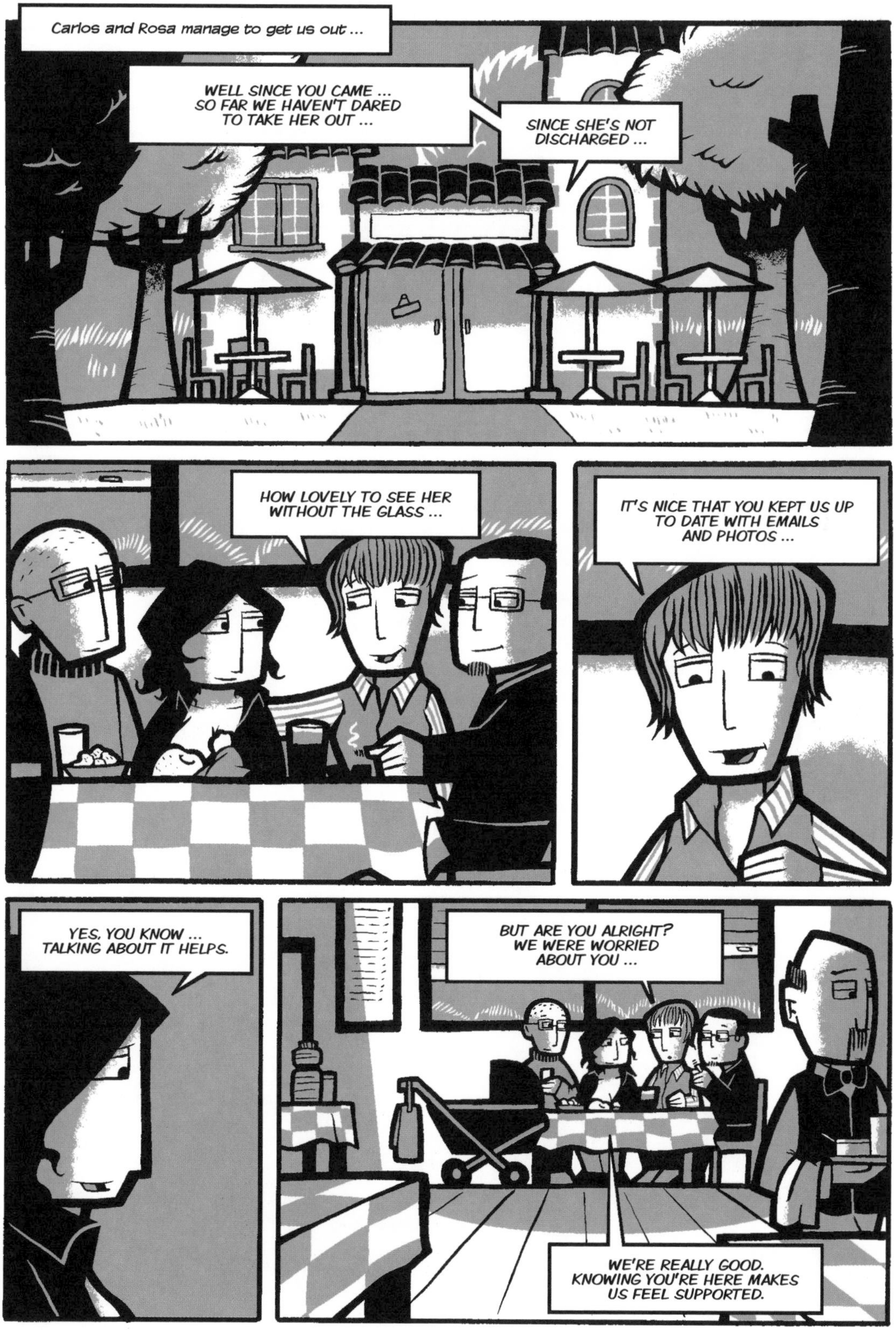
Carlos and Rosa manage to get us out ...
WELL SINCE YOU CAME ... SO FAR WE HAVEN'T DARED TO TAKE HER OUT ...
SINCE SHE'S NOT DISCHARGED ...
HOW LOVELY TO SEE HER WITHOUT THE GLASS ...
IT'S NICE THAT YOU KEPT US UP TO DATE WITH EMAILS AND PHOTOS ...
YES, YOU KNOW ... TALKING ABOUT IT HELPS.
BUT ARE YOU ALRIGHT? WE WERE WORRIED ABOUT YOU ...
WE'RE REALLY GOOD. KNOWING YOU'RE HERE MAKES US FEEL SUPPORTED.

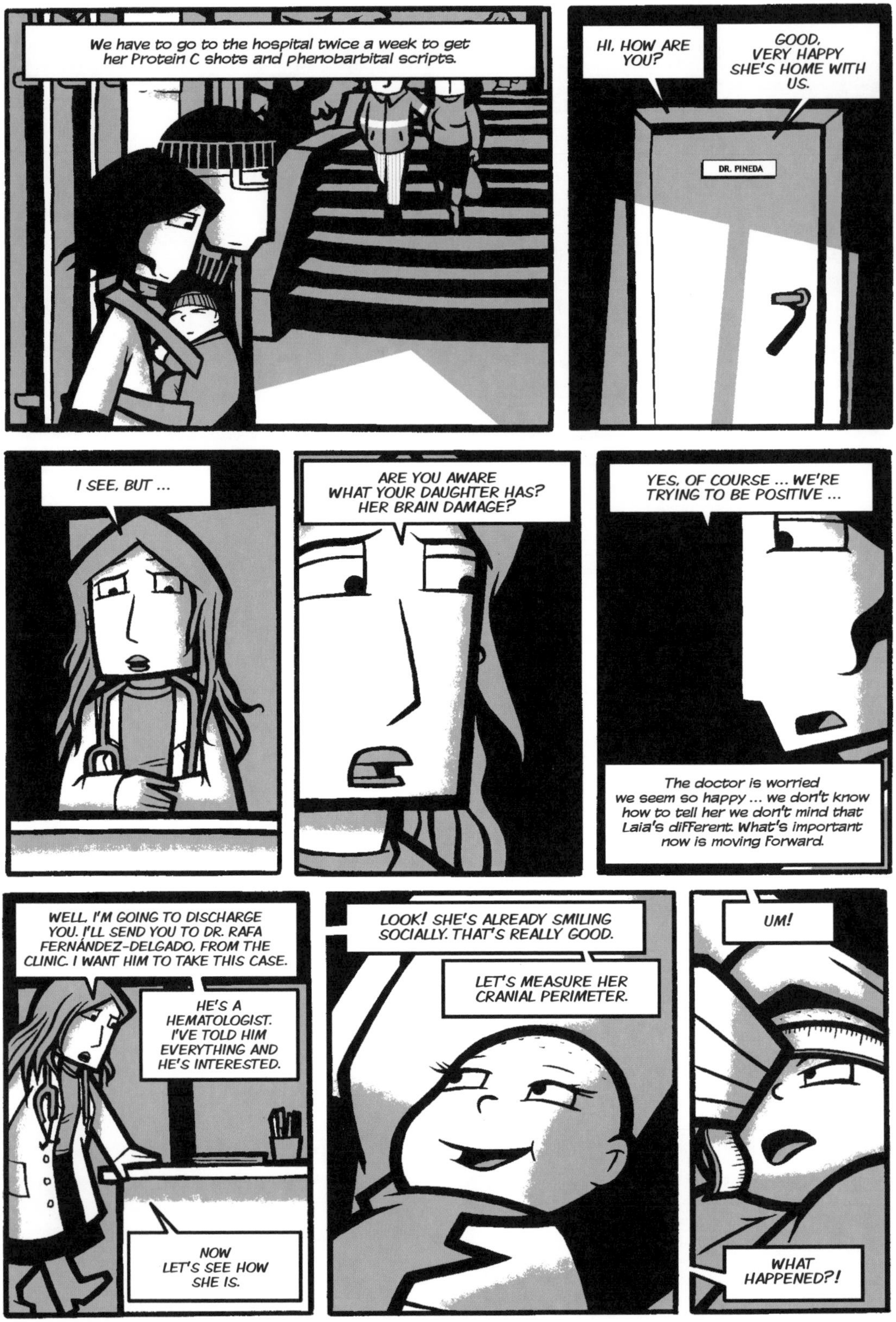

We have to go to the hospital twice a week to get her Protein C shots and phenobarbital scripts.
HI, HOW ARE YOU?
GOOD, VERY HAPPY SHE'S HOME WITH US.
DR. PINEDA
I SEE, BUT ...
ARE YOU AWARE WHAT YOUR DAUGHTER HAS? HER BRAIN DAMAGE?
YES, OF COURSE ... WE'RE TRYING TO BE POSITIVE ...
The doctor is worried we seem so happy ... we don't know how to tell her we don't mind that Laia's different. What's important now is moving forward.
WELL, I'M GOING TO DISCHARGE YOU. I'LL SEND YOU TO DR. RAFA FERNÁNDEZ-DELGADO, FROM THE CLINIC. I WANT HIM TO TAKE THIS CASE.
HE'S A HEMATOLOGIST. I'VE TOLD HIM EVERYTHING AND HE'S INTERESTED.
NOW LET'S SEE HOW SHE IS.
LOOK! SHE'S ALREADY SMILING SOCIALLY. THAT'S REALLY GOOD.
LET'S MEASURE HER CRANIAL PERIMETER.
UM!
WHAT HAPPENED?!

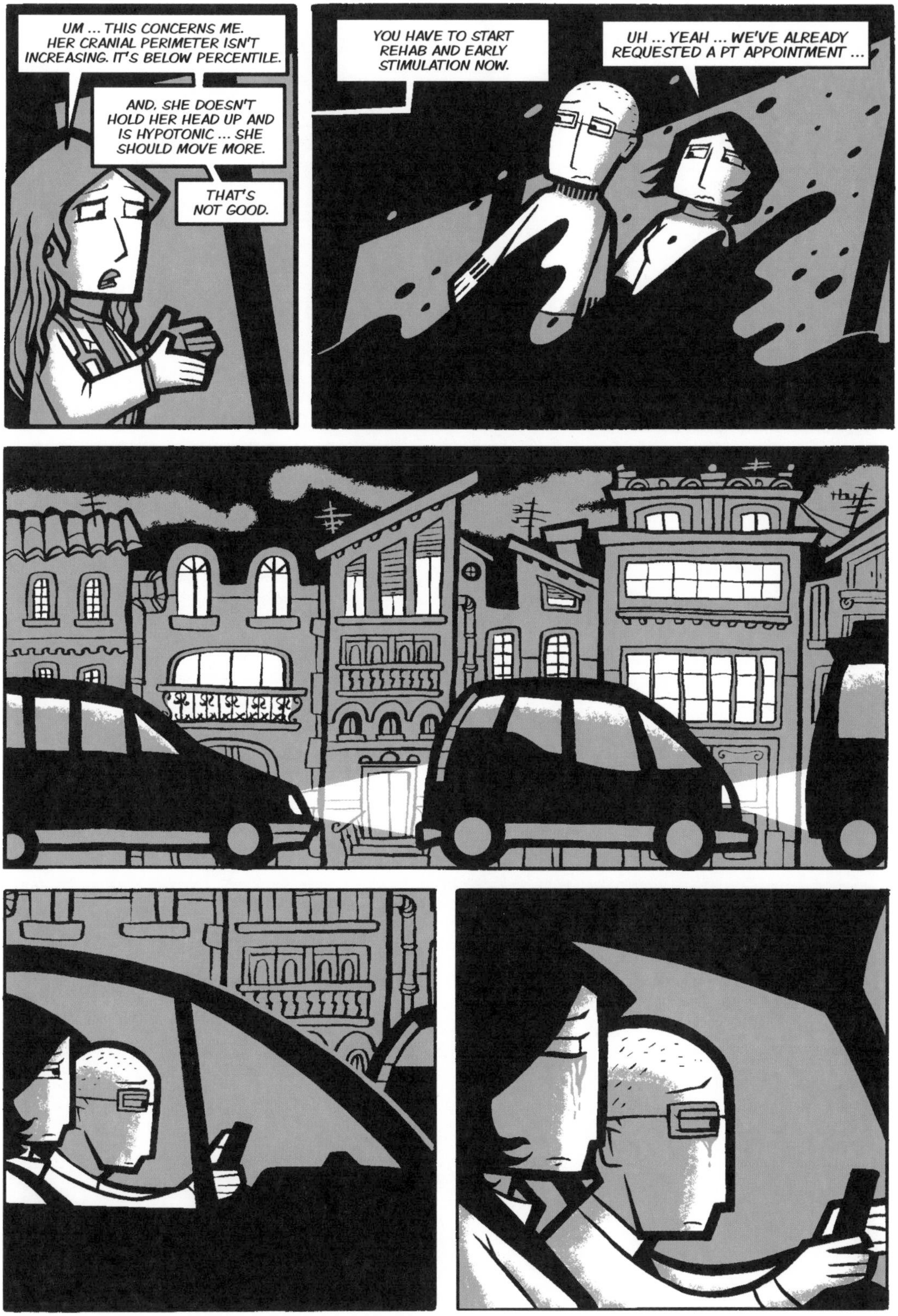
UM ... THIS CONCERNS ME. HER CRANIAL PERIMETER ISN'T INCREASING. IT'S BELOW PERCENTILE.
AND, SHE DOESN'T HOLD HER HEAD UP AND IS HYPOTONIC ... SHE SHOULD MOVE MORE.
THAT'S NOT GOOD.
YOU HAVE TO START REHAB AND EARLY STIMULATION NOW.
UH ... YEAH ... WE'VE ALREADY REQUESTED A PT APPOINTMENT ...

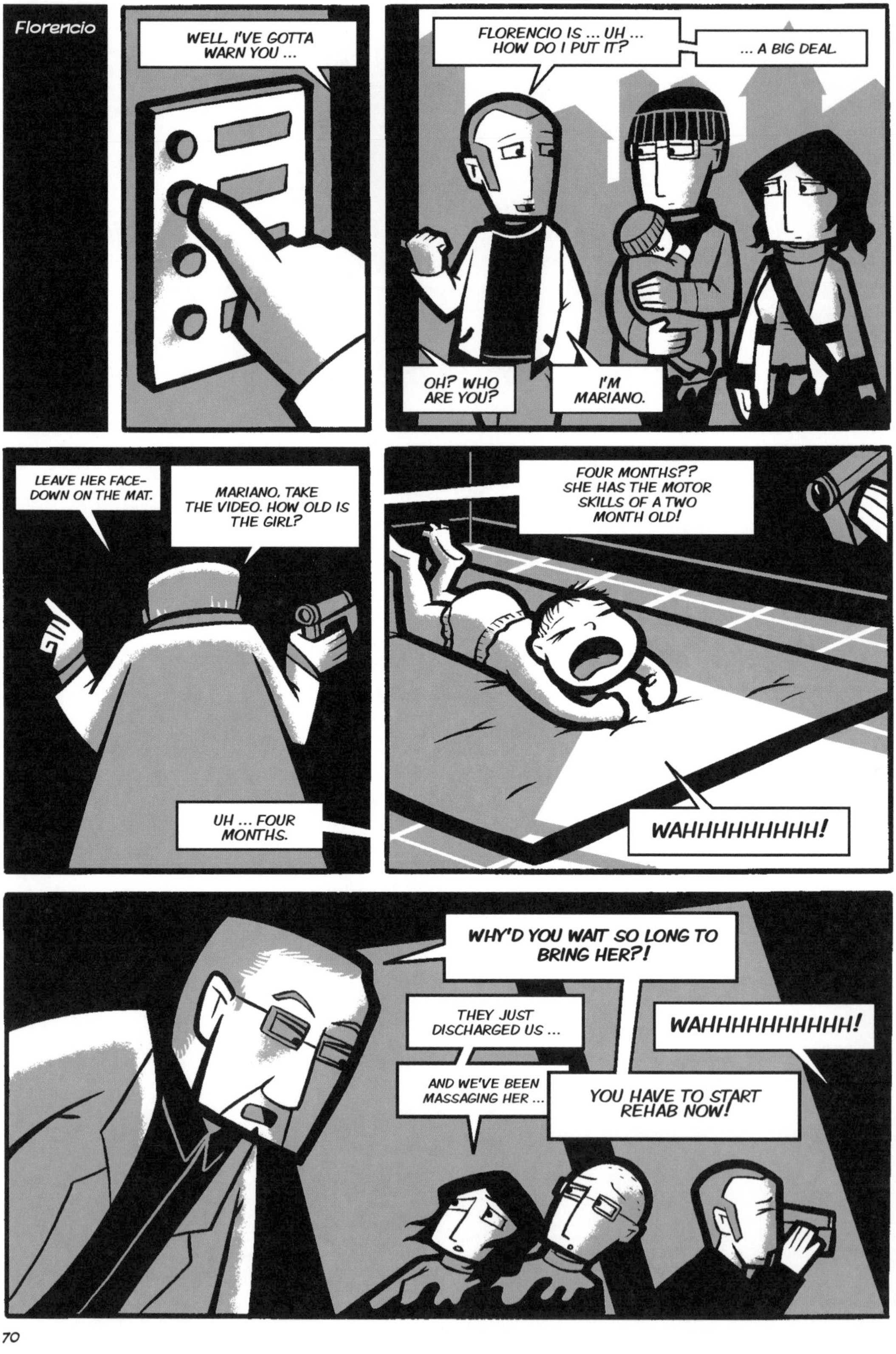
Florencio
WELL, I'VE GOTTA WARN YOU ...
FLORENCIO IS ... UH ... HOW DO I PUT IT?
... A BIG DEAL.
OH? WHO ARE YOU?
I'M MARIANO.
LEAVE HER FACE-DOWN ON THE MAT.
MARIANO, TAKE THE VIDEO. HOW OLD IS THE GIRL?
UH ... FOUR MONTHS.
FOUR MONTHS?? SHE HAS THE MOTOR SKILLS OF A TWO MONTH OLD!
WAHHHHHHHHHH!
WHY'D YOU WAIT SO LONG TO BRING HER?!
THEY JUST DISCHARGED US ...
AND WE'VE BEEN MASSAGING HER ...
WAHHHHHHHHHHH!
YOU HAVE TO START REHAB NOW!

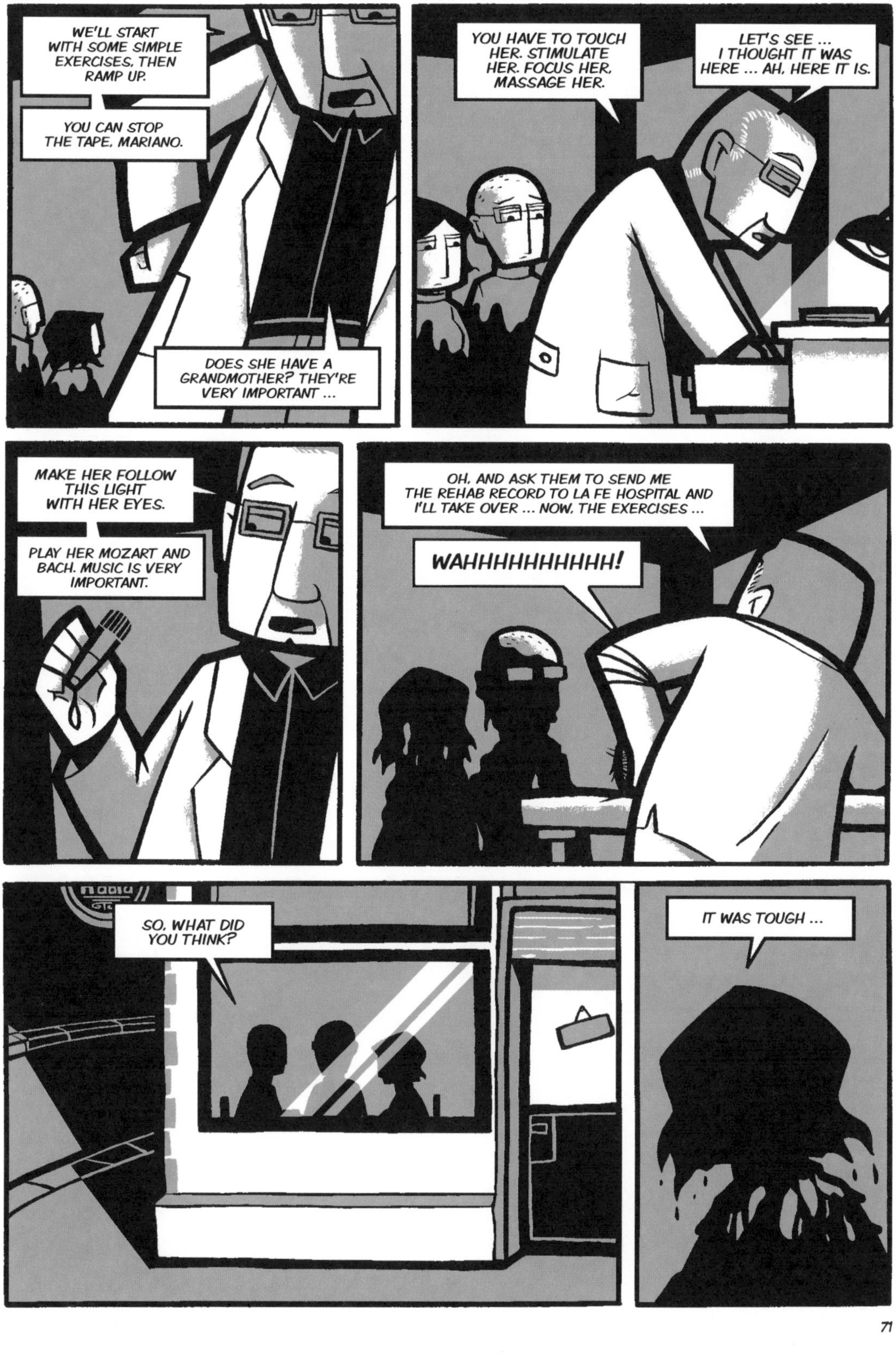
WE'LL START WITH SOME SIMPLE EXERCISES, THEN RAMP UP.
YOU CAN STOP THE TAPE, MARIANO.
DOES SHE HAVE A GRANDMOTHER? THEY'RE VERY IMPORTANT ...
YOU HAVE TO TOUCH HER. STIMULATE HER. FOCUS HER, MASSAGE HER.
LET'S SEE ... I THOUGHT IT WAS HERE ... AH, HERE IT IS.
MAKE HER FOLLOW THIS LIGHT WITH HER EYES.
PLAY HER MOZART AND BACH. MUSIC IS VERY IMPORTANT.
OH, AND ASK THEM TO SEND ME THE REHAB RECORD TO LA FE HOSPITAL AND I'LL TAKE OVER ... NOW, THE EXERCISES ...
WAHHHHHHHHHH!
SO, WHAT DID YOU THINK?
IT WAS TOUGH ...

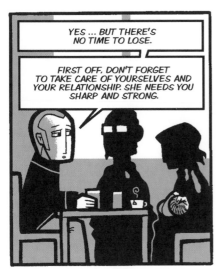

YES ... BUT THERE'S NO TIME TO LOSE.

FIRST OFF, DON'T FORGET TO TAKE CARE OF YOURSELVES AND YOUR RELATIONSHIP. SHE NEEDS YOU SHARP AND STRONG.

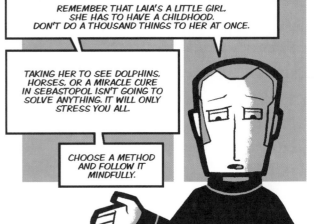

REMEMBER THAT LAIA'S A LITTLE GIRL. SHE HAS TO HAVE A CHILDHOOD. DON'T DO A THOUSAND THINGS TO HER AT ONCE.

TAKING HER TO SEE DOLPHINS, HORSES, OR A MIRACLE CURE IN SEBASTOPOL ISN'T GOING TO SOLVE ANYTHING. IT WILL ONLY STRESS YOU ALL.

CHOOSE A METHOD AND FOLLOW IT MINDFULLY.

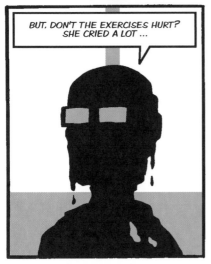

BUT, DON'T THE EXERCISES HURT? SHE CRIED A LOT ...

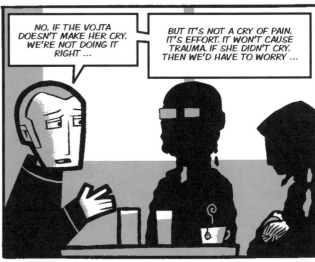

NO, IF THE VOJTA DOESN'T MAKE HER CRY, WE'RE NOT DOING IT RIGHT ...

BUT IT'S NOT A CRY OF PAIN, IT'S EFFORT. IT WON'T CAUSE TRAUMA. IF SHE DIDN'T CRY, THEN WE'D HAVE TO WORRY ...

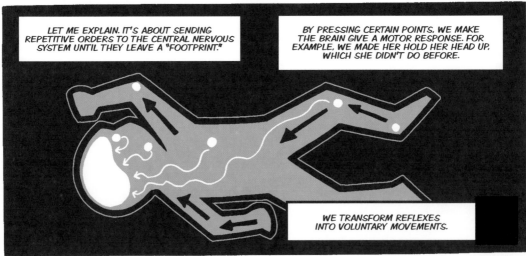

LET ME EXPLAIN. IT'S ABOUT SENDING REPETITIVE ORDERS TO THE CENTRAL NERVOUS SYSTEM UNTIL THEY LEAVE A "FOOTPRINT."

BY PRESSING CERTAIN POINTS, WE MAKE THE BRAIN GIVE A MOTOR RESPONSE. FOR EXAMPLE, WE MADE HER HOLD HER HEAD UP, WHICH SHE DIDN'T DO BEFORE.

WE TRANSFORM REFLEXES INTO VOLUNTARY MOVEMENTS.

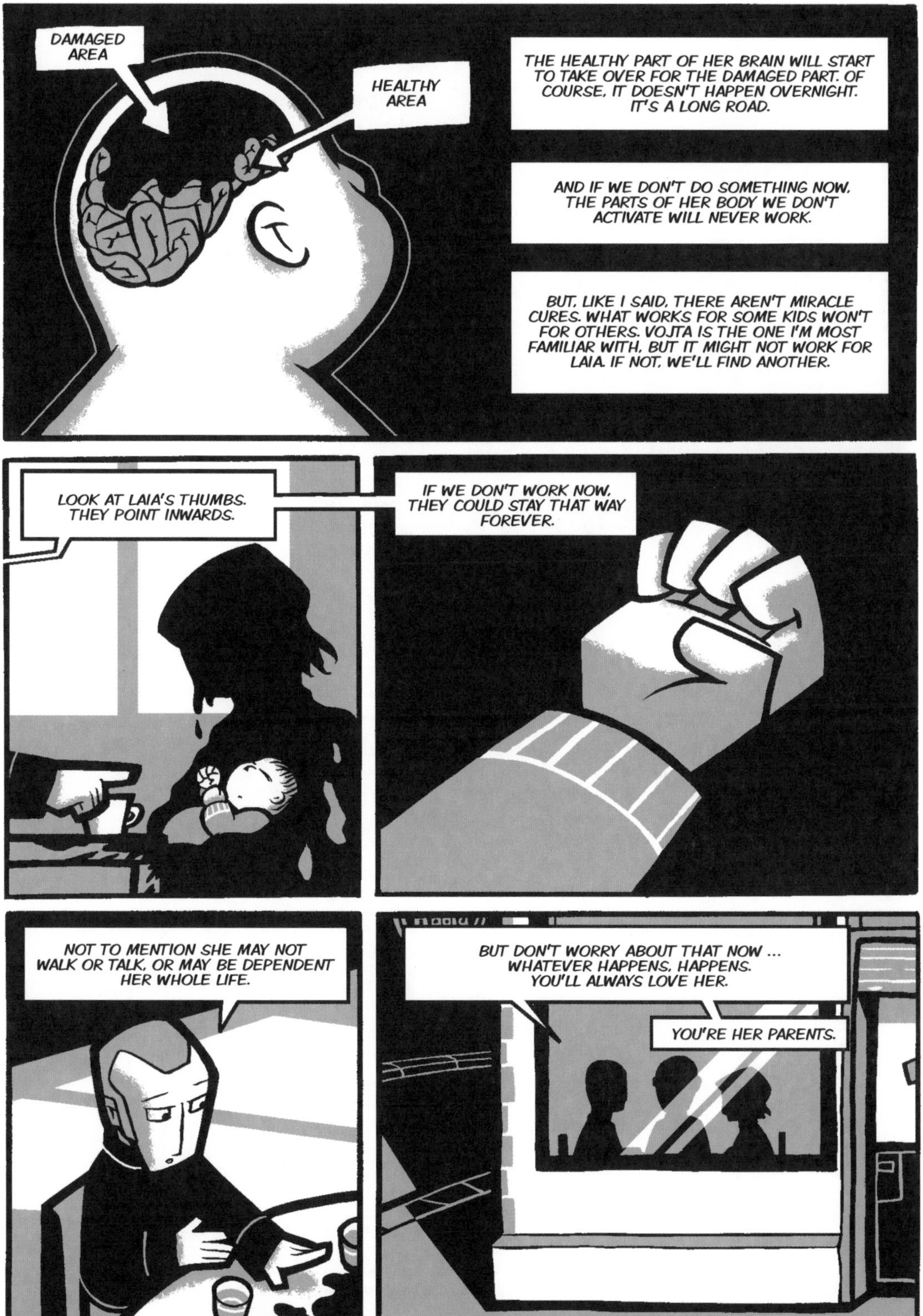
DAMAGED AREA
HEALTHY AREA
THE HEALTHY PART OF HER BRAIN WILL START TO TAKE OVER FOR THE DAMAGED PART. OF COURSE, IT DOESN'T HAPPEN OVERNIGHT. IT'S A LONG ROAD.
AND IF WE DON'T DO SOMETHING NOW, THE PARTS OF HER BODY WE DON'T ACTIVATE WILL NEVER WORK.
BUT, LIKE I SAID, THERE AREN'T MIRACLE CURES. WHAT WORKS FOR SOME KIDS WON'T FOR OTHERS. VOJTA IS THE ONE I'M MOST FAMILIAR WITH, BUT IT MIGHT NOT WORK FOR LAIA. IF NOT, WE'LL FIND ANOTHER.
LOOK AT LAIA'S THUMBS. THEY POINT INWARDS.
IF WE DON'T WORK NOW, THEY COULD STAY THAT WAY FOREVER.
NOT TO MENTION SHE MAY NOT WALK OR TALK, OR MAY BE DEPENDENT HER WHOLE LIFE.
BUT DON'T WORRY ABOUT THAT NOW ... WHATEVER HAPPENS, HAPPENS. YOU'LL ALWAYS LOVE HER.
YOU'RE HER PARENTS.

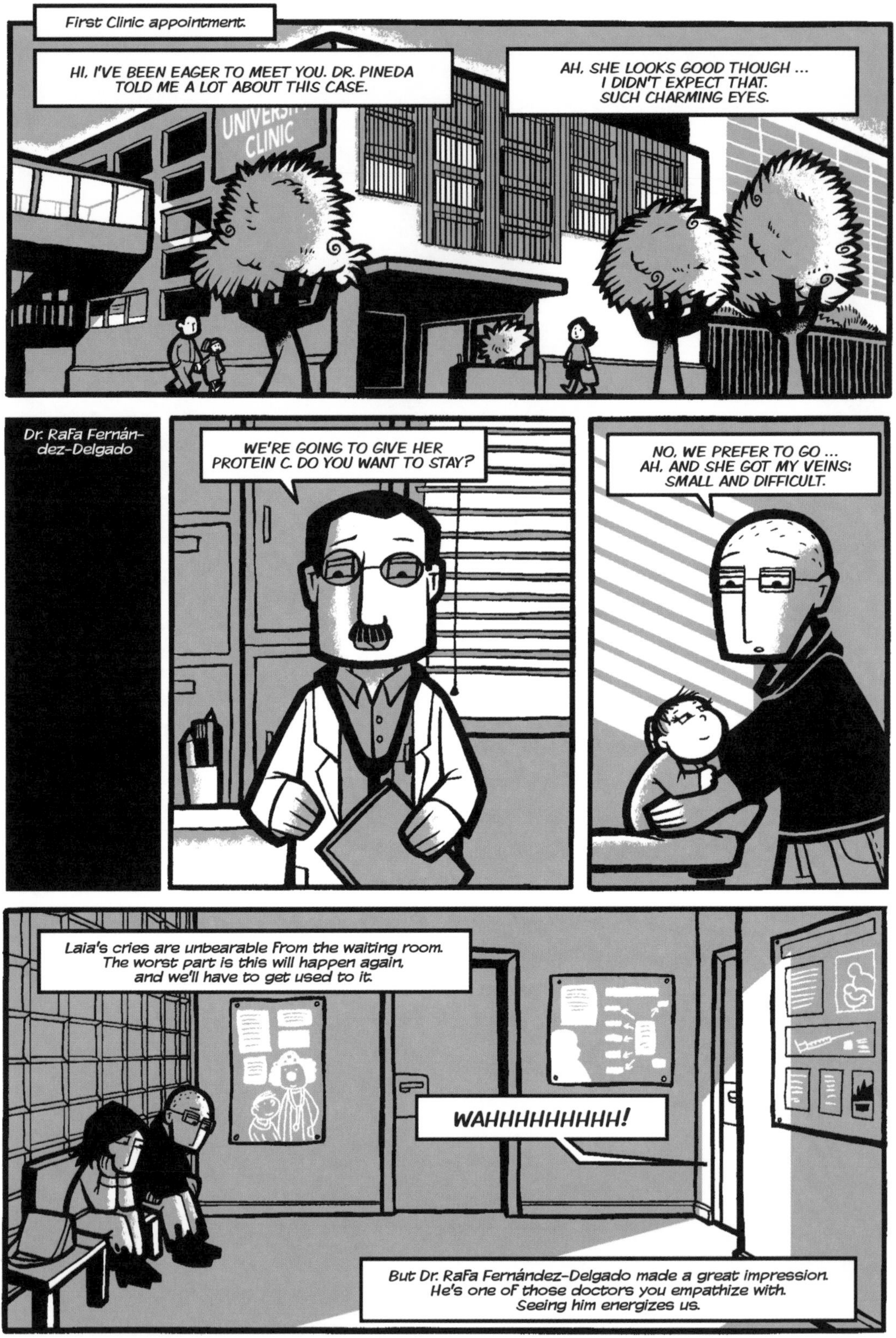
First Clinic appointment.
HI, I'VE BEEN EAGER TO MEET YOU. DR. PINEDA TOLD ME A LOT ABOUT THIS CASE.
AH, SHE LOOKS GOOD THOUGH ... I DIDN'T EXPECT THAT. SUCH CHARMING EYES.
CLINIC
Dr. RaFa Fernán-dez-Delgado
WE'RE GOING TO GIVE HER PROTEIN C. DO YOU WANT TO STAY?
NO, WE PREFER TO GO ... AH, AND SHE GOT MY VEINS: SMALL AND DIFFICULT.
Laia's cries are unbearable from the waiting room. The worst part is this will happen again, and we'll have to get used to it.
WAHHHHHHHHHH!
But Dr. RaFa Fernández-Delgado made a great impression. He's one of those doctors you empathize with. Seeing him energizes us.

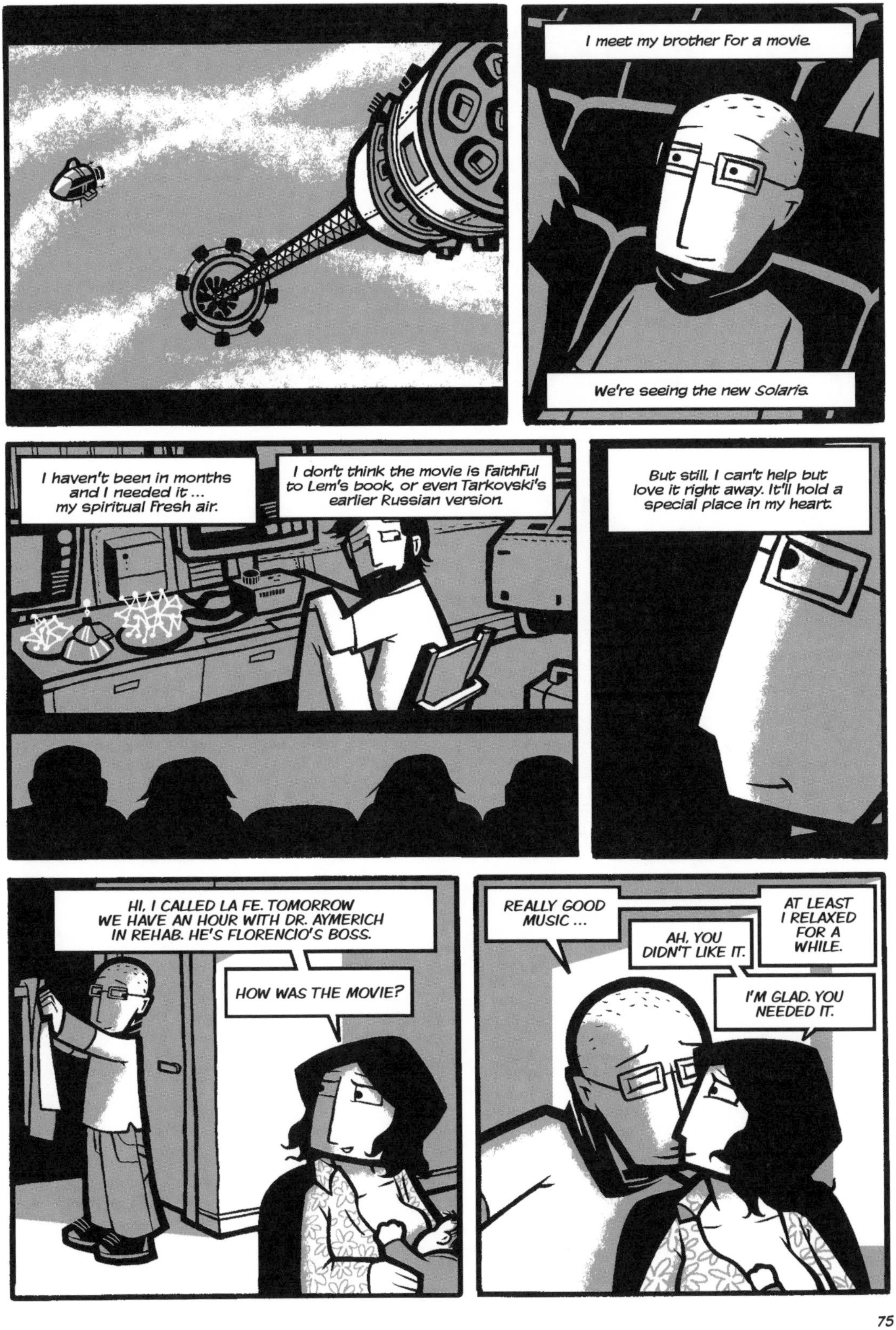
I meet my brother for a movie.
We're seeing the new Solaris.
I haven't been in months and I needed it ... my spiritual fresh air.
I don't think the movie is faithful to Lem's book, or even Tarkovski's earlier Russian version.
But still, I can't help but love it right away. It'll hold a special place in my heart.
HI, I CALLED LA FE. TOMORROW WE HAVE AN HOUR WITH DR. AYMERICH IN REHAB. HE'S FLORENCIO'S BOSS.
HOW WAS THE MOVIE?
REALLY GOOD MUSIC ...
AH, YOU DIDN'T LIKE IT.
AT LEAST I RELAXED FOR A WHILE.
I'M GLAD. YOU NEEDED IT.

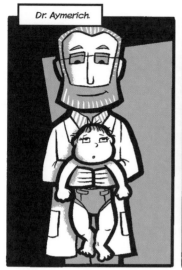

Dr. Aymerich.

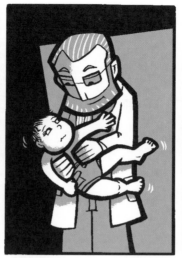

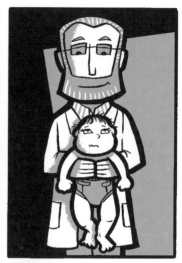

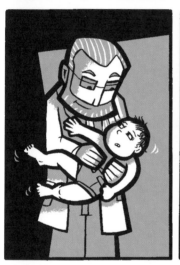

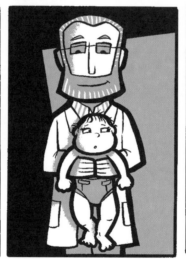

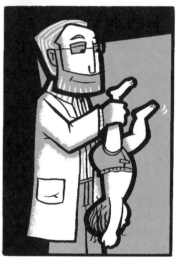

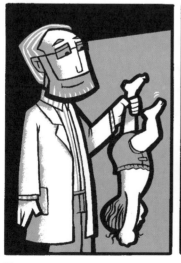

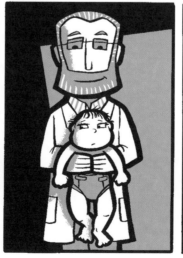

GOOD, SHE DOESN'T HAVE HER PRIMITIVE REFLEXES ANYMORE. THAT'S GREAT. BUT ...

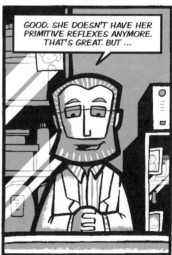

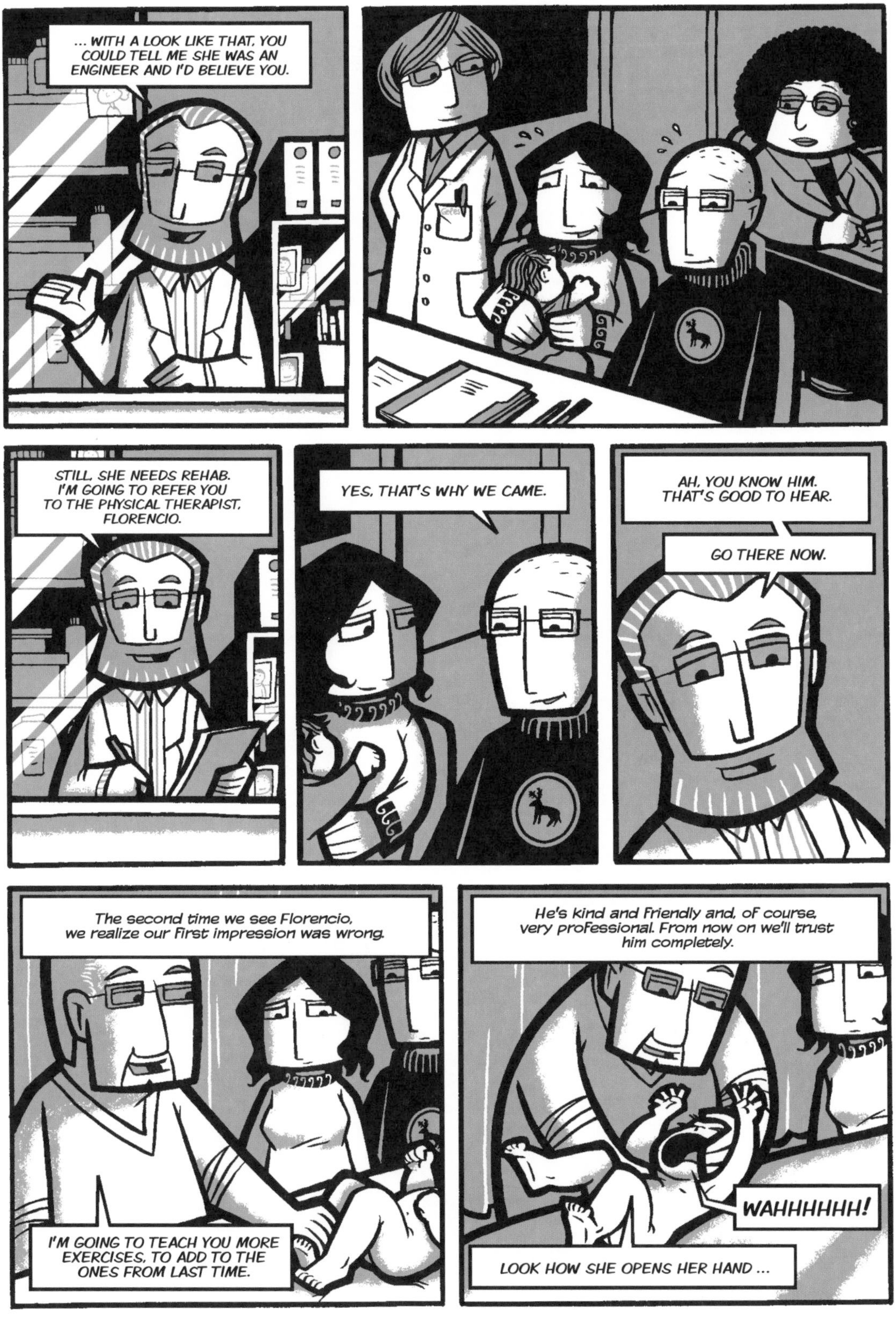
... WITH A LOOK LIKE THAT, YOU COULD TELL ME SHE WAS AN ENGINEER AND I'D BELIEVE YOU.
STILL, SHE NEEDS REHAB. I'M GOING TO REFER YOU TO THE PHYSICAL THERAPIST, FLORENCIO.
YES, THAT'S WHY WE CAME.
AH, YOU KNOW HIM. THAT'S GOOD TO HEAR.
GO THERE NOW.
The second time we see Florencio, we realize our first impression was wrong.
I'M GOING TO TEACH YOU MORE EXERCISES, TO ADD TO THE ONES FROM LAST TIME.
He's kind and friendly and, of course, very professional. From now on we'll trust him completely.
WAHHHHHH!
LOOK HOW SHE OPENS HER HAND ...

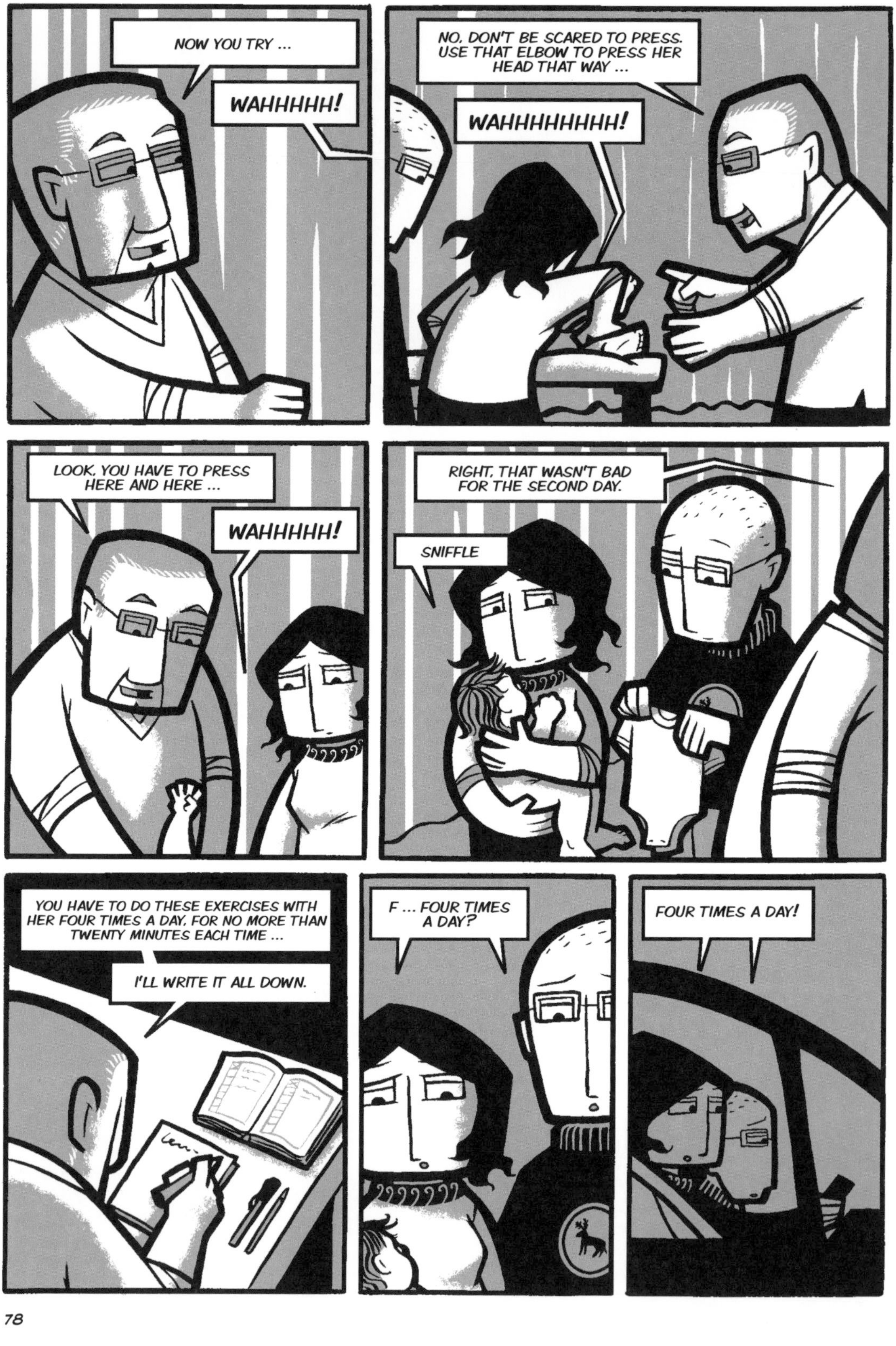
NOW YOU TRY ...
WAHHHHH!
NO, DON'T BE SCARED TO PRESS. USE THAT ELBOW TO PRESS HER HEAD THAT WAY ...
WAHHHHHHHHH!
LOOK, YOU HAVE TO PRESS HERE AND HERE ...
WAHHHHH!
RIGHT, THAT WASN'T BAD FOR THE SECOND DAY.
SNIFFLE
YOU HAVE TO DO THESE EXERCISES WITH HER FOUR TIMES A DAY, FOR NO MORE THAN TWENTY MINUTES EACH TIME ...
I'LL WRITE IT ALL DOWN.
F ... FOUR TIMES A DAY?
FOUR TIMES A DAY!

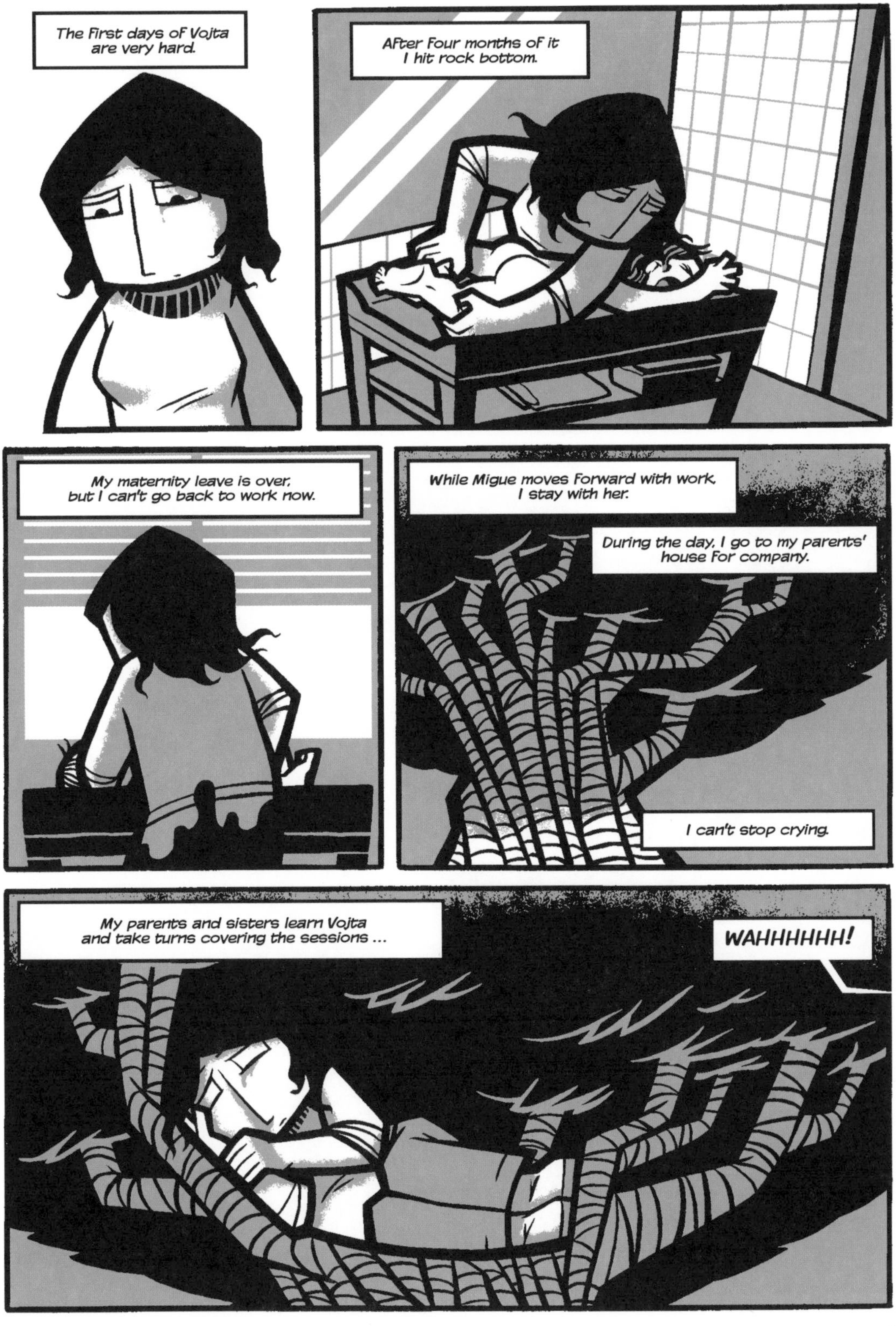
The First days of Vojta are very hard.
After Four months of it I hit rock bottom.
My maternity leave is over, but I can't go back to work now.
While Migue moves Forward with work, I stay with her.
During the day, I go to my parents' house for company.
I can't stop crying.
My parents and sisters learn Vojta and take turns covering the sessions ...
WAHHHHHH!

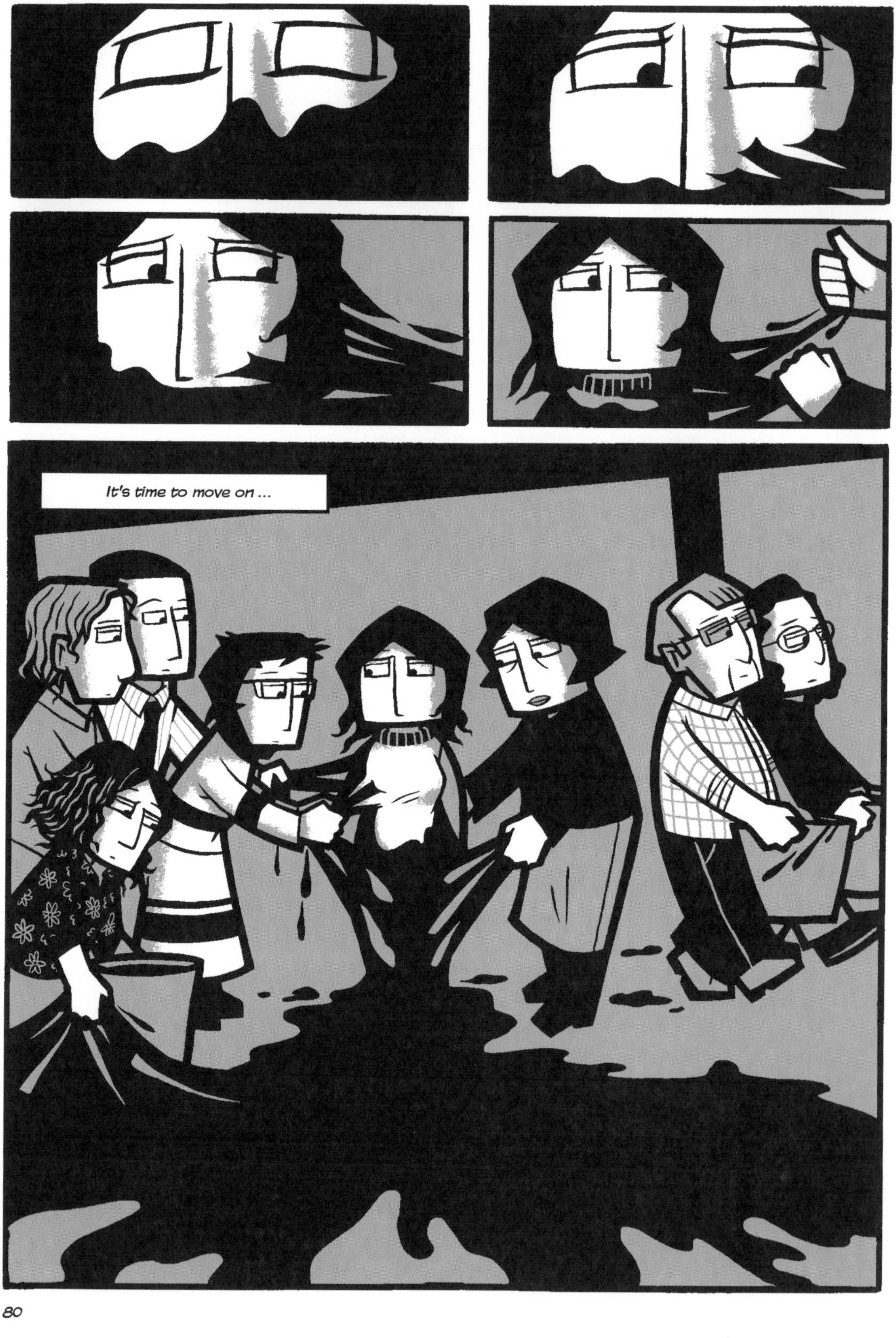
It's time to move on ...

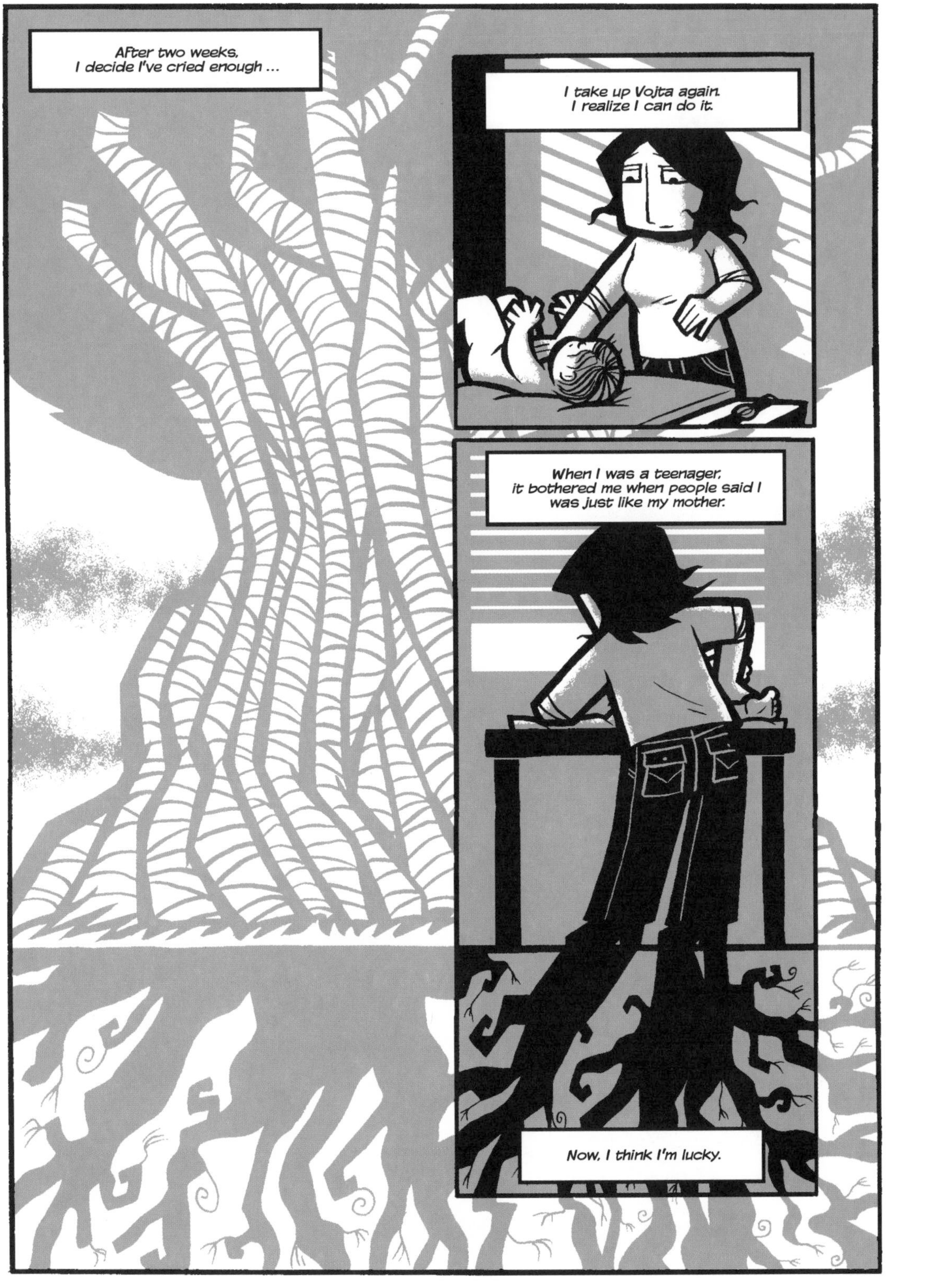
After two weeks, I decide I've cried enough ...
I take up Vojta again. I realize I can do it.
When I was a teenager, it bothered me when people said I was just like my mother.
Now, I think I'm lucky.

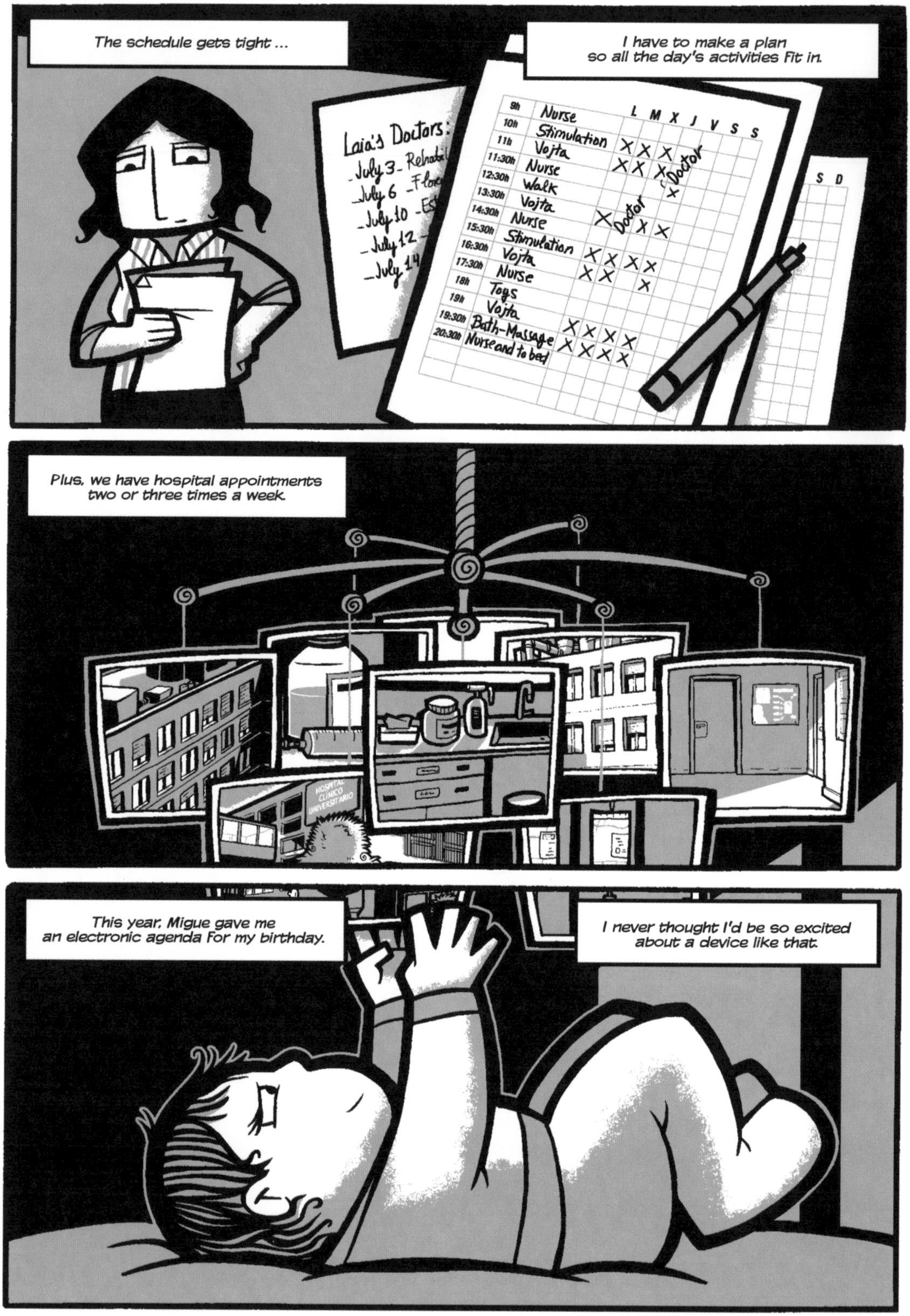
The schedule gets tight ...
I have to make a plan so all the day's activities fit in.
Laia's Doctors:
-July 3
-July 6
-July 10
-July 12
-July 14
L M X J V S S
9h Nurse
10h Stimulation
11h Vojta
11:30h Nurse
12:30h Walk
13:30h Vojta
14:30h Nurse
15:30h Stimulation
16:30h Vojta
17:30h Nurse
18h Toys
19h Vojta
19:30h Bath-Massage
20:30h Nurse and to bed
Doctor
Doctor
S D
Plus, we have hospital appointments two or three times a week.
HOSPITAL CLINICO UNIVERSITARIO
This year, Migue gave me an electronic agenda for my birthday.
I never thought I'd be so excited about a device like that.

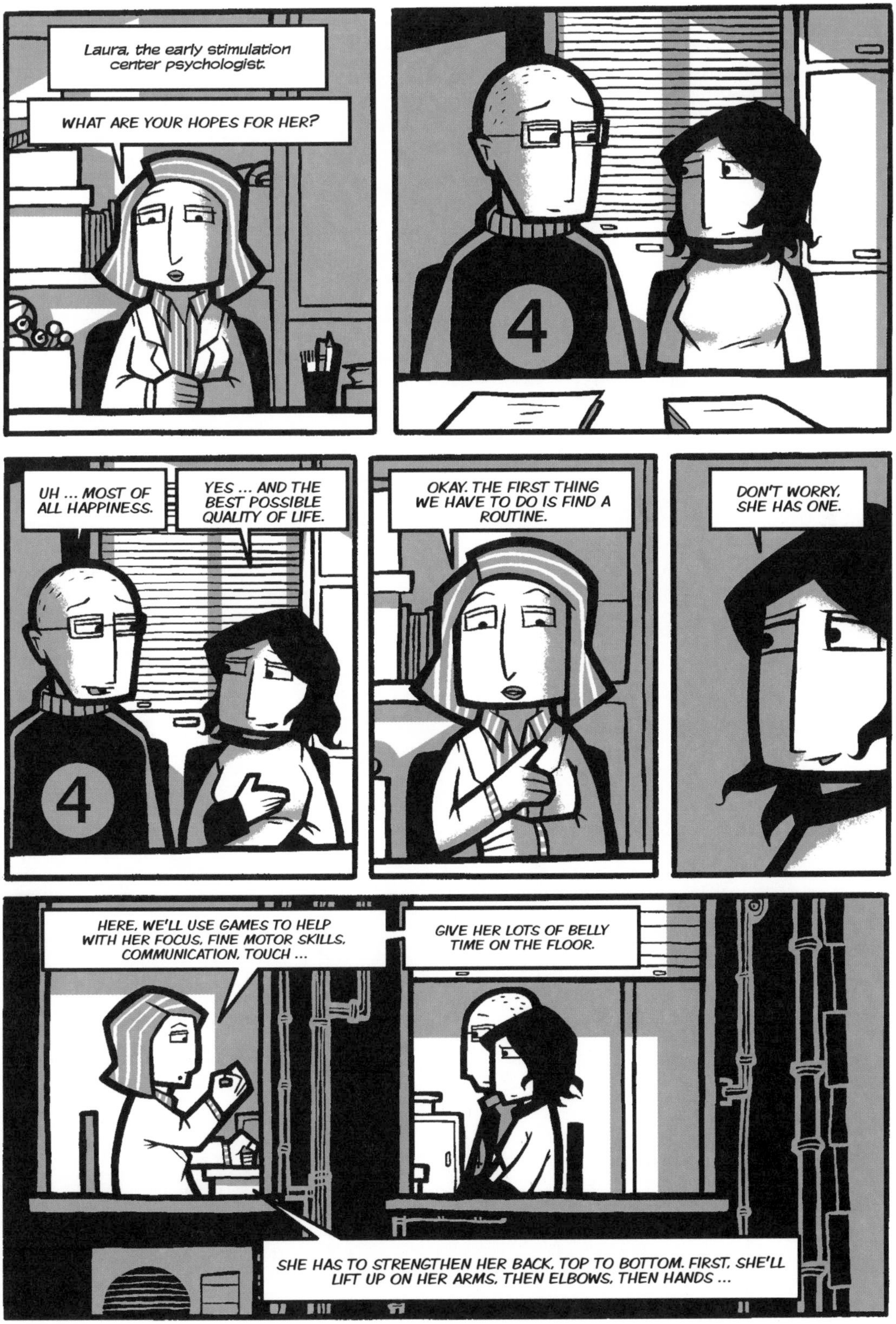
Laura, the early stimulation center psychologist.
WHAT ARE YOUR HOPES FOR HER?
UH ... MOST OF ALL HAPPINESS.
YES ... AND THE BEST POSSIBLE QUALITY OF LIFE.
OKAY. THE FIRST THING WE HAVE TO DO IS FIND A ROUTINE.
DON'T WORRY. SHE HAS ONE.
HERE, WE'LL USE GAMES TO HELP WITH HER FOCUS, FINE MOTOR SKILLS, COMMUNICATION, TOUCH ...
GIVE HER LOTS OF BELLY TIME ON THE FLOOR.
SHE HAS TO STRENGTHEN HER BACK, TOP TO BOTTOM. FIRST, SHE'LL LIFT UP ON HER ARMS, THEN ELBOWS, THEN HANDS ...

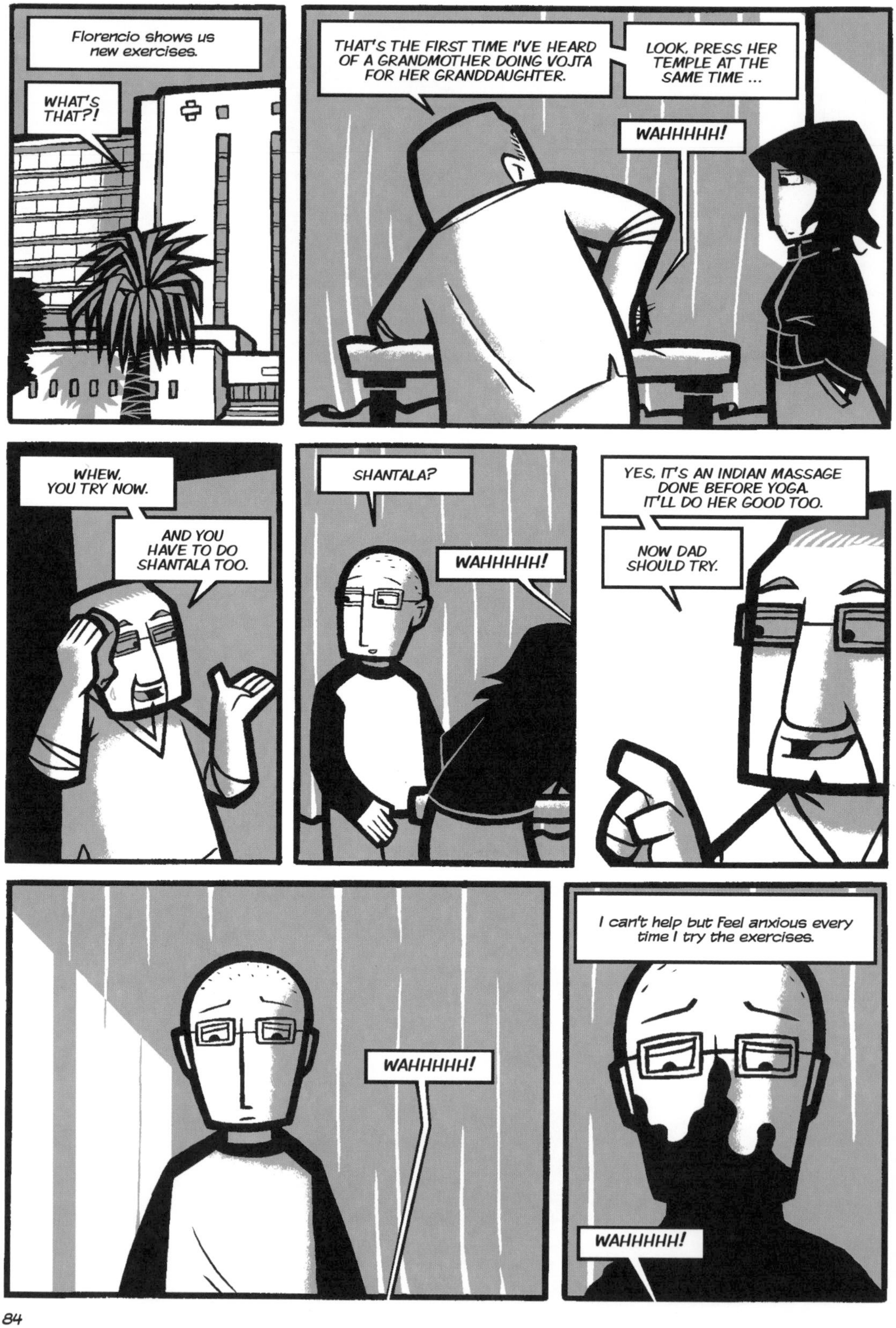
Florencio shows us new exercises.
WHAT'S THAT?!
THAT'S THE FIRST TIME I'VE HEARD OF A GRANDMOTHER DOING VOJTA FOR HER GRANDDAUGHTER.
LOOK, PRESS HER TEMPLE AT THE SAME TIME ...
WAHHHHH!
WHEW, YOU TRY NOW.
AND YOU HAVE TO DO SHANTALA TOO.
SHANTALA?
WAHHHHH!
YES, IT'S AN INDIAN MASSAGE DONE BEFORE YOGA. IT'LL DO HER GOOD TOO.
NOW DAD SHOULD TRY.
WAHHHHH!
I can't help but feel anxious every time I try the exercises.
WAHHHHH!

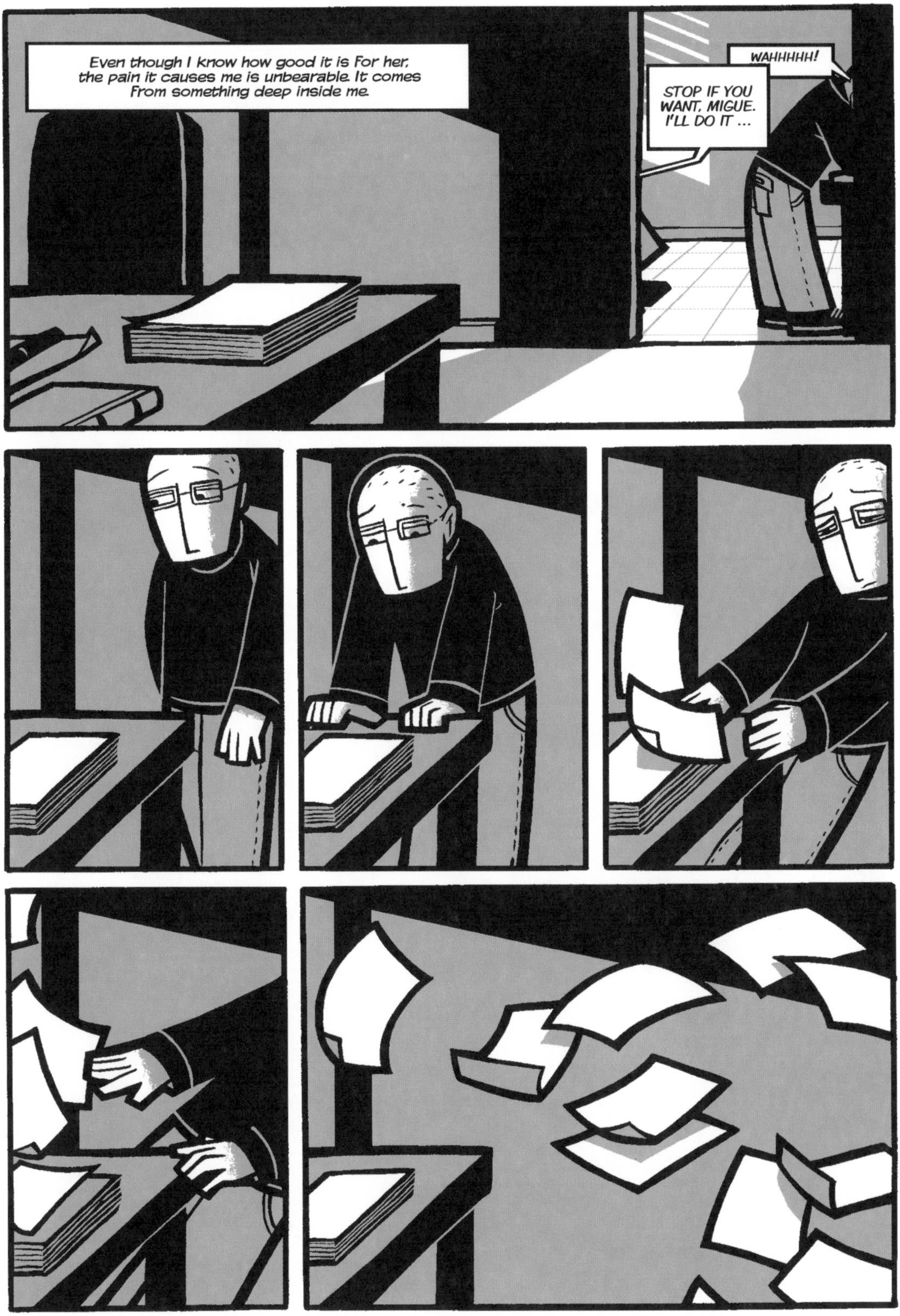
Even though I know how good it is for her, the pain it causes me is unbearable. It comes from something deep inside me.
WAHHHHH!
STOP IF YOU WANT, MIGUE. I'LL DO IT ...

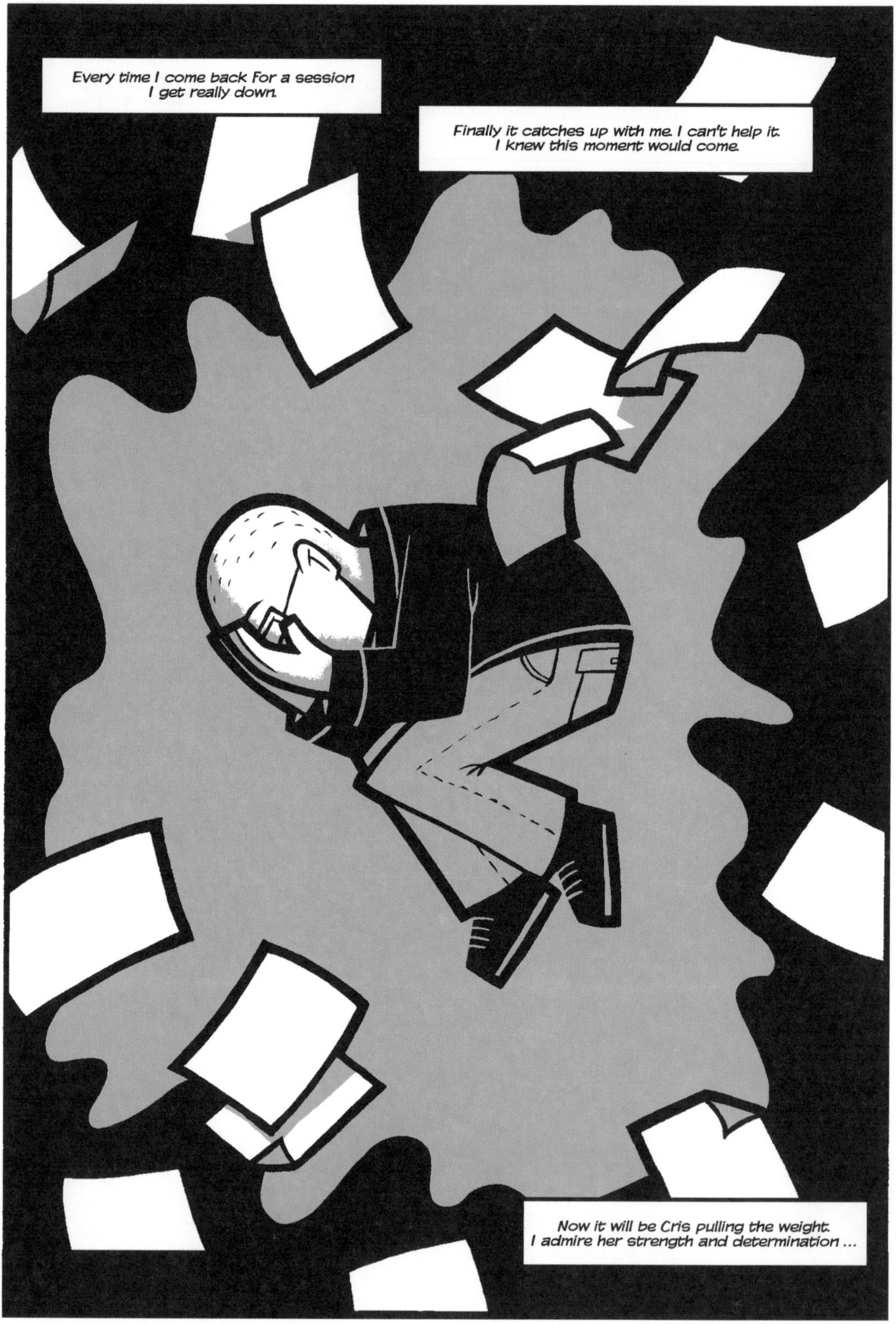
Every time I come back for a session
I get really down.
Finally it catches up with me. I can't help it.
I knew this moment would come.
Now it will be Cris pulling the weight.
I admire her strength and determination ...

5.
THE CHANCE

**É melhor ser alegre que
ser triste.
Alegria é la melhor coisa
que existe.**

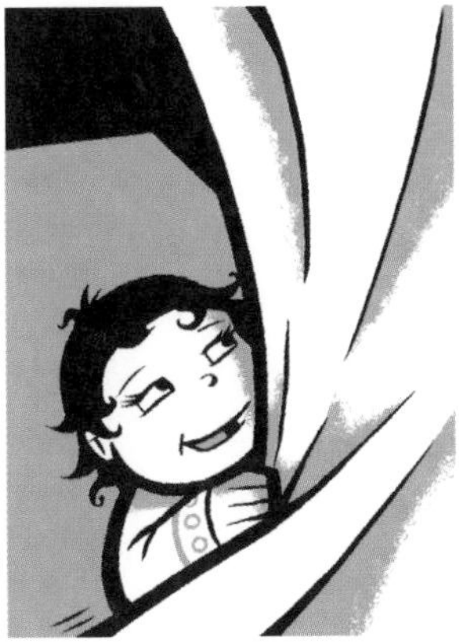

"Samba da bênção,"
Vinicius de Moraes
Baden Powell

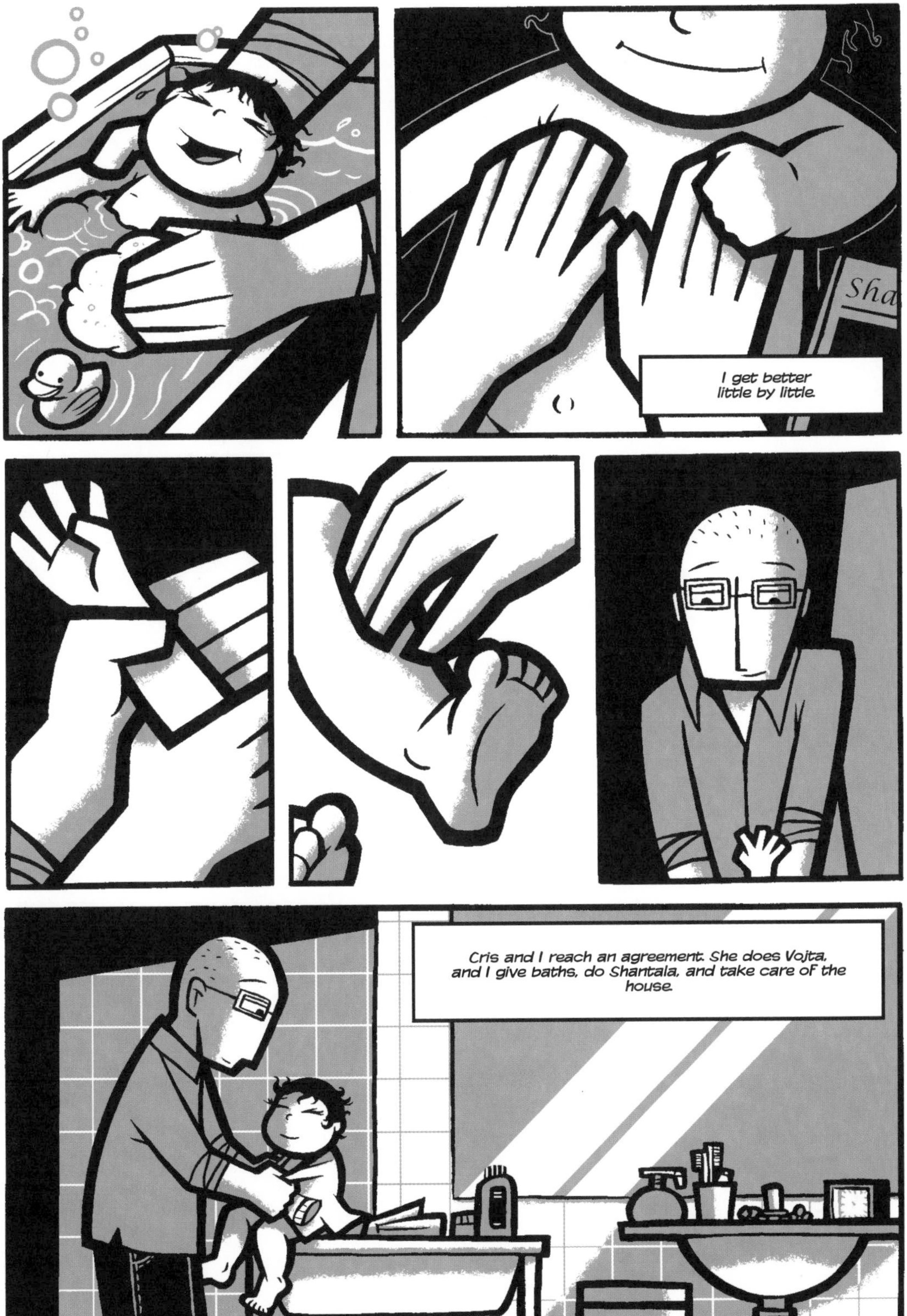
I get better little by little.
Cris and I reach an agreement. She does Vojta, and I give baths, do Shantala, and take care of the house.

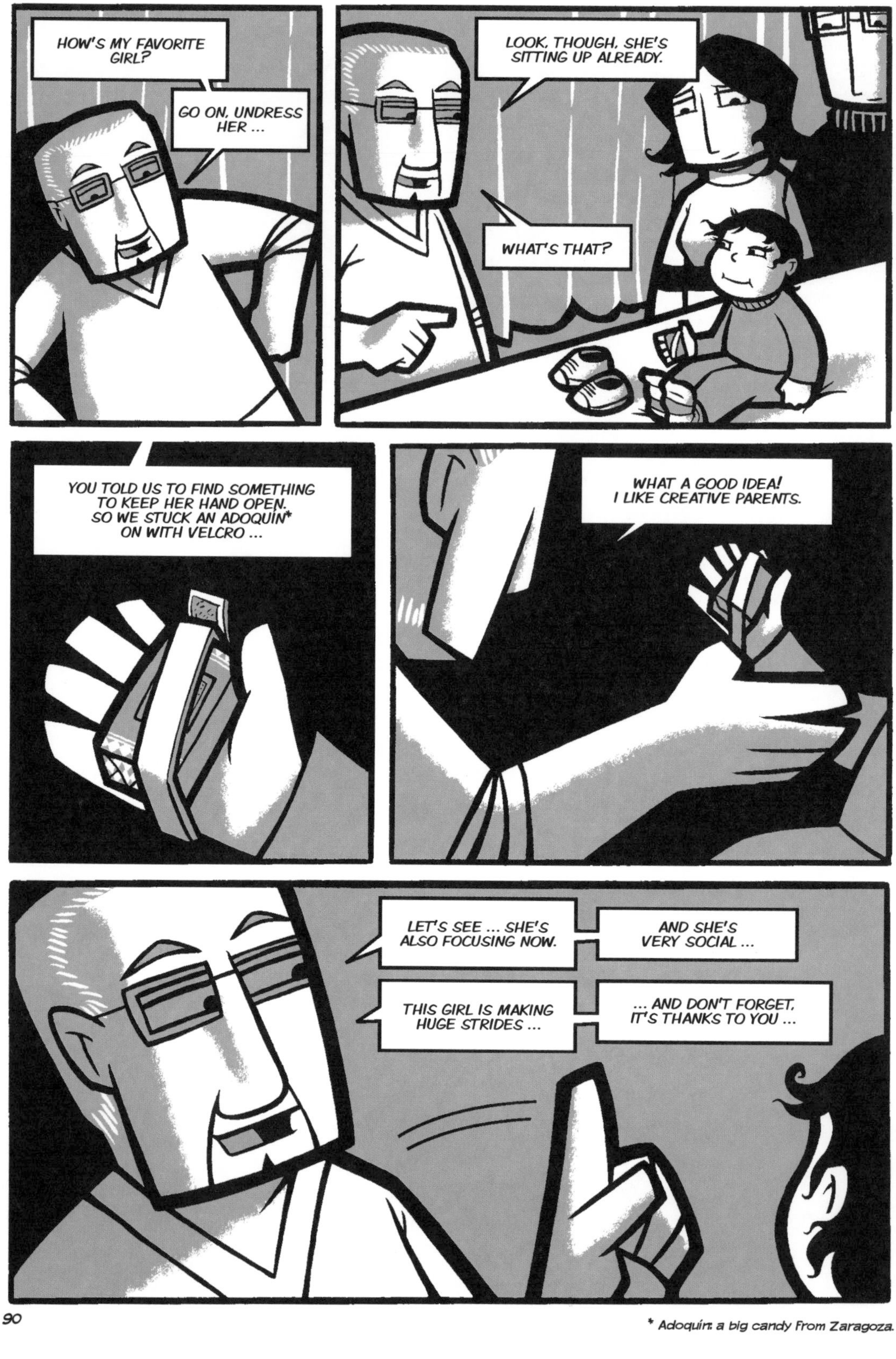
HOW'S MY FAVORITE GIRL?
GO ON, UNDRESS HER ...
LOOK, THOUGH, SHE'S SITTING UP ALREADY.
WHAT'S THAT?
YOU TOLD US TO FIND SOMETHING TO KEEP HER HAND OPEN. SO WE STUCK AN ADOQUÍN* ON WITH VELCRO ...
WHAT A GOOD IDEA! I LIKE CREATIVE PARENTS.
LET'S SEE ... SHE'S ALSO FOCUSING NOW.
AND SHE'S VERY SOCIAL ...
THIS GIRL IS MAKING HUGE STRIDES ...
... AND DON'T FORGET, IT'S THANKS TO YOU ...

* Adoquín: a big candy from Zaragoza.

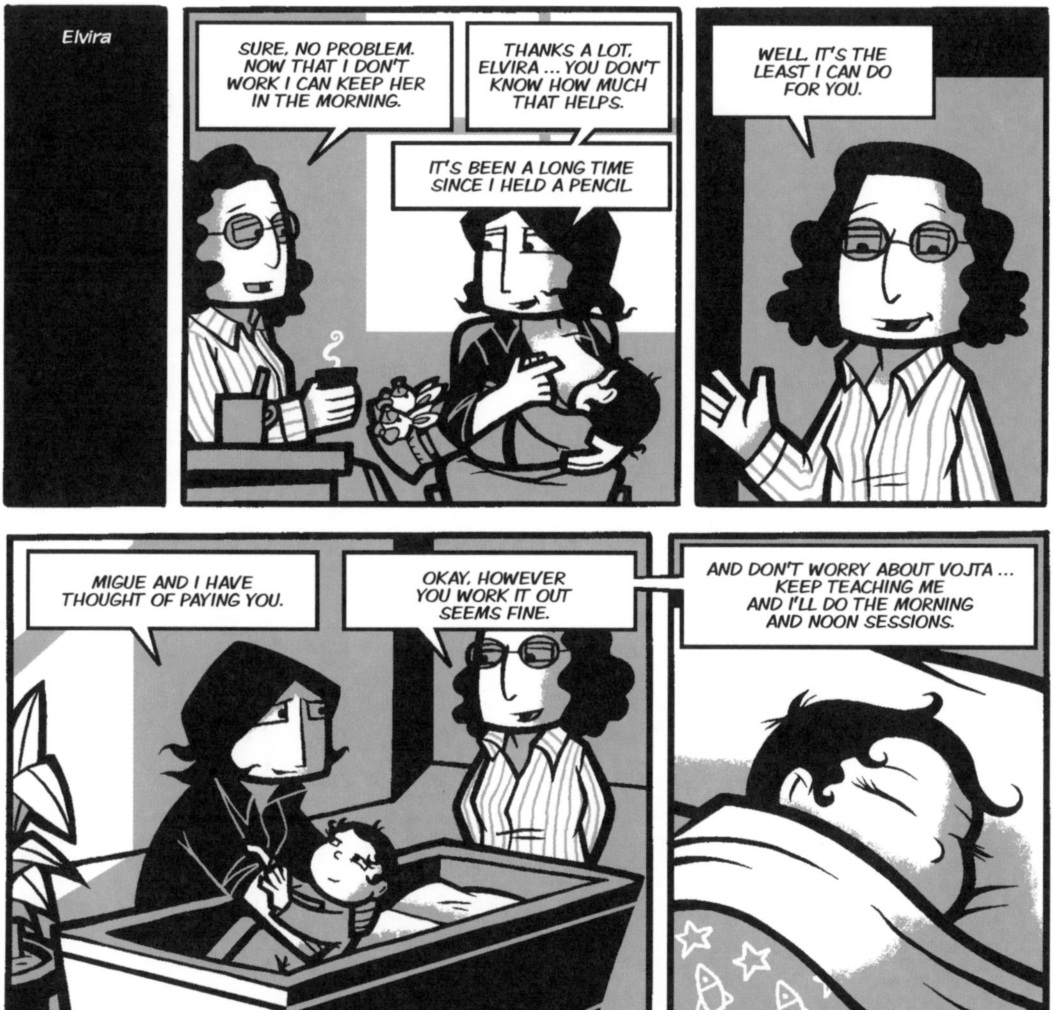
Elvira
SURE, NO PROBLEM. NOW THAT I DON'T WORK I CAN KEEP HER IN THE MORNING.
THANKS A LOT, ELVIRA ... YOU DON'T KNOW HOW MUCH THAT HELPS.
IT'S BEEN A LONG TIME SINCE I HELD A PENCIL.
WELL, IT'S THE LEAST I CAN DO FOR YOU.
MIGUE AND I HAVE THOUGHT OF PAYING YOU.
OKAY, HOWEVER YOU WORK IT OUT SEEMS FINE.
AND DON'T WORRY ABOUT VOJTA ... KEEP TEACHING ME AND I'LL DO THE MORNING AND NOON SESSIONS.
OH, THAT WOULD BE GREAT. BUT YOU SHOULD KNOW IT'S HARD ...
NO WORRIES ...
I'M JUST HER AUNT. IT WON'T AFFECT ME LIKE YOU.

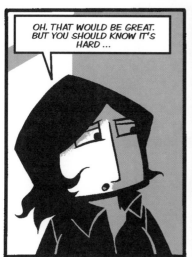

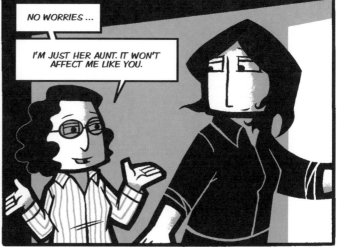

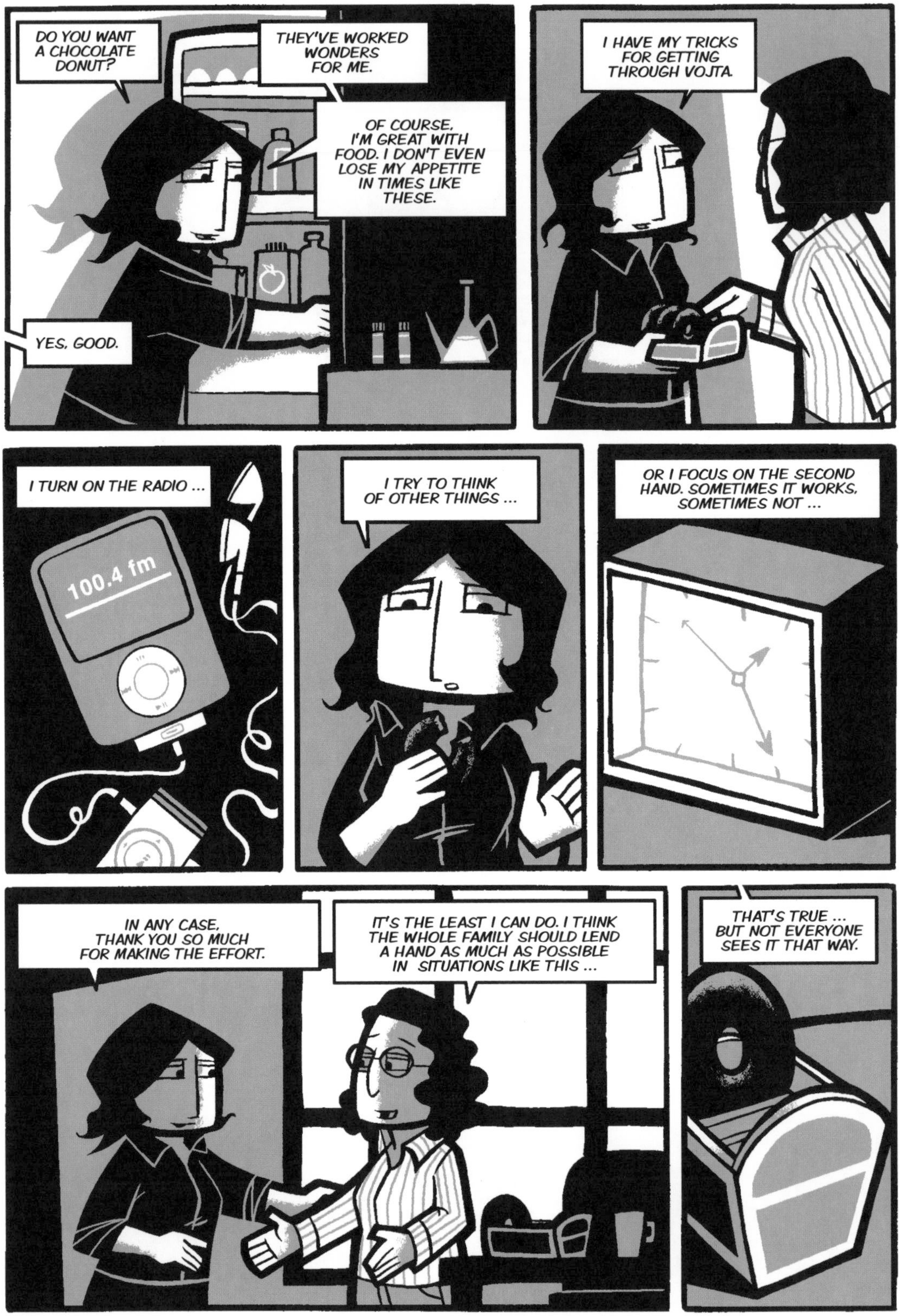
DO YOU WANT A CHOCOLATE DONUT?
THEY'VE WORKED WONDERS FOR ME.
OF COURSE, I'M GREAT WITH FOOD. I DON'T EVEN LOSE MY APPETITE IN TIMES LIKE THESE.
YES, GOOD.
I HAVE MY TRICKS FOR GETTING THROUGH VOJTA.
I TURN ON THE RADIO ...
100.4 fm
I TRY TO THINK OF OTHER THINGS ...
OR I FOCUS ON THE SECOND HAND. SOMETIMES IT WORKS, SOMETIMES NOT ...
IN ANY CASE, THANK YOU SO MUCH FOR MAKING THE EFFORT.
IT'S THE LEAST I CAN DO. I THINK THE WHOLE FAMILY SHOULD LEND A HAND AS MUCH AS POSSIBLE IN SITUATIONS LIKE THIS ...
THAT'S TRUE ... BUT NOT EVERYONE SEES IT THAT WAY.

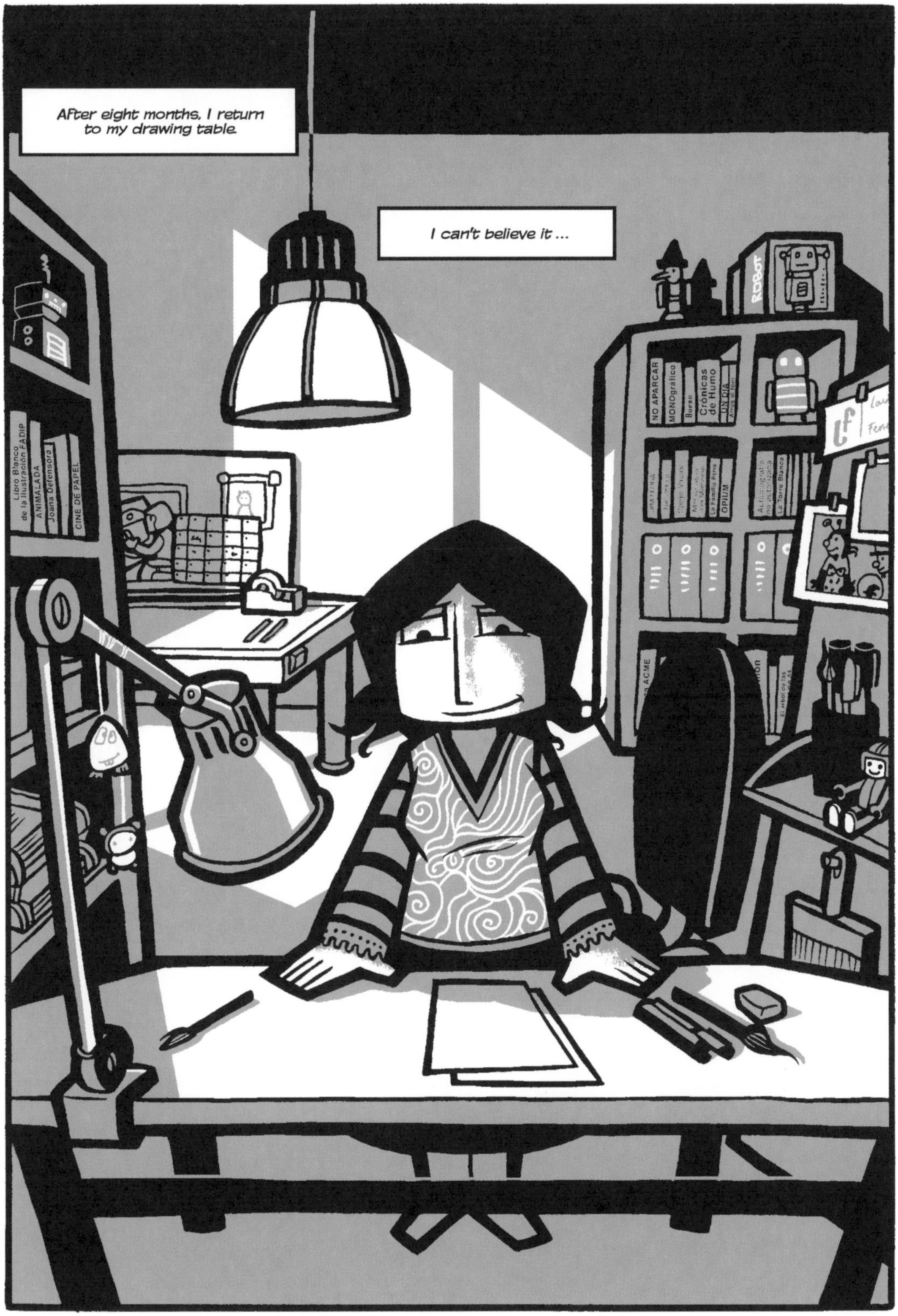
After eight months, I return to my drawing table.
I can't believe it ...
Libro Blanco de la ilustración FADIP
ANIMALADA
Joana Defensora
CINE DE PAPEL
NO APARCAR
MONOgrafico
Crónicas de Humo
UN DIA
OPIUM
La Torre Blanca
ACME
ROBOT

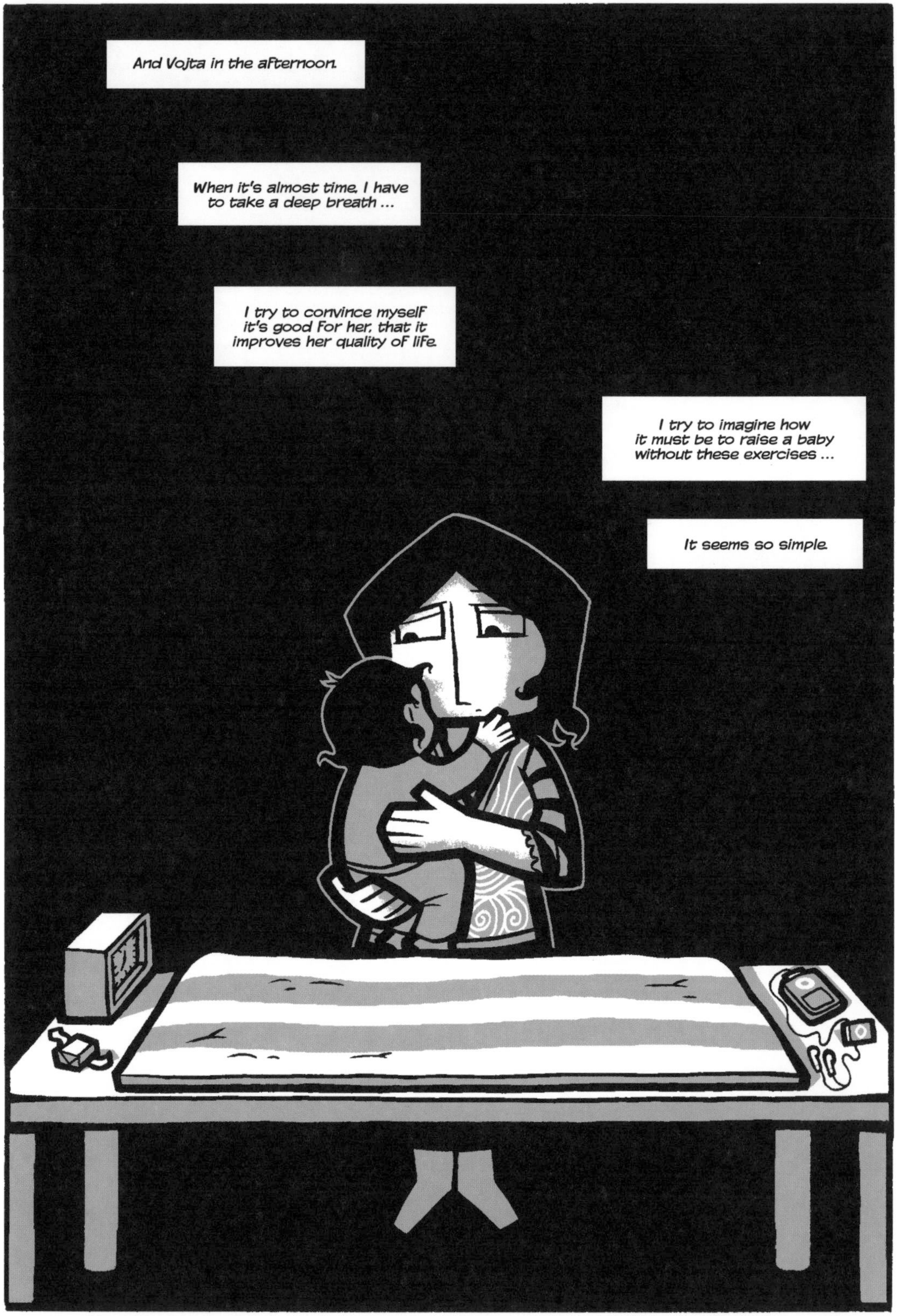
And Vojta in the afternoon.
When it's almost time, I have to take a deep breath ...
I try to convince myself it's good for her, that it improves her quality of life.
I try to imagine how it must be to raise a baby without these exercises ...
It seems so simple.

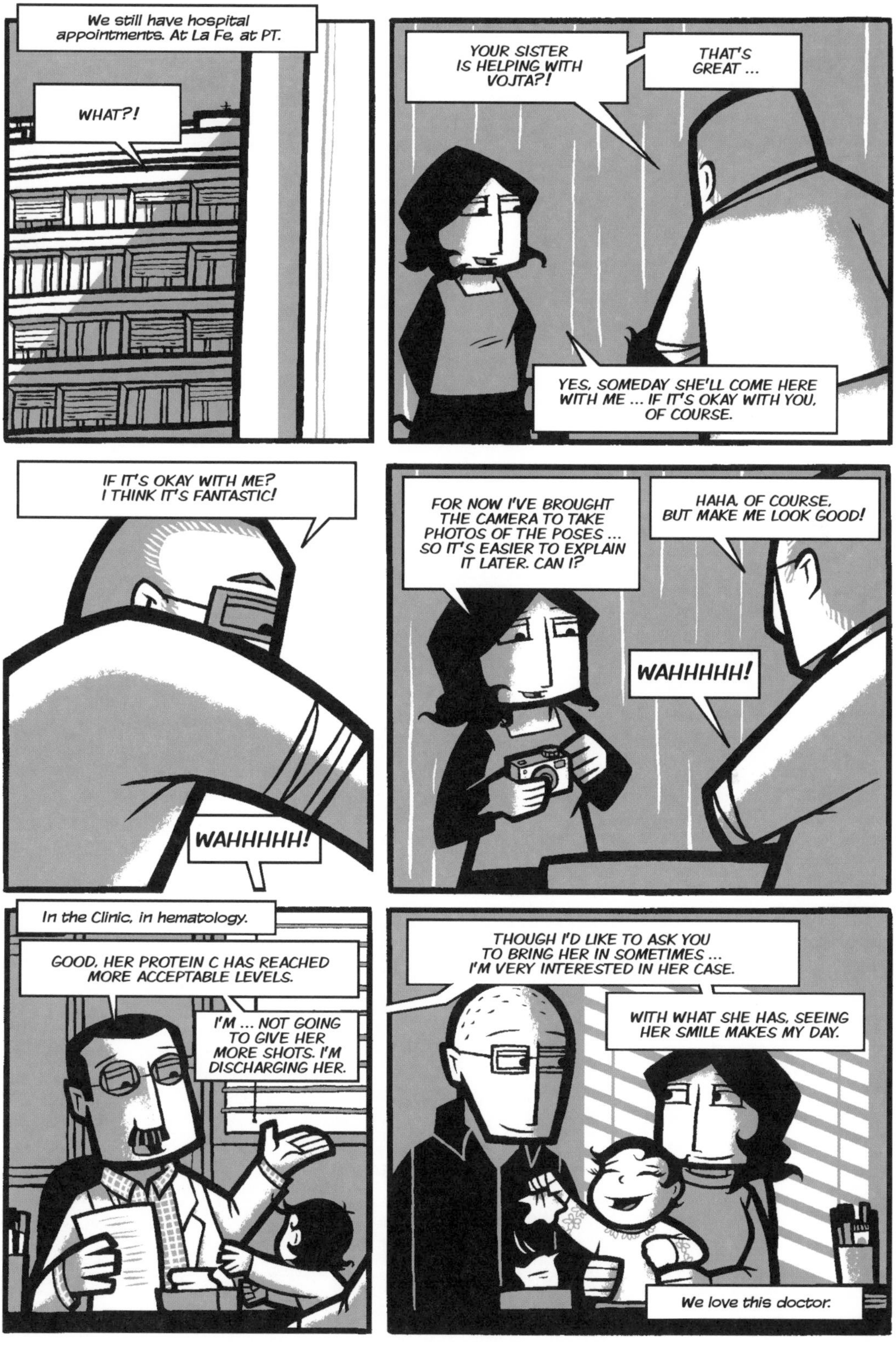
We still have hospital appointments. At La Fe, at PT.
WHAT?!
YOUR SISTER IS HELPING WITH VOJTA?!
THAT'S GREAT ...
YES, SOMEDAY SHE'LL COME HERE WITH ME ... IF IT'S OKAY WITH YOU, OF COURSE.
IF IT'S OKAY WITH ME? I THINK IT'S FANTASTIC!
WAHHHHH!
FOR NOW I'VE BROUGHT THE CAMERA TO TAKE PHOTOS OF THE POSES ... SO IT'S EASIER TO EXPLAIN IT LATER. CAN I?
HAHA, OF COURSE, BUT MAKE ME LOOK GOOD!
WAHHHHH!
In the Clinic, in hematology.
GOOD, HER PROTEIN C HAS REACHED MORE ACCEPTABLE LEVELS.
I'M ... NOT GOING TO GIVE HER MORE SHOTS. I'M DISCHARGING HER.
THOUGH I'D LIKE TO ASK YOU TO BRING HER IN SOMETIMES ... I'M VERY INTERESTED IN HER CASE.
WITH WHAT SHE HAS, SEEING HER SMILE MAKES MY DAY.
We love this doctor.

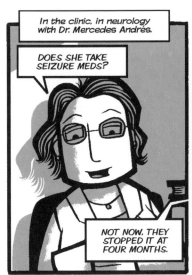

In the clinic, in neurology with Dr. Mercedes Andrés.

DOES SHE TAKE SEIZURE MEDS?

NOT NOW. THEY STOPPED IT AT FOUR MONTHS.

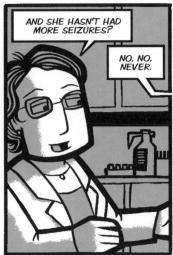

AND SHE HASN'T HAD MORE SEIZURES?

NO, NO, NEVER.

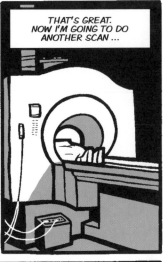

THAT'S GREAT. NOW I'M GOING TO DO ANOTHER SCAN ...

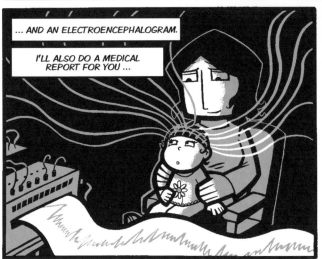

... AND AN ELECTROENCEPHALOGRAM.

I'LL ALSO DO A MEDICAL REPORT FOR YOU ...

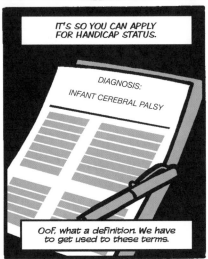

IT'S SO YOU CAN APPLY FOR HANDICAP STATUS.

DIAGNOSIS:

INFANT CEREBRAL PALSY

Oof, what a definition. We have to get used to these terms.

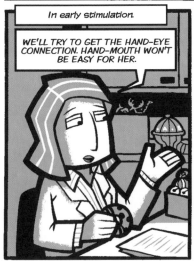

In early stimulation.

WE'LL TRY TO GET THE HAND–EYE CONNECTION. HAND–MOUTH WON'T BE EASY FOR HER.

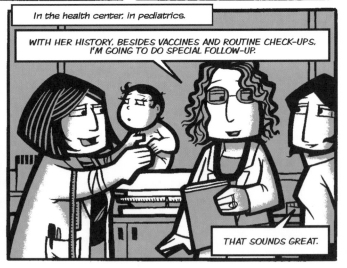

In the health center, in pediatrics.

WITH HER HISTORY, BESIDES VACCINES AND ROUTINE CHECK-UPS, I'M GOING TO DO SPECIAL FOLLOW-UP.

THAT SOUNDS GREAT.

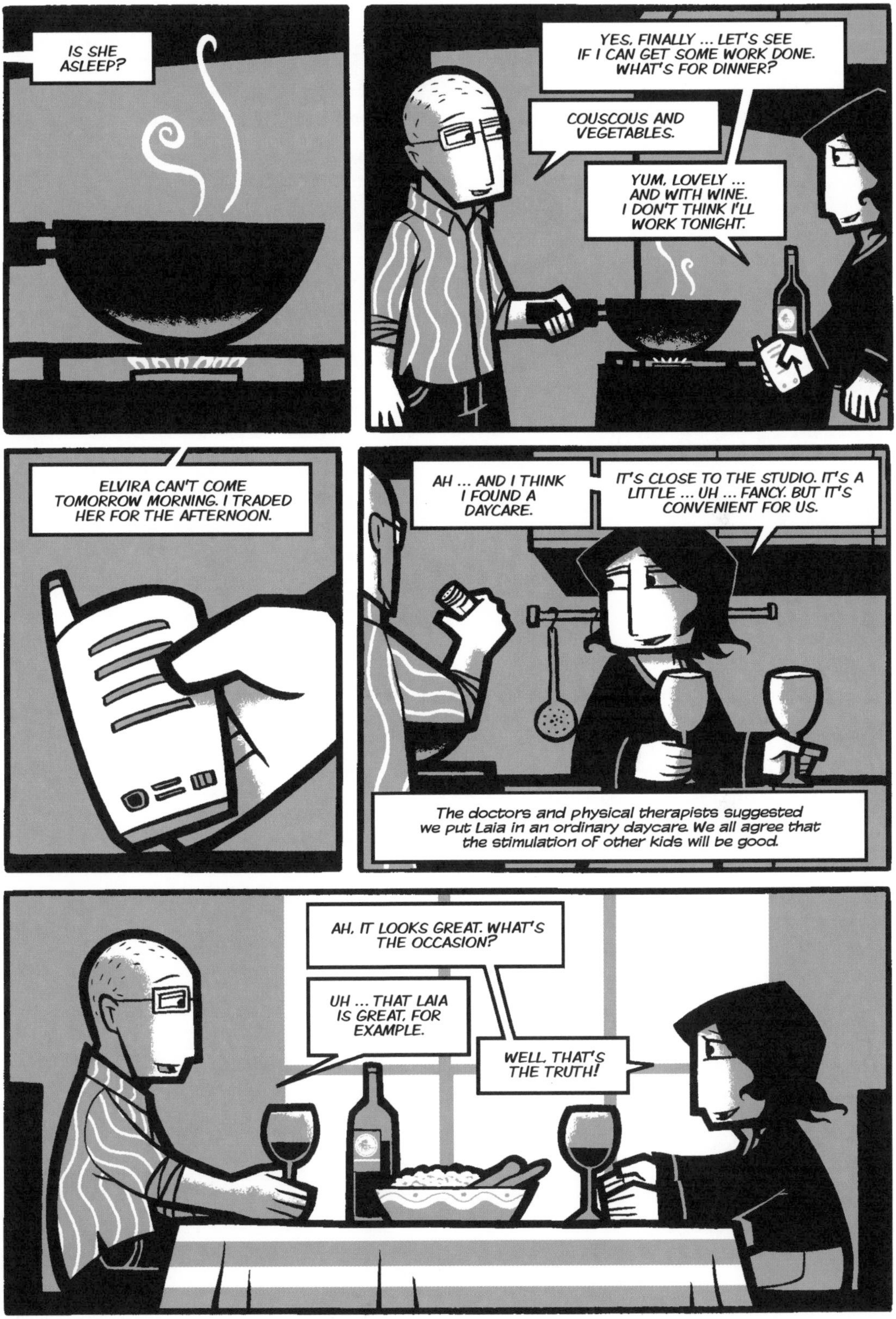
IS SHE ASLEEP?
YES, FINALLY ... LET'S SEE IF I CAN GET SOME WORK DONE. WHAT'S FOR DINNER?
COUSCOUS AND VEGETABLES.
YUM, LOVELY ... AND WITH WINE. I DON'T THINK I'LL WORK TONIGHT.
ELVIRA CAN'T COME TOMORROW MORNING. I TRADED HER FOR THE AFTERNOON.
AH ... AND I THINK I FOUND A DAYCARE.
IT'S CLOSE TO THE STUDIO. IT'S A LITTLE ... UH ... FANCY. BUT IT'S CONVENIENT FOR US.
The doctors and physical therapists suggested we put Laia in an ordinary daycare. We all agree that the stimulation of other kids will be good.
AH, IT LOOKS GREAT. WHAT'S THE OCCASION?
UH ... THAT LAIA IS GREAT, FOR EXAMPLE.
WELL, THAT'S THE TRUTH!

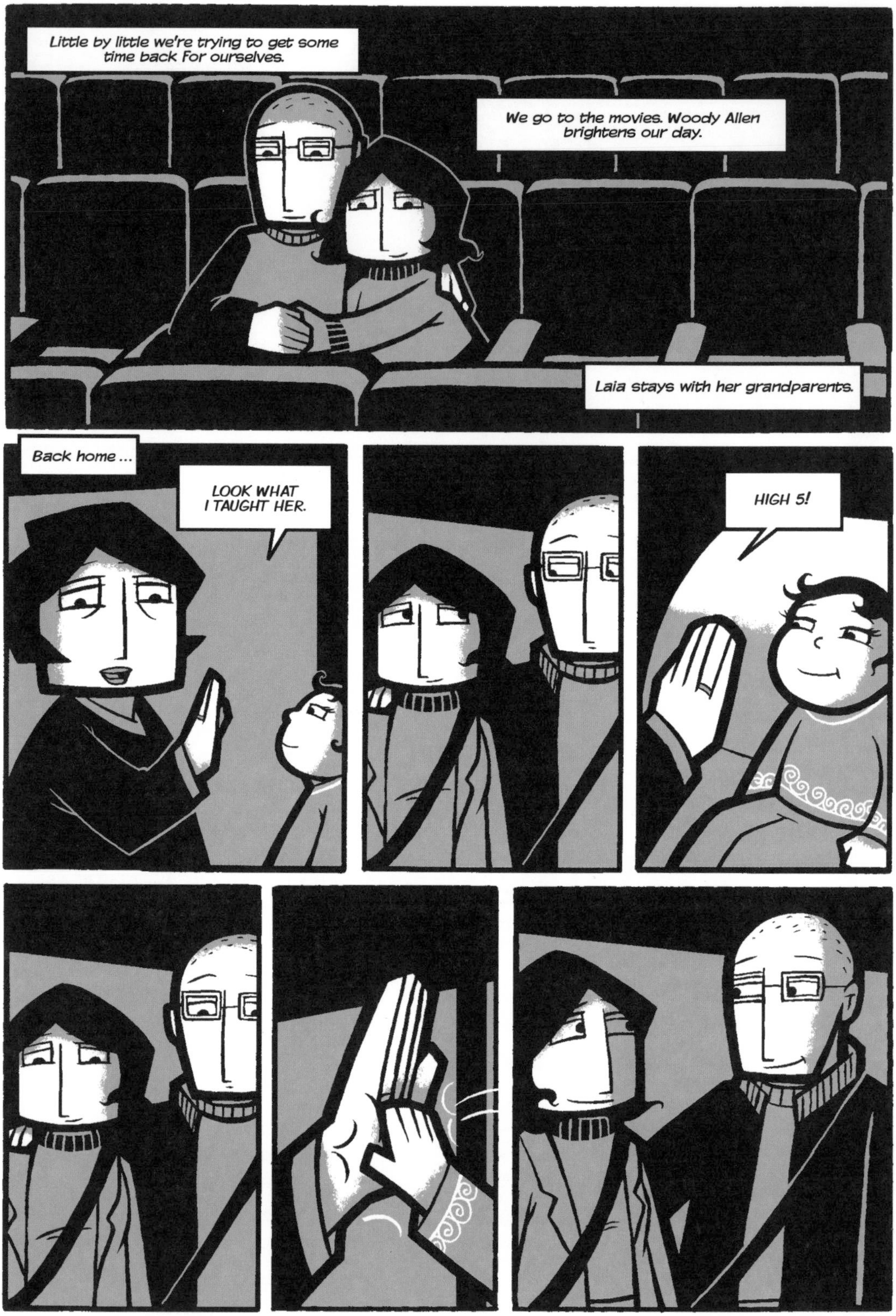
Little by little we're trying to get some time back for ourselves.
We go to the movies. Woody Allen brightens our day.
Laia stays with her grandparents.
Back home ...
LOOK WHAT I TAUGHT HER.
HIGH 5!

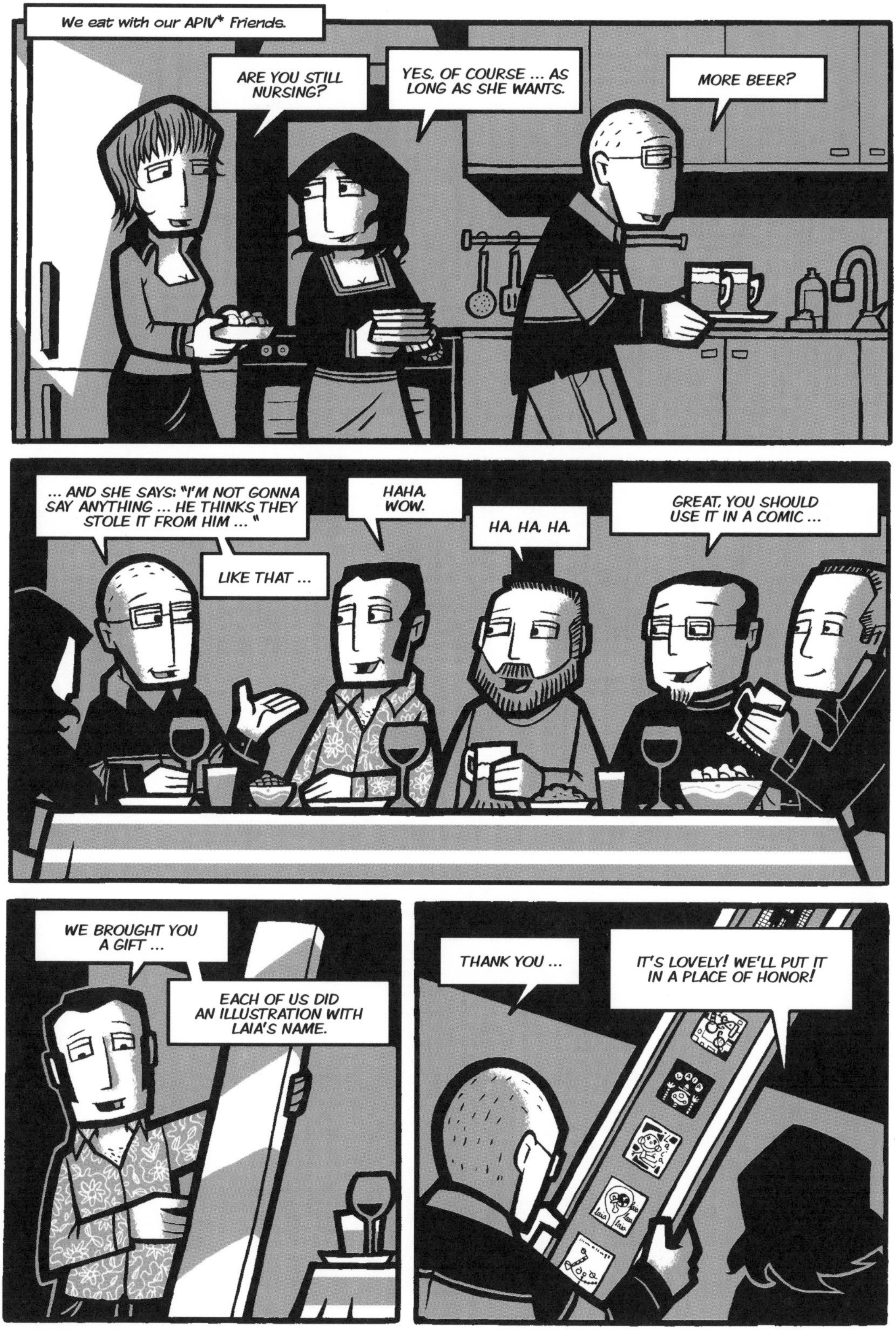
We eat with our APIV* Friends.
ARE YOU STILL NURSING?
YES, OF COURSE ... AS LONG AS SHE WANTS.
MORE BEER?
... AND SHE SAYS: "I'M NOT GONNA SAY ANYTHING ... HE THINKS THEY STOLE IT FROM HIM ..."
LIKE THAT ...
HAHA. WOW.
HA. HA. HA.
GREAT. YOU SHOULD USE IT IN A COMIC ...
WE BROUGHT YOU A GIFT ...
EACH OF US DID AN ILLUSTRATION WITH LAIA'S NAME.
THANK YOU ...
IT'S LOVELY! WE'LL PUT IT IN A PLACE OF HONOR!

* APIV: Valencia Association of Professional Illustrators

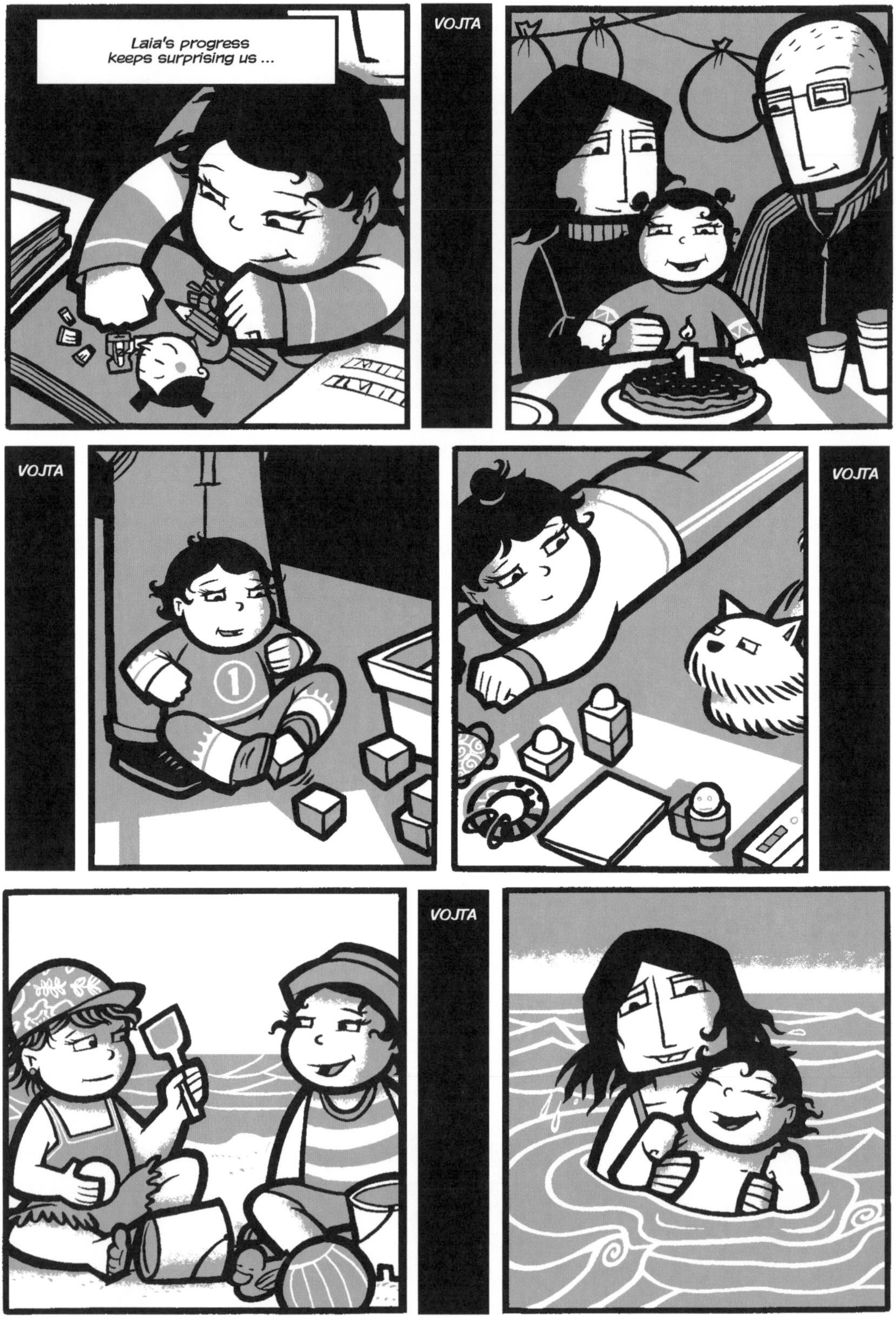
Laia's progress keeps surprising us ...
VOJTA
VOJTA
VOJTA
VOJTA
VOJTA

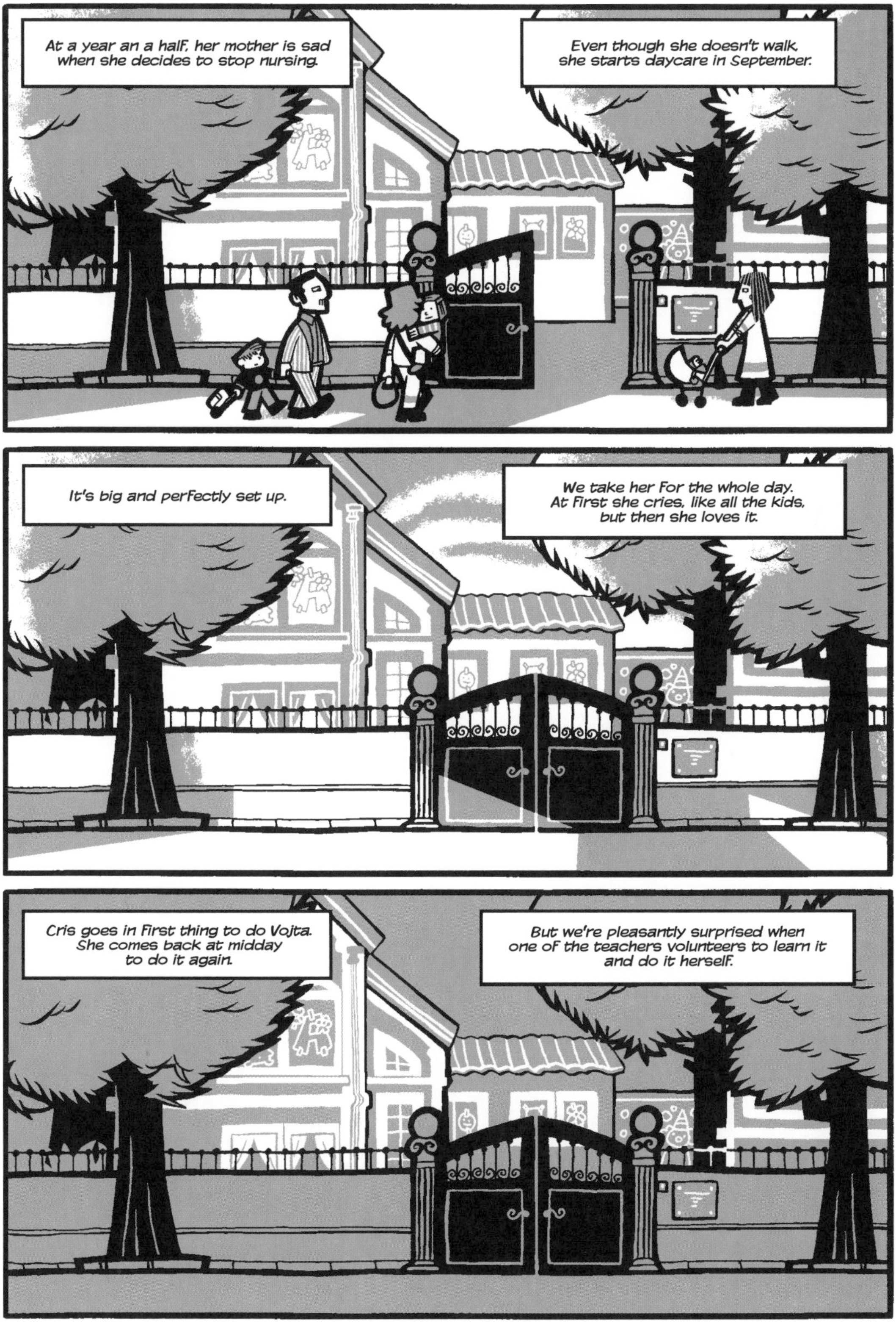
At a year an a half, her mother is sad when she decides to stop nursing.
Even though she doesn't walk, she starts daycare in September.
It's big and perfectly set up.
We take her for the whole day. At first she cries, like all the kids, but then she loves it.
Cris goes in first thing to do Vojta. She comes back at midday to do it again.
But we're pleasantly surprised when one of the teachers volunteers to learn it and do it herself.

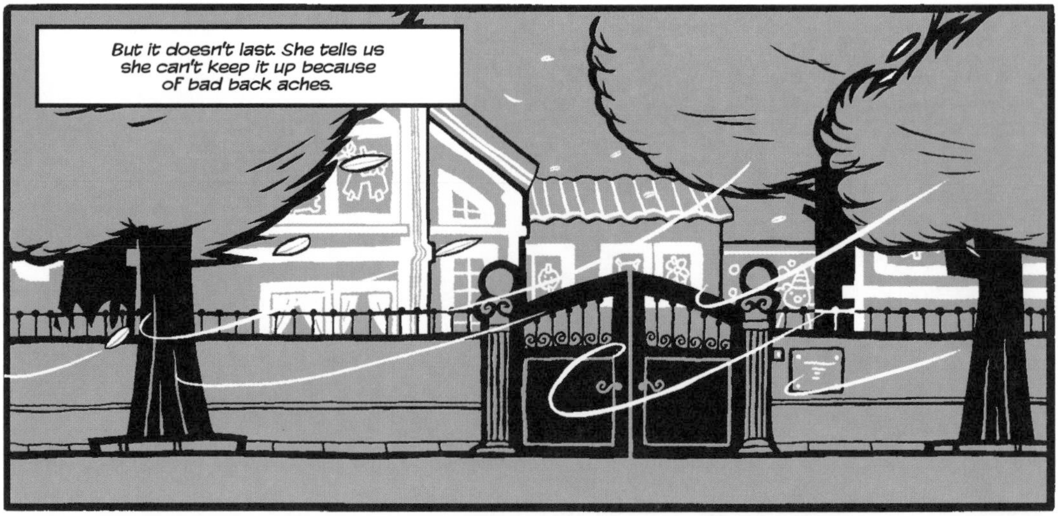
But it doesn't last. She tells us she can't keep it up because of bad back aches.

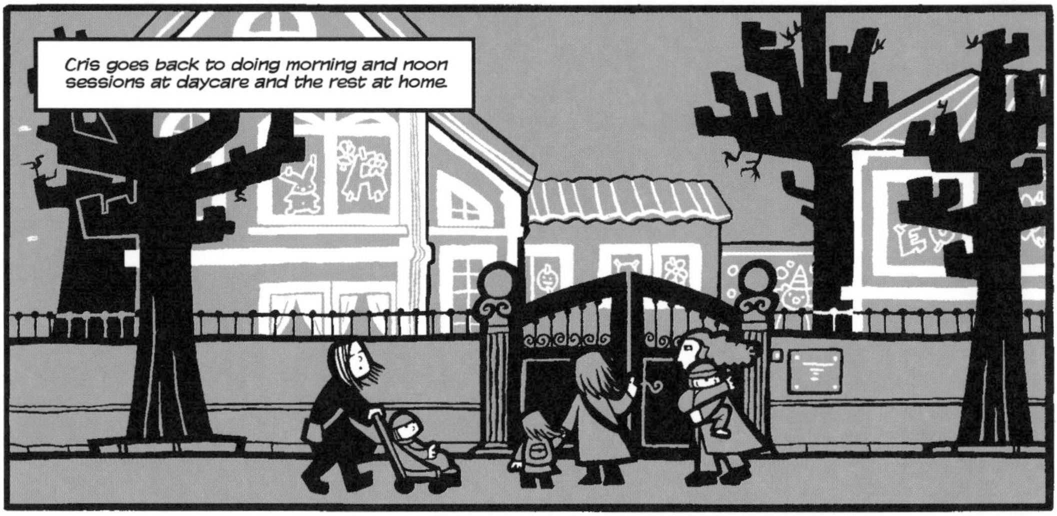
Cris goes back to doing morning and noon sessions at daycare and the rest at home.

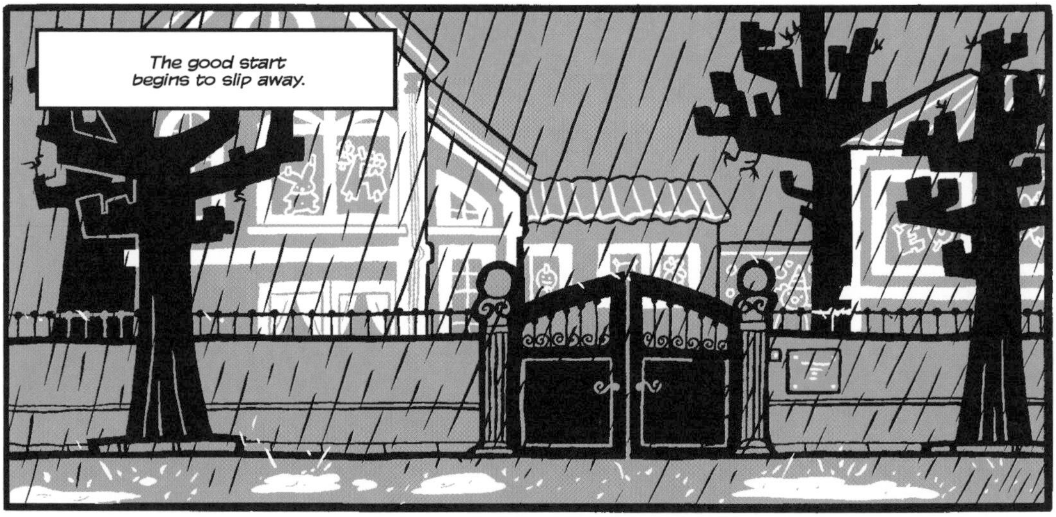
The good start begins to slip away.

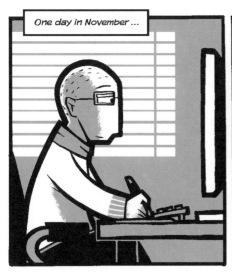

One day in November ...

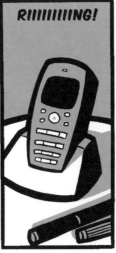

RIIIIIIIING!

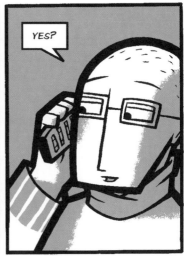

YES?

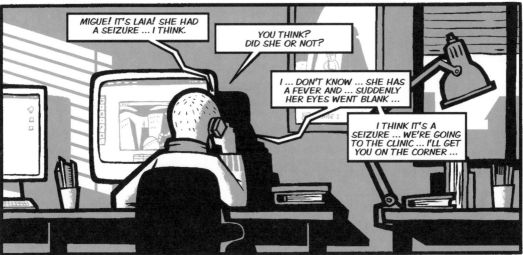

MIGUE! IT'S LAIA! SHE HAD A SEIZURE ... I THINK.

YOU THINK? DID SHE OR NOT?

I ... DON'T KNOW ... SHE HAS A FEVER AND ... SUDDENLY HER EYES WENT BLANK ...

I THINK IT'S A SEIZURE ... WE'RE GOING TO THE CLINIC ... I'LL GET YOU ON THE CORNER ...

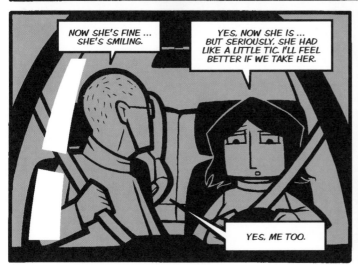

NOW SHE'S FINE ... SHE'S SMILING.

YES, NOW SHE IS ... BUT SERIOUSLY, SHE HAD LIKE A LITTLE TIC. I'LL FEEL BETTER IF WE TAKE HER.

YES, ME TOO.

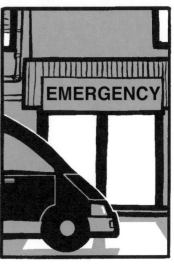

EMERGENCY

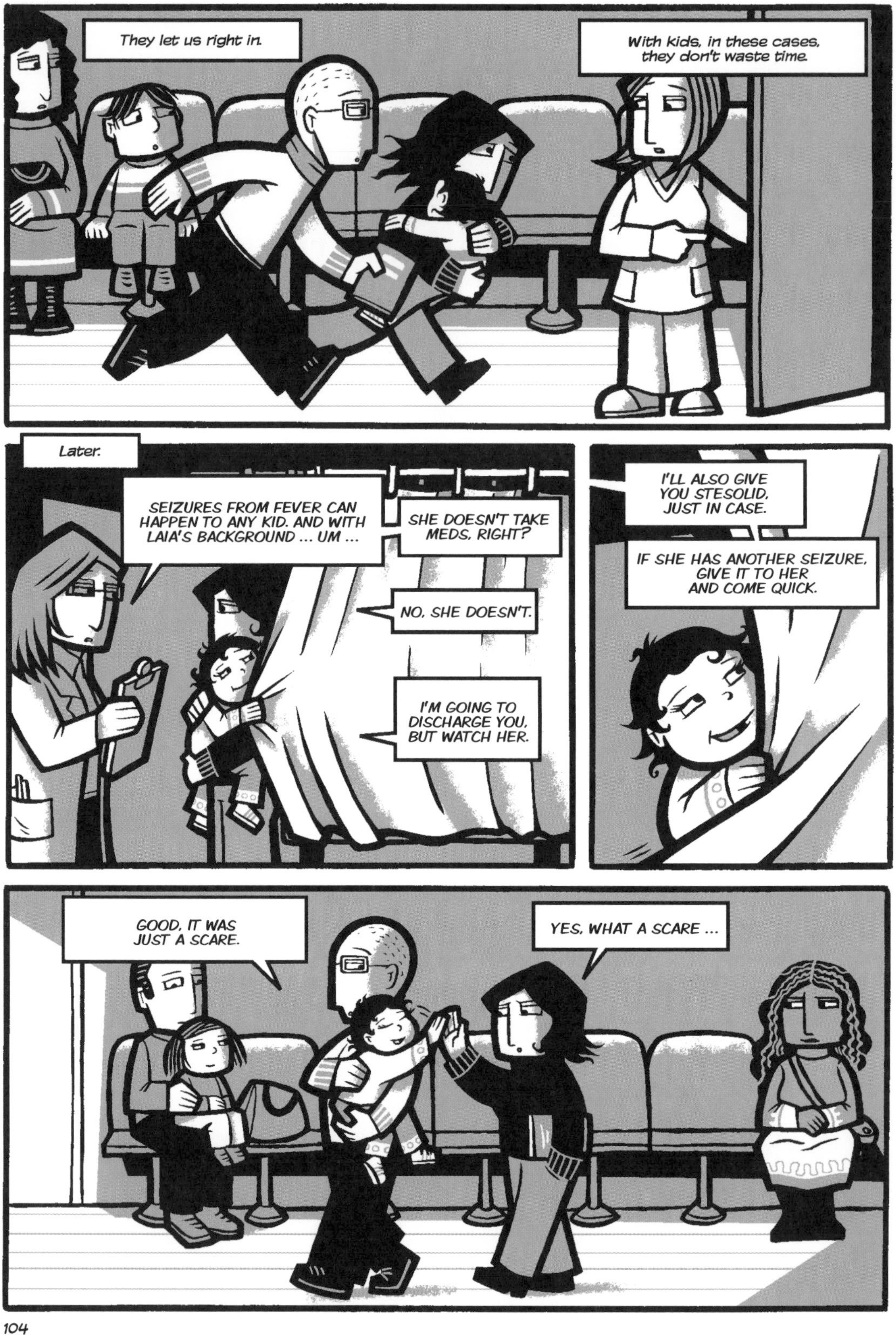
They let us right in.
With kids, in these cases, they don't waste time.
Later.
SEIZURES FROM FEVER CAN HAPPEN TO ANY KID. AND WITH LAIA'S BACKGROUND ... UM ...
SHE DOESN'T TAKE MEDS, RIGHT?
NO, SHE DOESN'T.
I'M GOING TO DISCHARGE YOU, BUT WATCH HER.
I'LL ALSO GIVE YOU STESOLID, JUST IN CASE.
IF SHE HAS ANOTHER SEIZURE, GIVE IT TO HER AND COME QUICK.
GOOD, IT WAS JUST A SCARE.
YES, WHAT A SCARE ...

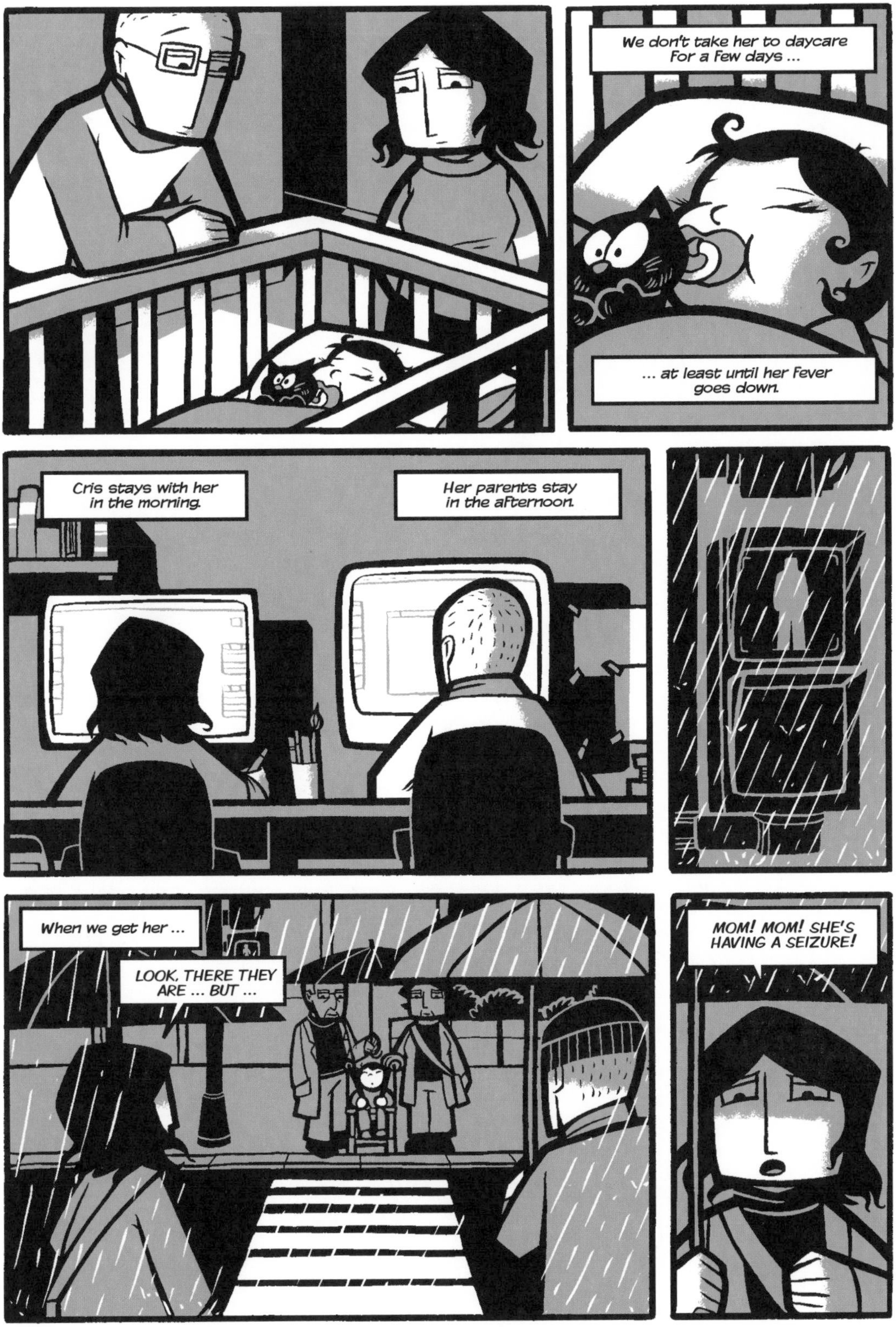
We don't take her to daycare for a few days ...
... at least until her fever goes down.
Cris stays with her in the morning.
Her parents stay in the afternoon.
When we get her ...
LOOK, THERE THEY ARE ... BUT ...
MOM! MOM! SHE'S HAVING A SEIZURE!

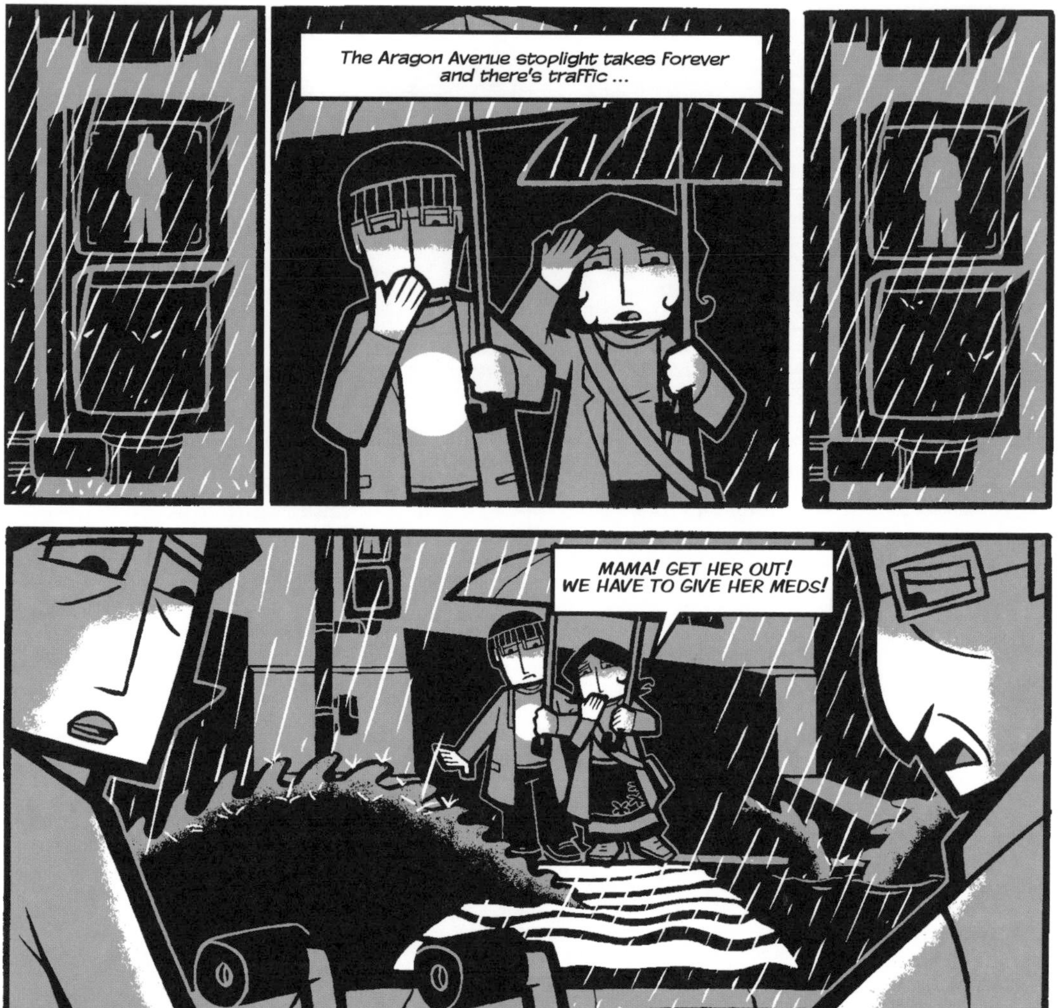
The Aragon Avenue stoplight takes forever and there's traffic ...
MAMA! GET HER OUT! WE HAVE TO GIVE HER MEDS!
I GAVE HER ALL OF IT AND THE SEIZURE ISN'T STOPPING.
LET'S GO TO THE CLINIC NOW.

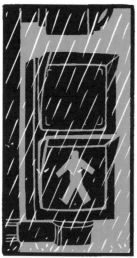

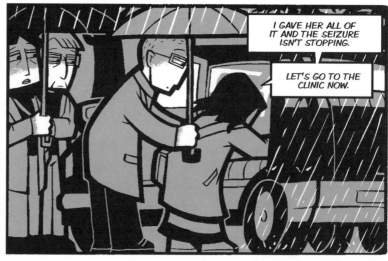

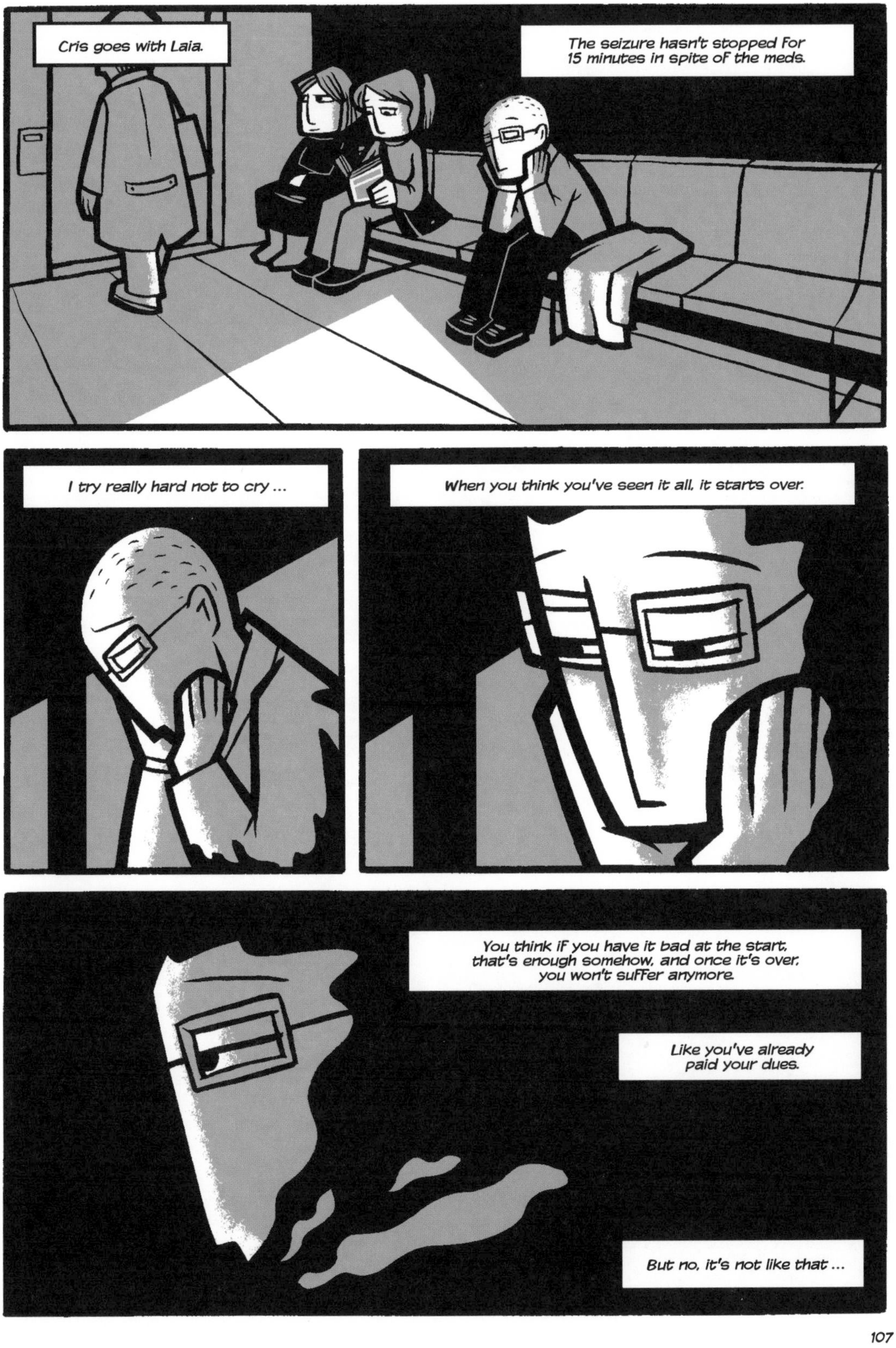
Cris goes with Laia.
The seizure hasn't stopped for 15 minutes in spite of the meds.
I try really hard not to cry ...
When you think you've seen it all, it starts over.
You think if you have it bad at the start, that's enough somehow, and once it's over, you won't suffer anymore.
Like you've already paid your dues.
But no, it's not like that ...

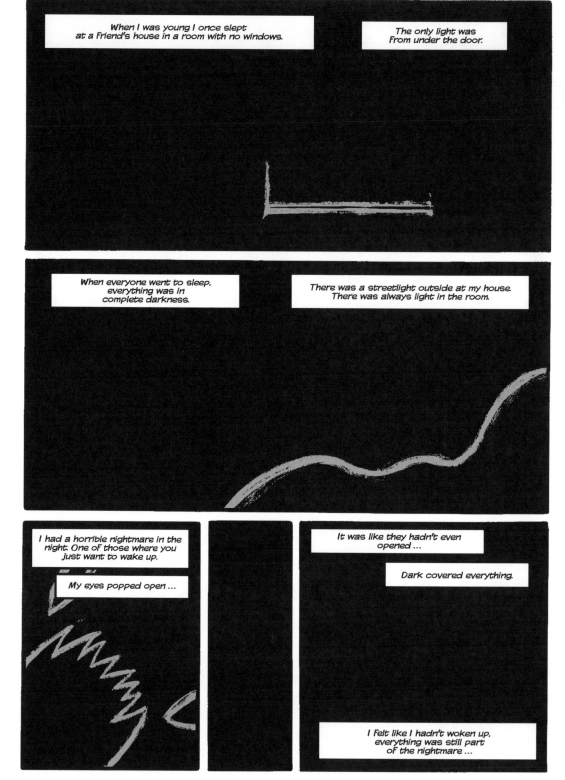

When I was young I once slept
at a friend's house in a room with no windows.

The only light was
From under the door.

When everyone went to sleep,
everything was in
complete darkness.

There was a streetlight outside at my house.
There was always light in the room.

I had a horrible nightmare in the
night. One of those where you
just want to wake up.

My eyes popped open ...

It was like they hadn't even
opened ...

Dark covered everything.

I felt like I hadn't woken up,
everything was still part
of the nightmare ...

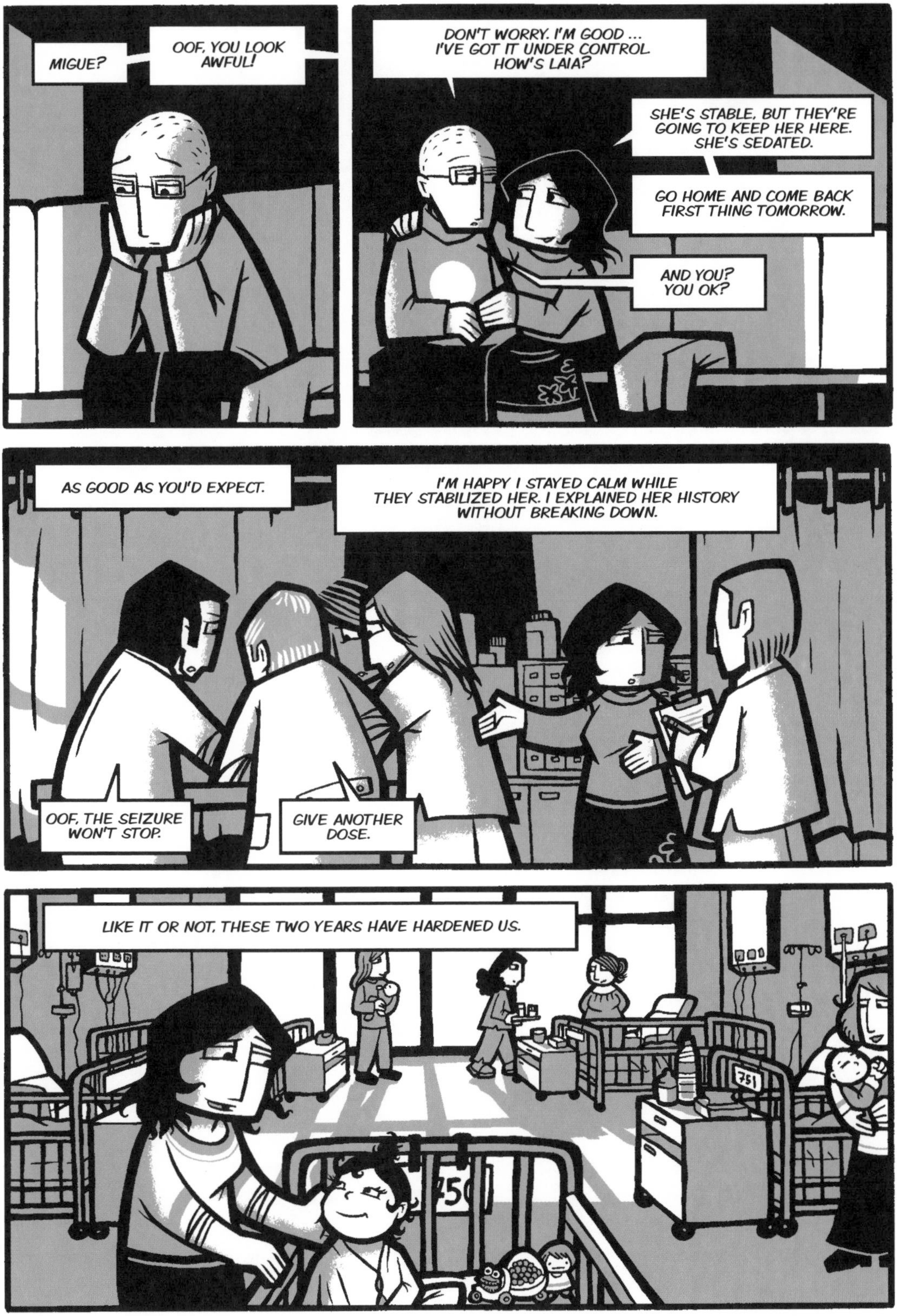
MIGUE?
OOF, YOU LOOK AWFUL!
DON'T WORRY. I'M GOOD ... I'VE GOT IT UNDER CONTROL HOW'S LAIA?
SHE'S STABLE, BUT THEY'RE GOING TO KEEP HER HERE. SHE'S SEDATED.
GO HOME AND COME BACK FIRST THING TOMORROW.
AND YOU? YOU OK?
AS GOOD AS YOU'D EXPECT.
I'M HAPPY I STAYED CALM WHILE THEY STABILIZED HER. I EXPLAINED HER HISTORY WITHOUT BREAKING DOWN.
OOF, THE SEIZURE WON'T STOP.
GIVE ANOTHER DOSE.
LIKE IT OR NOT, THESE TWO YEARS HAVE HARDENED US.
751
450

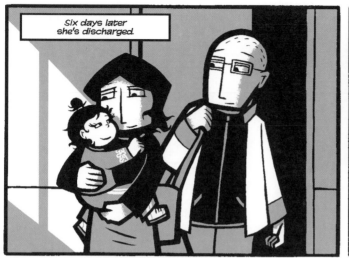

Six days later she's discharged.

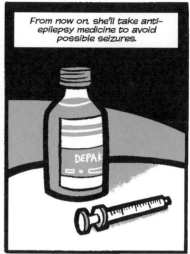

From now on, she'll take anti-epilepsy medicine to avoid possible seizures.

DEPAK

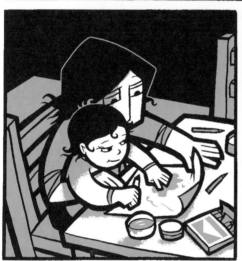

VOJTA

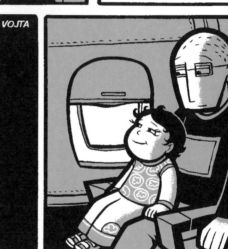

VOJTA

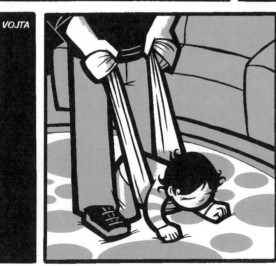

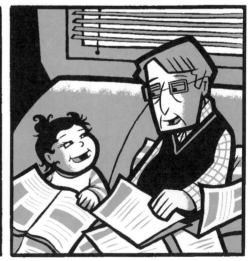

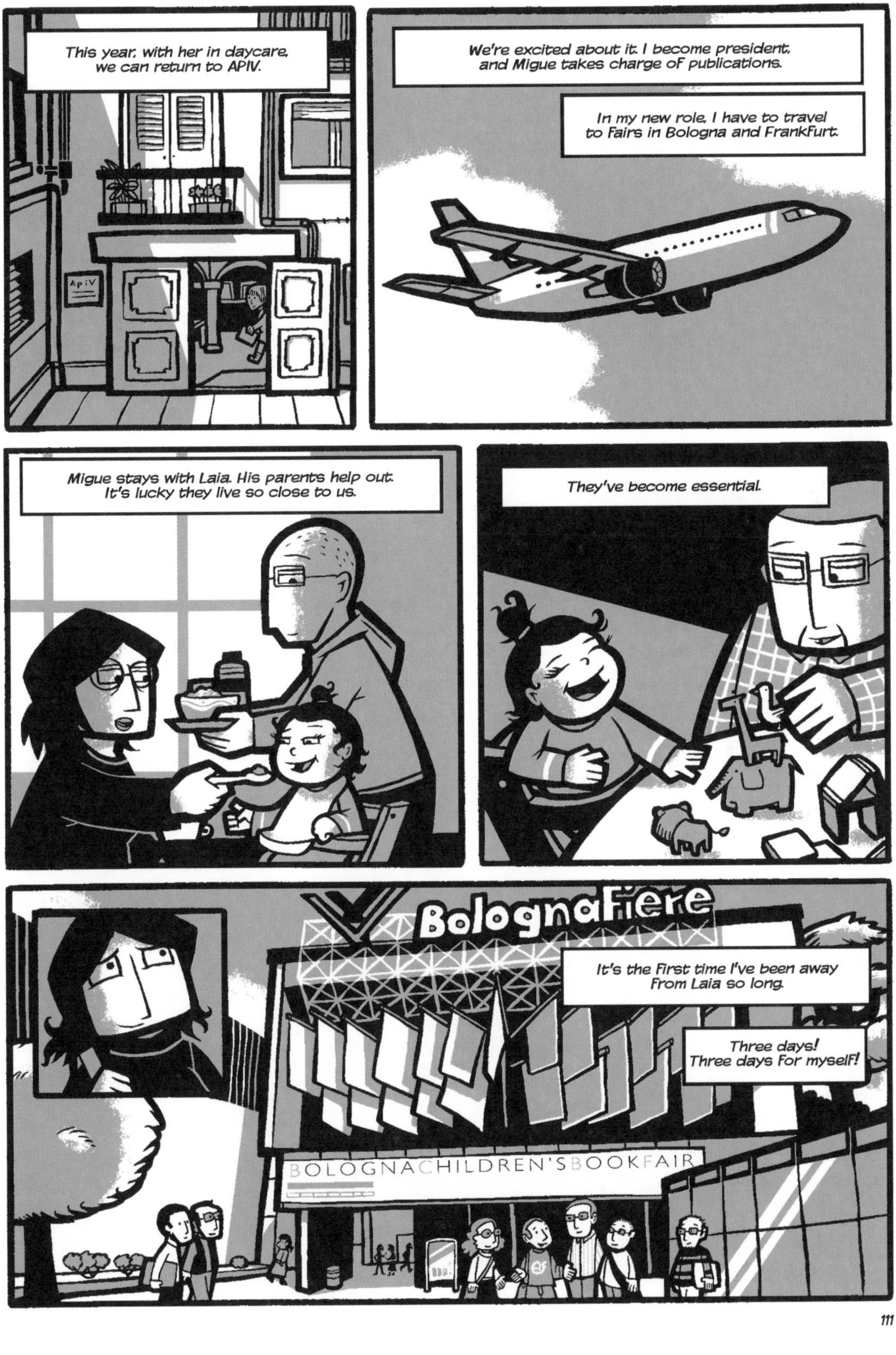
This year, with her in daycare, we can return to APIV.
ApiV
We're excited about it. I become president, and Migue takes charge of publications.
In my new role, I have to travel to Fairs in Bologna and Frankfurt.
Migue stays with Laia. His parents help out. It's lucky they live so close to us.
They've become essential.
BolognaFiere
It's the first time I've been away from Laia so long.
Three days! Three days for myself!
BOLOGNACHILDREN'SBOOKFAIR

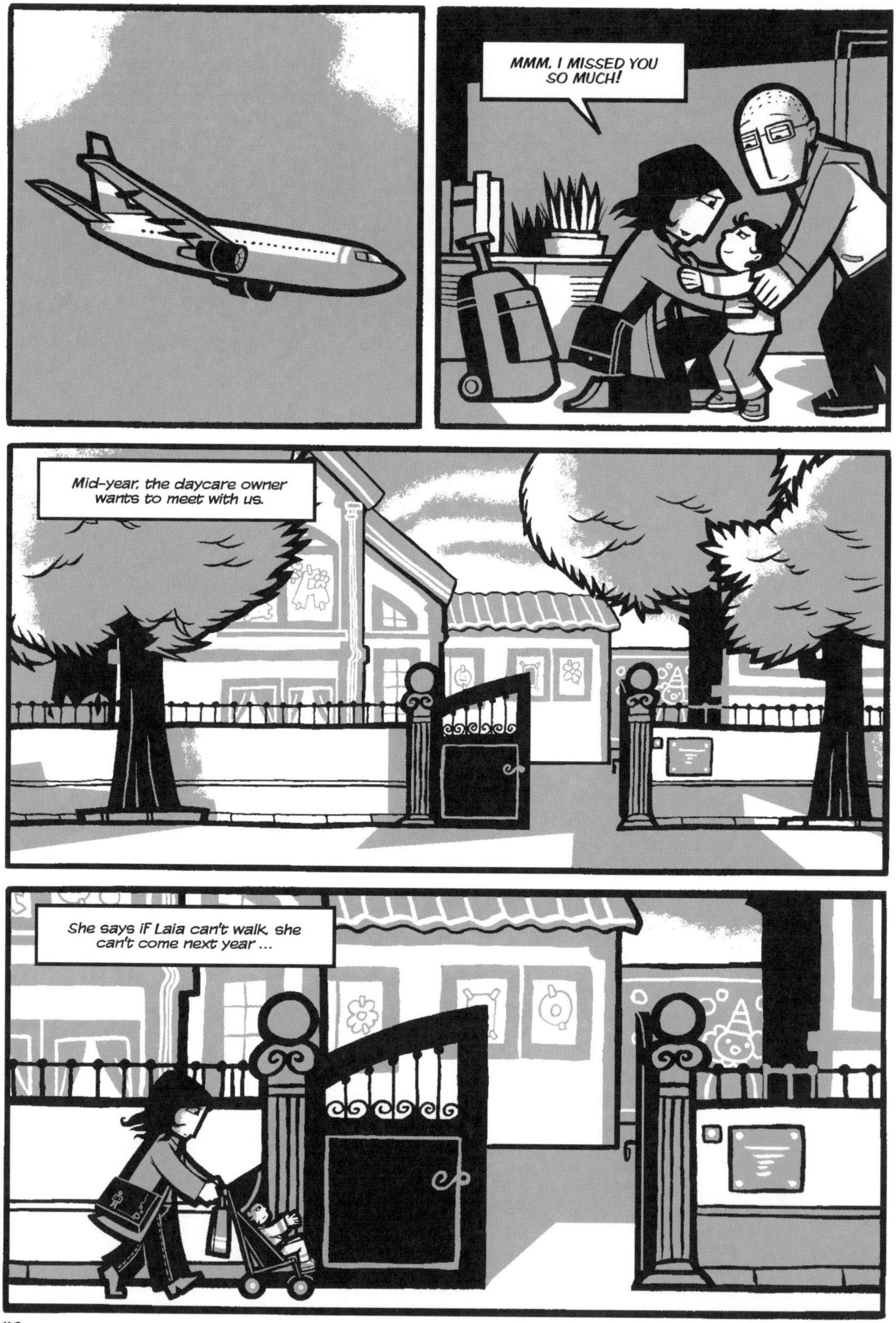
MMM, I MISSED YOU SO MUCH!
Mid-year, the daycare owner wants to meet with us.
She says if Laia can't walk, she can't come next year ...

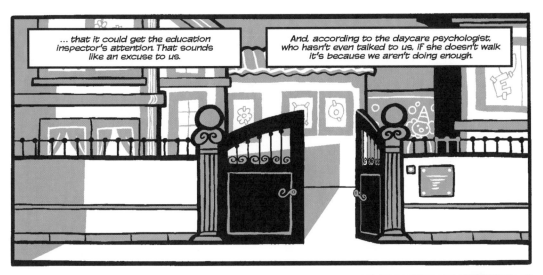

... that it could get the education inspector's attention. That sounds like an excuse to us.

And, according to the daycare psychologist, who hasn't even talked to us, if she doesn't walk it's because we aren't doing enough.

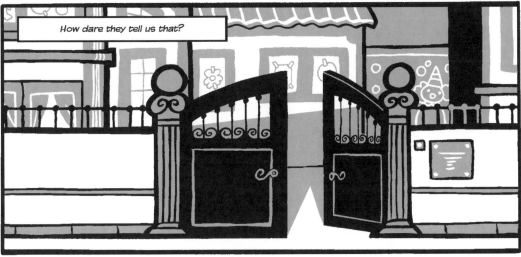

How dare they tell us that?

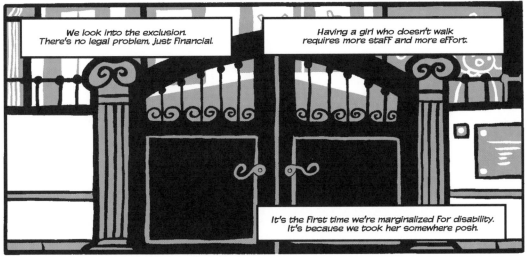

We look into the exclusion. There's no legal problem, just financial.

Having a girl who doesn't walk requires more staff and more effort.

It's the first time we're marginalized for disability. It's because we took her somewhere posh.

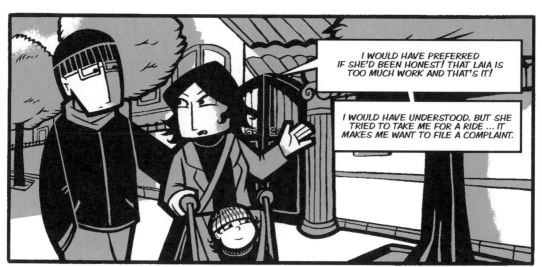

I WOULD HAVE PREFERRED IF SHE'D BEEN HONEST! THAT LAIA IS TOO MUCH WORK AND THAT'S IT!

I WOULD HAVE UNDERSTOOD, BUT SHE TRIED TO TAKE ME FOR A RIDE ... IT MAKES ME WANT TO FILE A COMPLAINT.

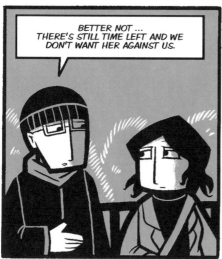

BETTER NOT ... THERE'S STILL TIME LEFT AND WE DON'T WANT HER AGAINST US.

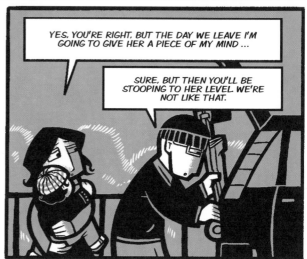

YES, YOU'RE RIGHT, BUT THE DAY WE LEAVE I'M GOING TO GIVE HER A PIECE OF MY MIND ...

SURE, BUT THEN YOU'LL BE STOOPING TO HER LEVEL WE'RE NOT LIKE THAT.

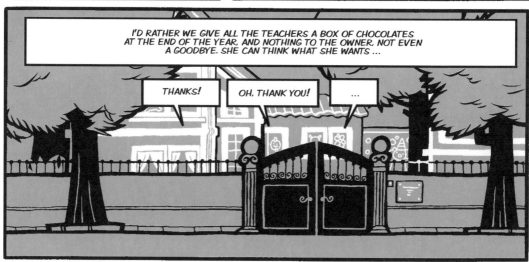

I'D RATHER WE GIVE ALL THE TEACHERS A BOX OF CHOCOLATES AT THE END OF THE YEAR, AND NOTHING TO THE OWNER, NOT EVEN A GOODBYE. SHE CAN THINK WHAT SHE WANTS ...

THANKS!

OH, THANK YOU!

...

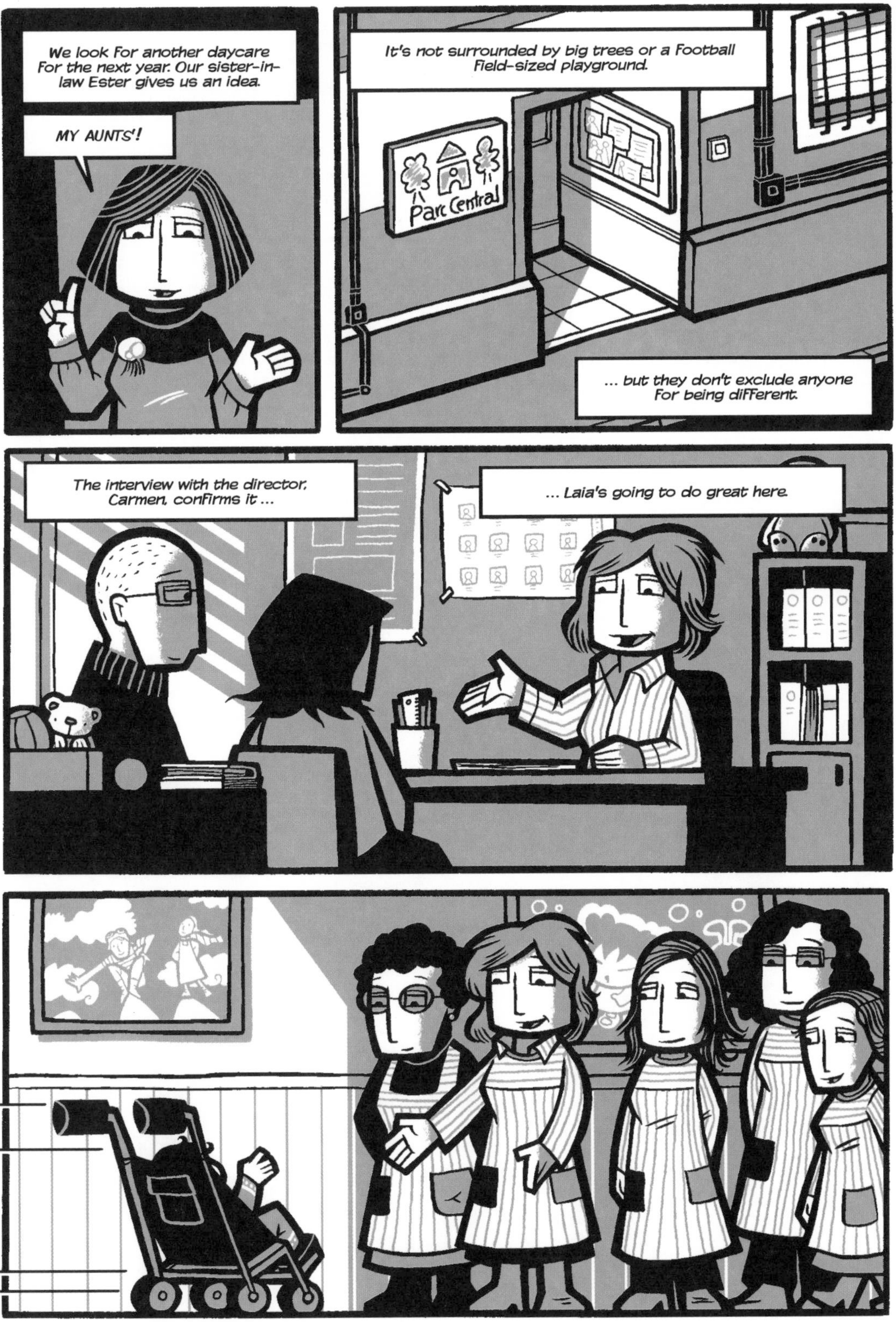
We look for another daycare for the next year. Our sister-in-law Ester gives us an idea.
MY AUNTS'!
It's not surrounded by big trees or a football field-sized playground.
Parc Central
... but they don't exclude anyone for being different.
The interview with the director, Carmen, confirms it ...
... Laia's going to do great here.

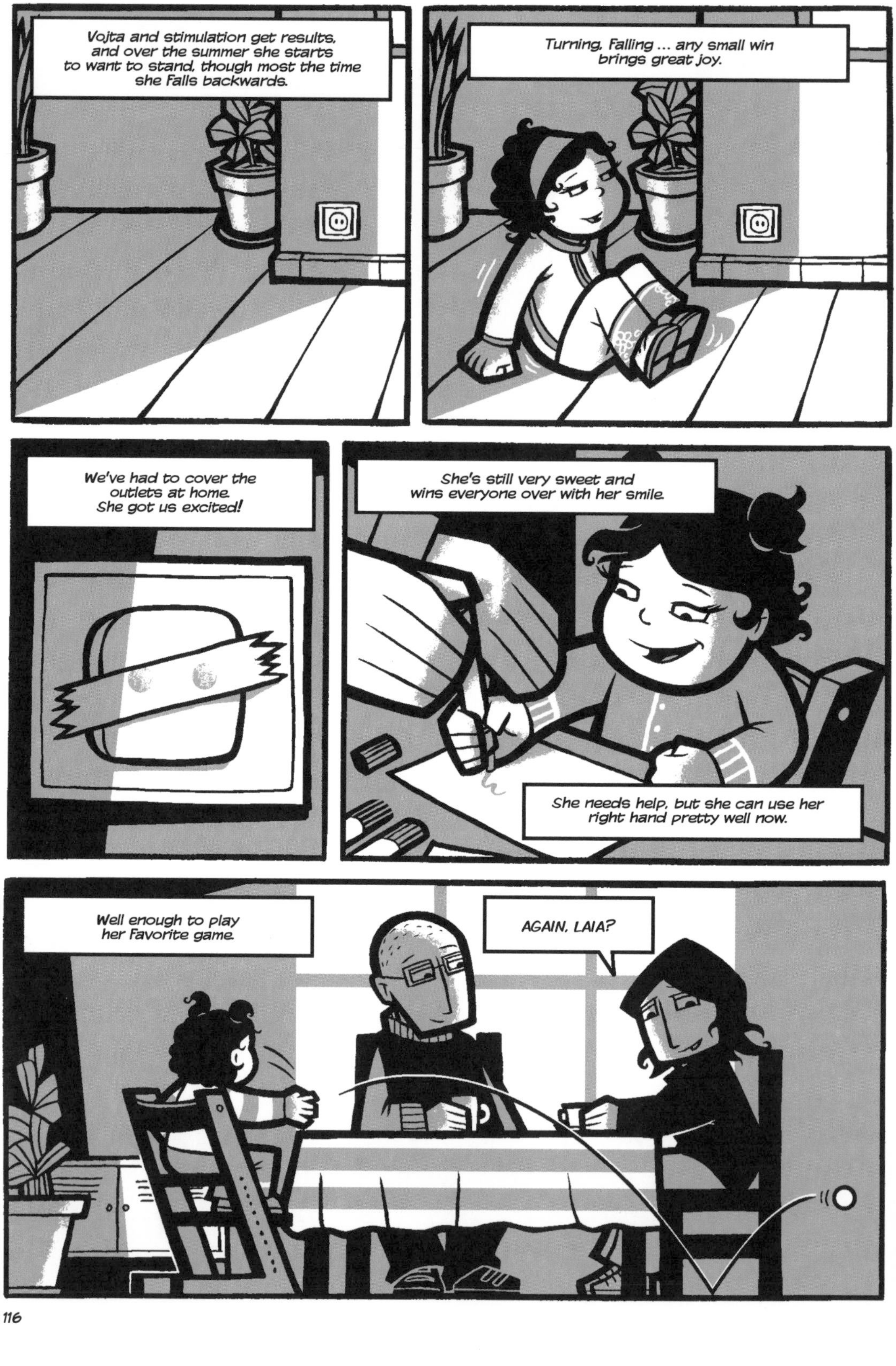
Vojta and stimulation get results, and over the summer she starts to want to stand, though most the time she falls backwards.
Turning, falling ... any small win brings great joy.
We've had to cover the outlets at home. She got us excited!
She's still very sweet and wins everyone over with her smile.
She needs help, but she can use her right hand pretty well now.
Well enough to play her favorite game.
AGAIN, LAIA?

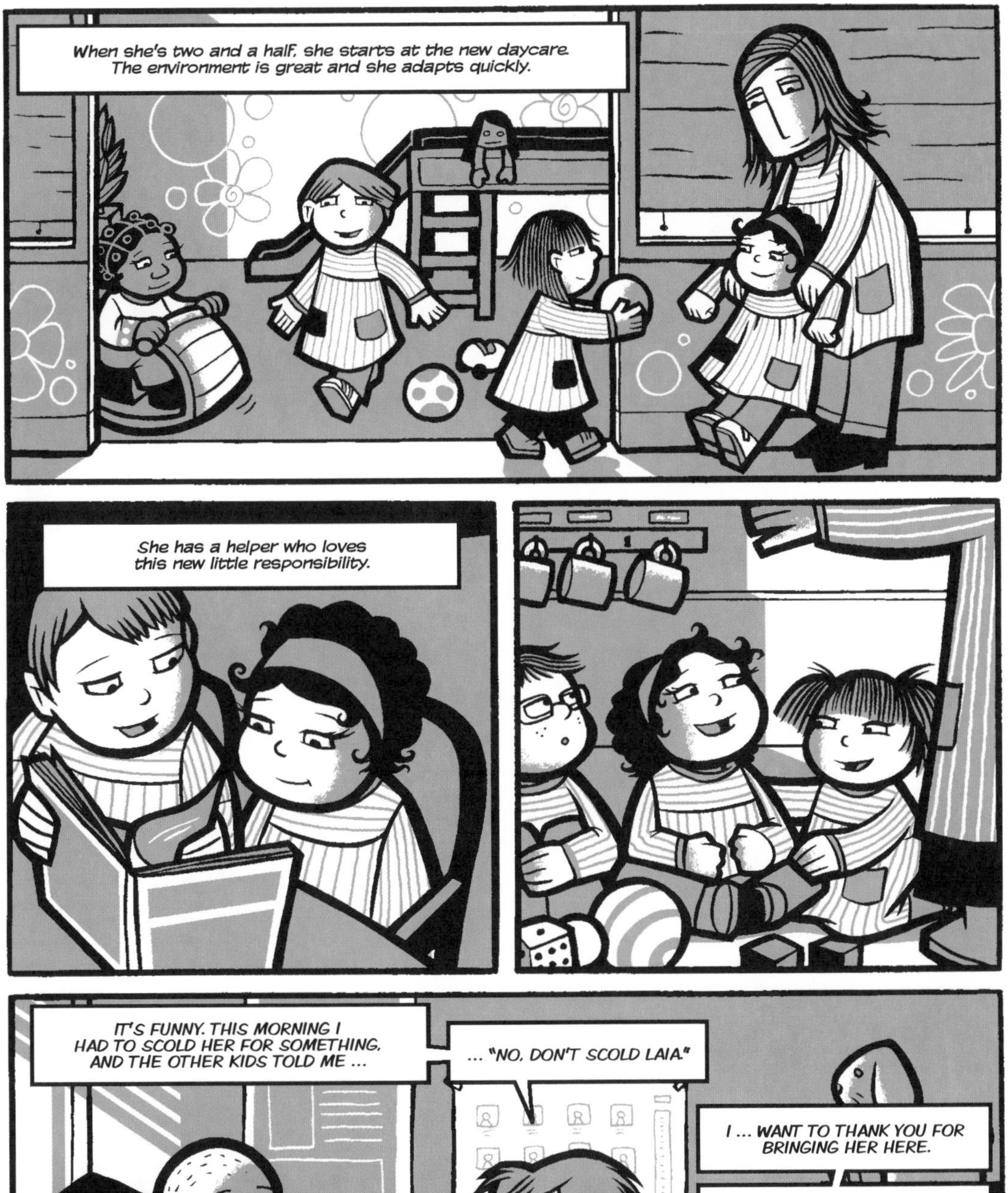
When she's two and a half, she starts at the new daycare. The environment is great and she adapts quickly.
She has a helper who loves this new little responsibility.
IT'S FUNNY. THIS MORNING I HAD TO SCOLD HER FOR SOMETHING, AND THE OTHER KIDS TOLD ME ...
... "NO, DON'T SCOLD LAIA."
I ... WANT TO THANK YOU FOR BRINGING HER HERE.
IT'S NOT JUST GOOD FOR HER, BUT IMPORTANT FOR EVERYONE. ESPECIALLY THE OTHER CHILDREN ...
LEARNING ABOUT INCLUSION FROM A YOUNG AGE.

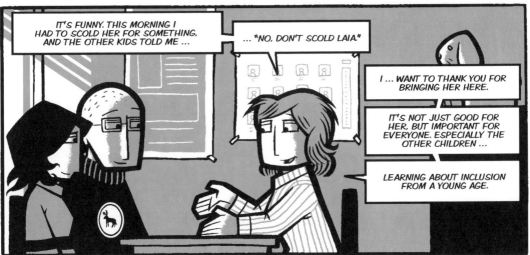

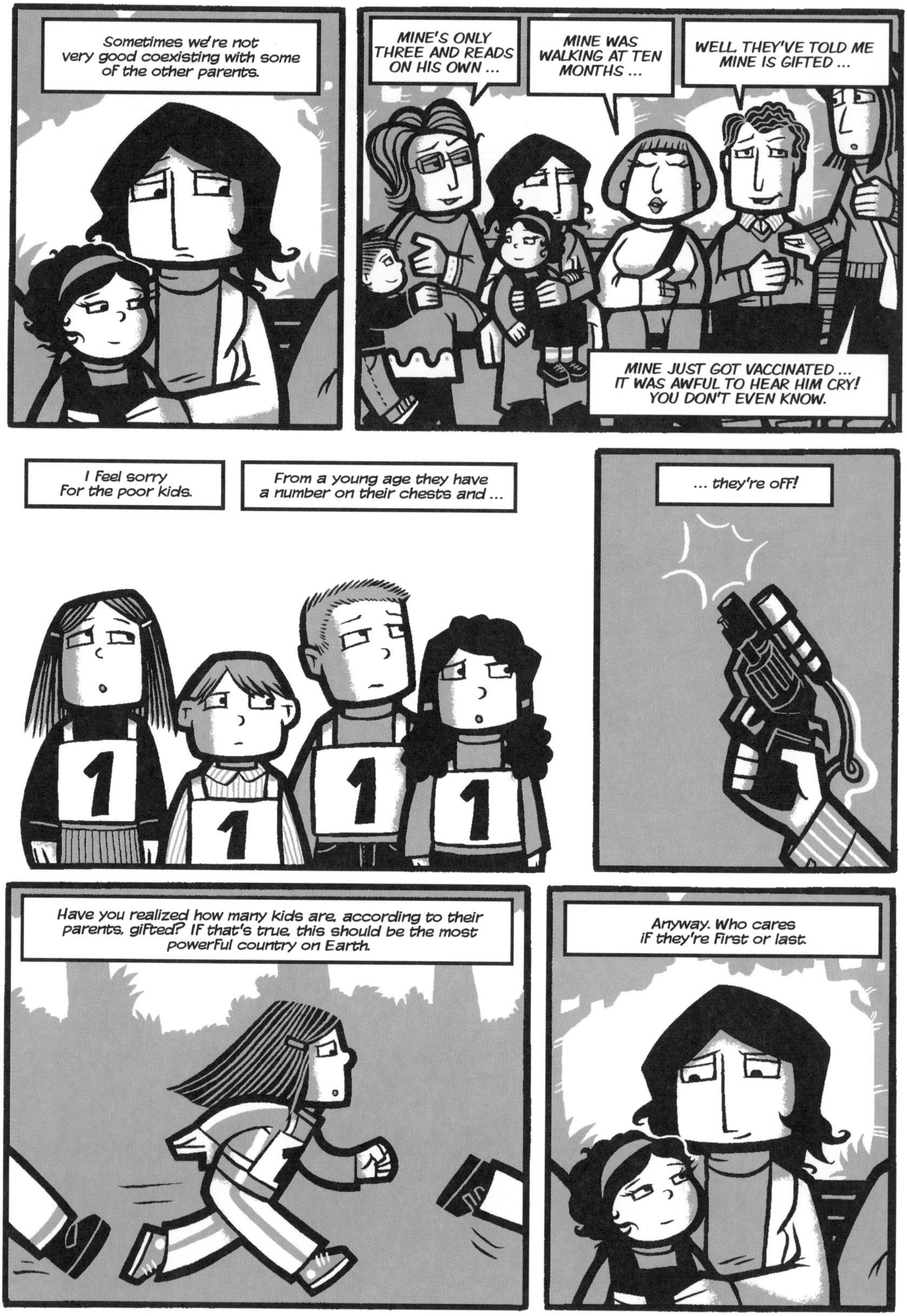
Sometimes we're not very good coexisting with some of the other parents.
MINE'S ONLY THREE AND READS ON HIS OWN ...
MINE WAS WALKING AT TEN MONTHS ...
WELL, THEY'VE TOLD ME MINE IS GIFTED ...
MINE JUST GOT VACCINATED ... IT WAS AWFUL TO HEAR HIM CRY! YOU DON'T EVEN KNOW.
I feel sorry for the poor kids.
From a young age they have a number on their chests and ...
1
1
1
1
... they're off!
Have you realized how many kids are, according to their parents, gifted? If that's true, this should be the most powerful country on Earth.
Anyway. Who cares if they're first or last.

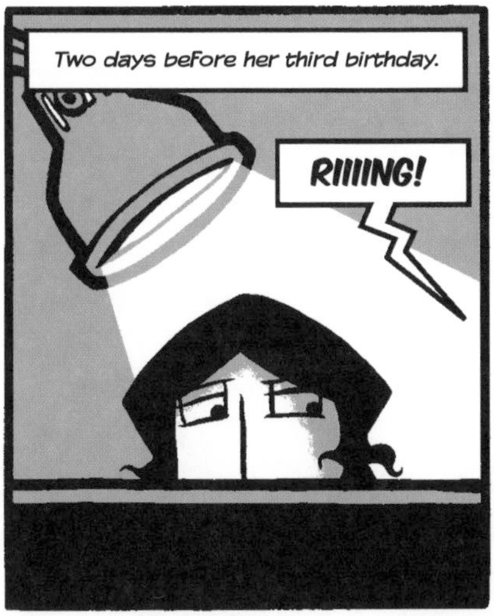
Two days before her third birthday.
RIIIING!
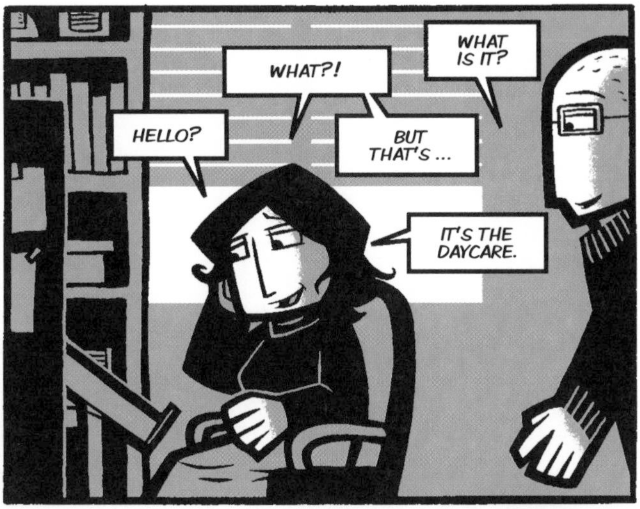
HELLO?
WHAT?!
BUT THAT'S ...
WHAT IS IT?
IT'S THE DAYCARE.
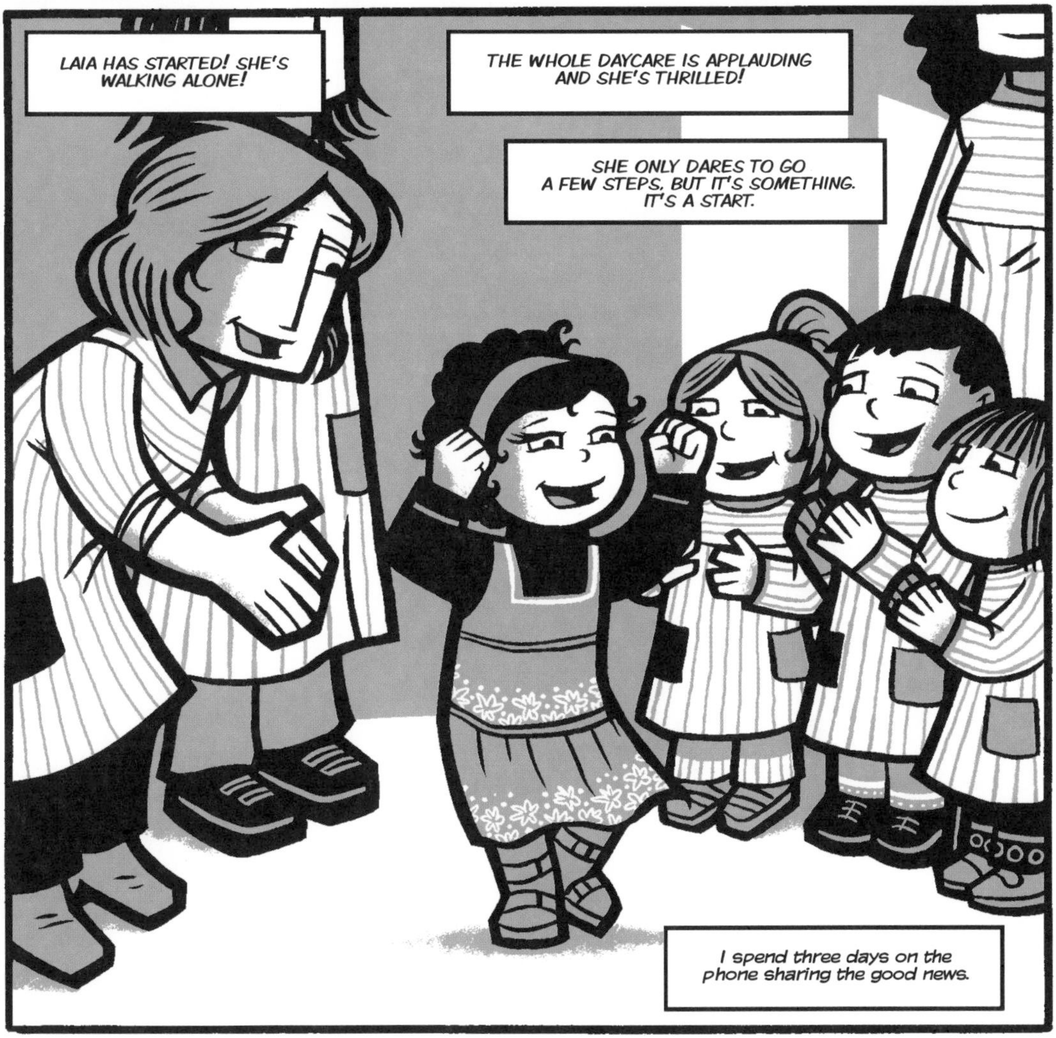
LAIA HAS STARTED! SHE'S WALKING ALONE!
THE WHOLE DAYCARE IS APPLAUDING AND SHE'S THRILLED!
SHE ONLY DARES TO GO A FEW STEPS, BUT IT'S SOMETHING. IT'S A START.
I spend three days on the phone sharing the good news.

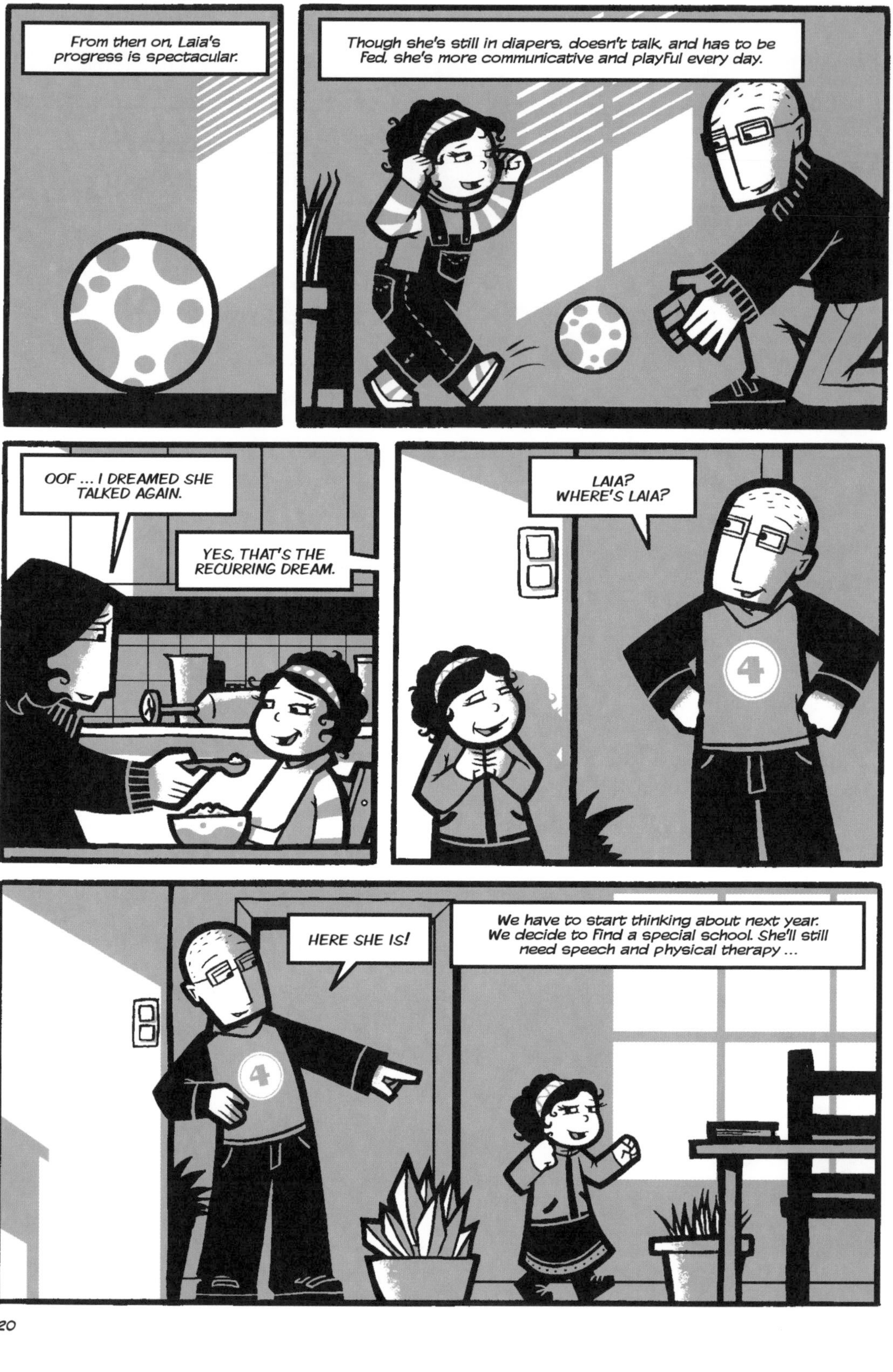
From then on, Laia's progress is spectacular.
Though she's still in diapers, doesn't talk, and has to be fed, she's more communicative and playful every day.
OOF ... I DREAMED SHE TALKED AGAIN.
YES, THAT'S THE RECURRING DREAM.
LAIA? WHERE'S LAIA?
HERE SHE IS!
We have to start thinking about next year. We decide to find a special school. She'll still need speech and physical therapy ...

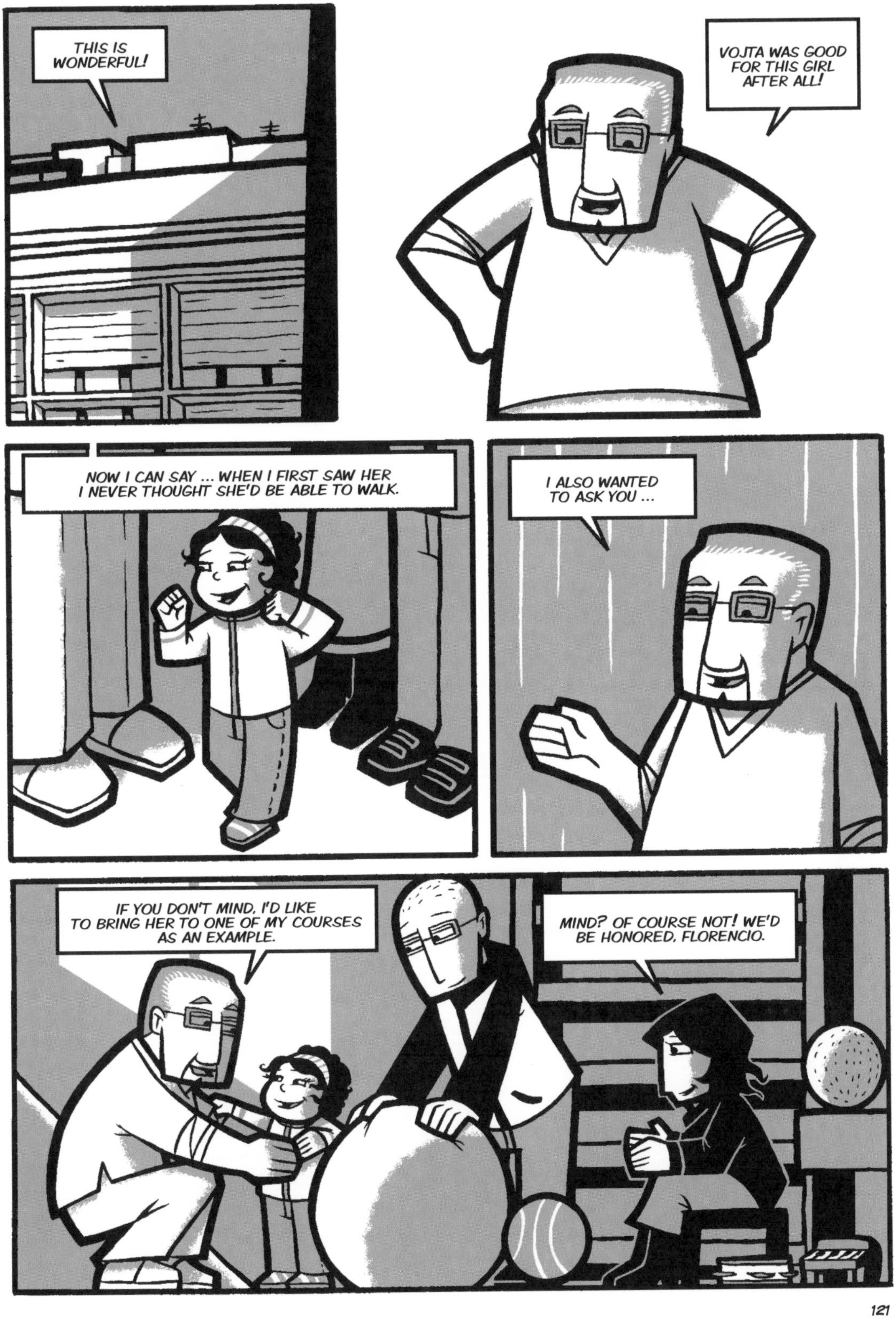
THIS IS WONDERFUL!
VOJTA WAS GOOD FOR THIS GIRL AFTER ALL!
NOW I CAN SAY ... WHEN I FIRST SAW HER I NEVER THOUGHT SHE'D BE ABLE TO WALK.
I ALSO WANTED TO ASK YOU ...
IF YOU DON'T MIND, I'D LIKE TO BRING HER TO ONE OF MY COURSES AS AN EXAMPLE.
MIND? OF COURSE NOT! WE'D BE HONORED, FLORENCIO.

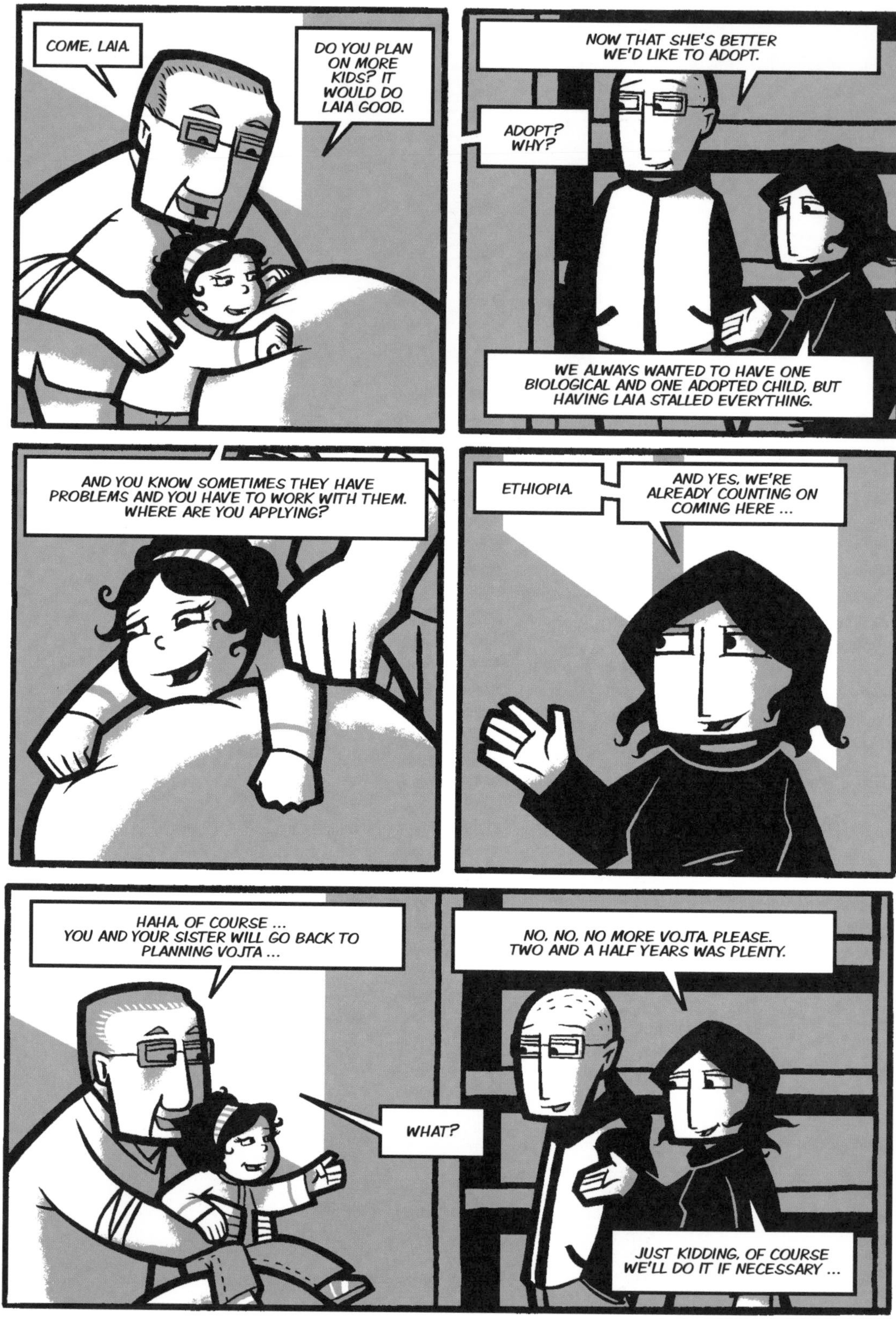
COME, LAIA.
DO YOU PLAN ON MORE KIDS? IT WOULD DO LAIA GOOD.
NOW THAT SHE'S BETTER WE'D LIKE TO ADOPT.
ADOPT? WHY?
WE ALWAYS WANTED TO HAVE ONE BIOLOGICAL AND ONE ADOPTED CHILD, BUT HAVING LAIA STALLED EVERYTHING.
AND YOU KNOW SOMETIMES THEY HAVE PROBLEMS AND YOU HAVE TO WORK WITH THEM. WHERE ARE YOU APPLYING?
ETHIOPIA.
AND YES, WE'RE ALREADY COUNTING ON COMING HERE ...
HAHA, OF COURSE ... YOU AND YOUR SISTER WILL GO BACK TO PLANNING VOJTA ...
WHAT?
NO, NO, NO MORE VOJTA. PLEASE. TWO AND A HALF YEARS WAS PLENTY.
JUST KIDDING, OF COURSE WE'LL DO IT IF NECESSARY ...

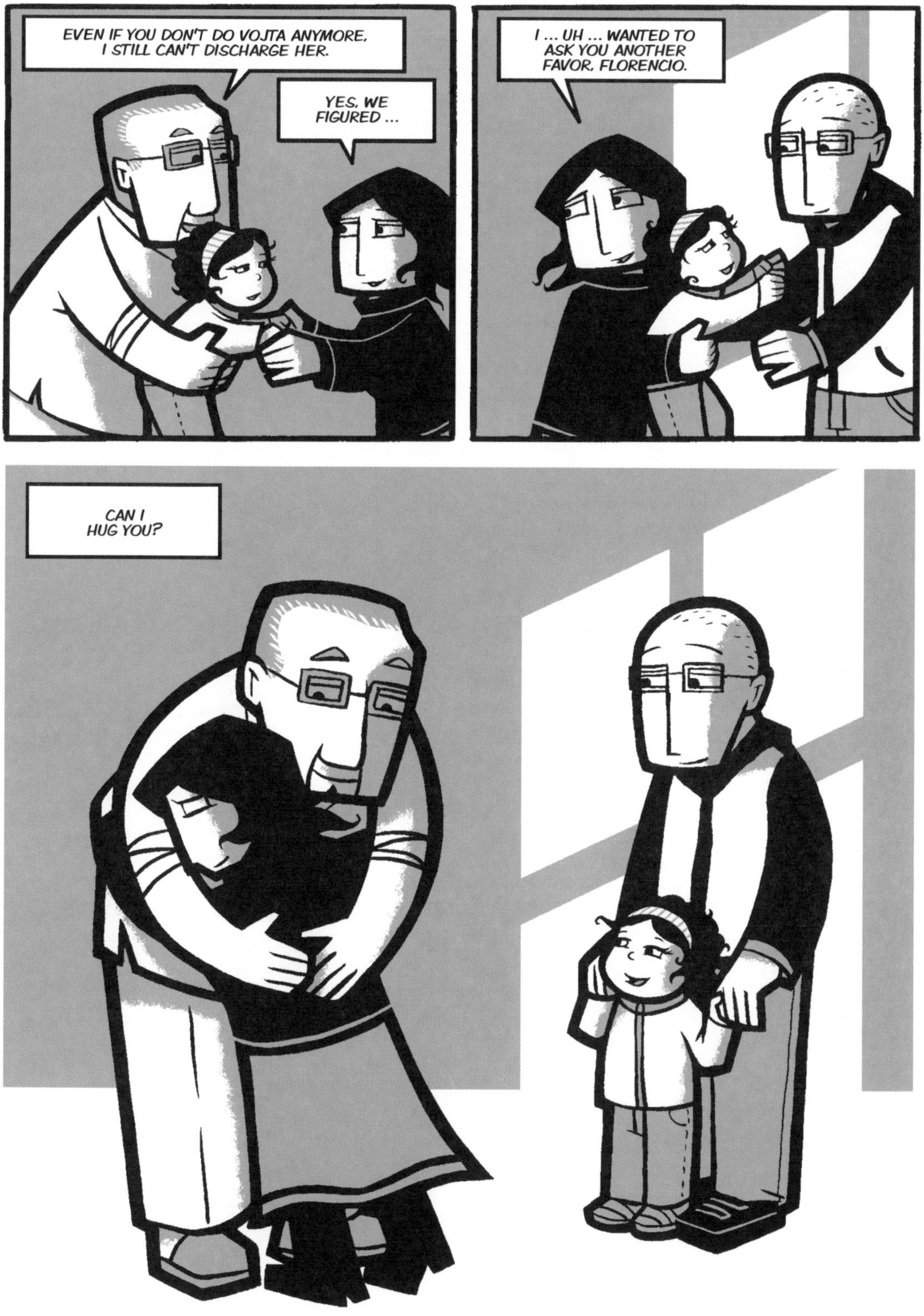
EVEN IF YOU DON'T DO VOJTA ANYMORE, I STILL CAN'T DISCHARGE HER.
YES, WE FIGURED ...
I ... UH ... WANTED TO ASK YOU ANOTHER FAVOR, FLORENCIO.
CAN I HUG YOU?

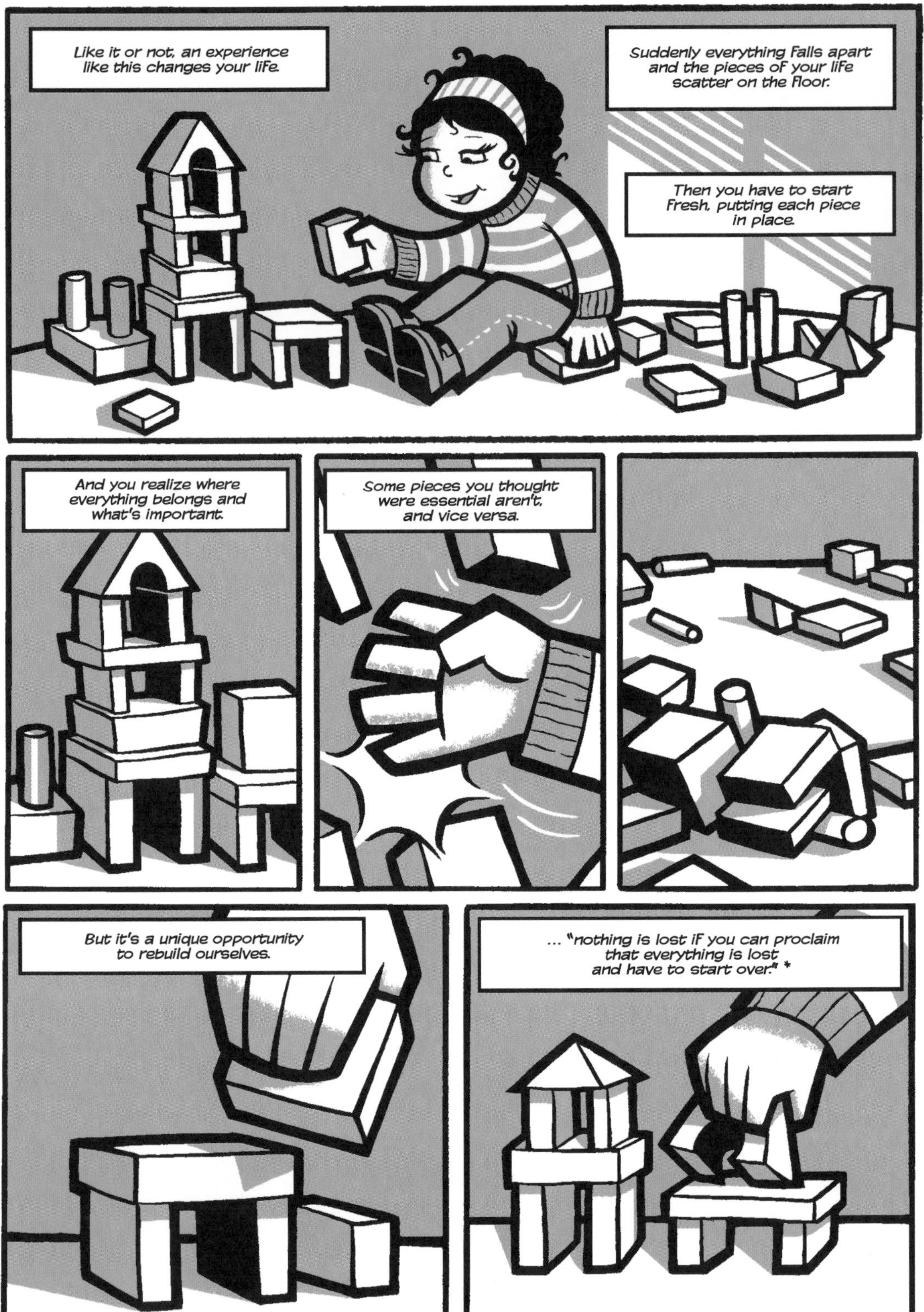
Like it or not, an experience like this changes your life.
Suddenly everything falls apart and the pieces of your life scatter on the floor.
Then you have to start fresh, putting each piece in place.
And you realize where everything belongs and what's important.
Some pieces you thought were essential aren't, and vice versa.
But it's a unique opportunity to rebuild ourselves.
... "nothing is lost if you can proclaim that everything is lost and have to start over." *

* Julio Cortázar.

Book 2

EFRÉN'S
MACHINE

Chapter I
THE DECISION

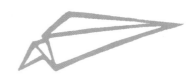

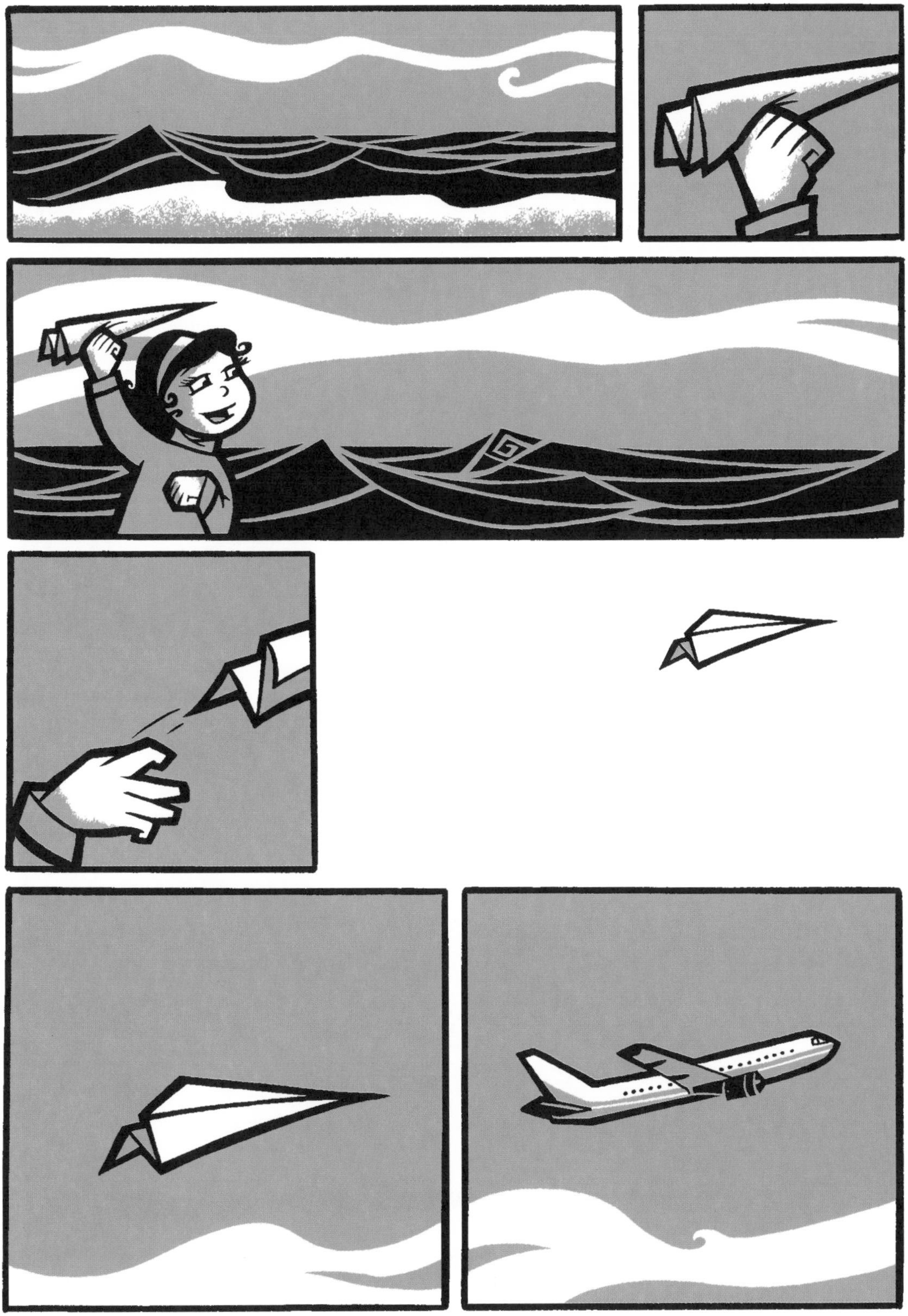

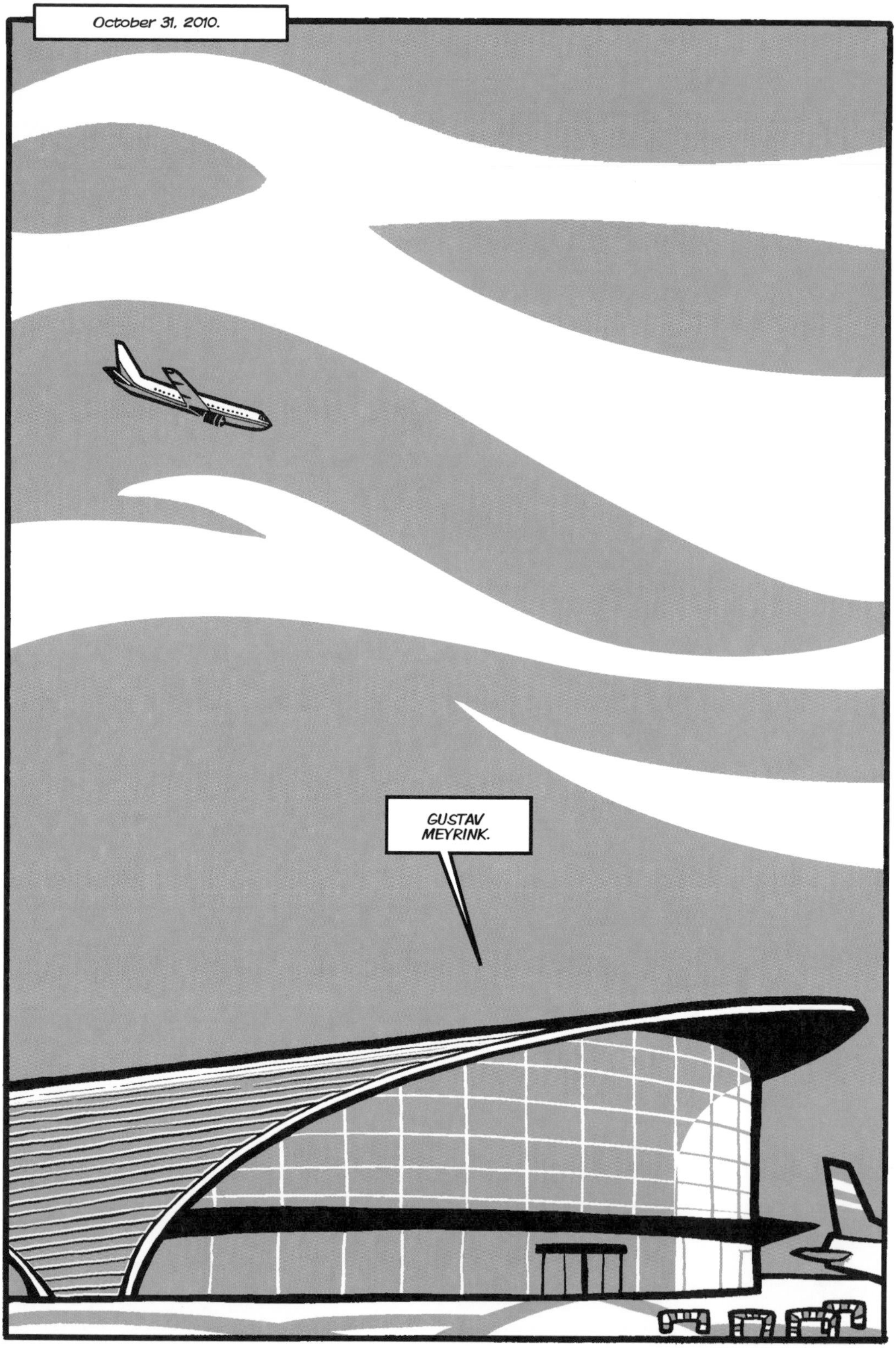
October 31, 2010.
GUSTAV MEYRINK.

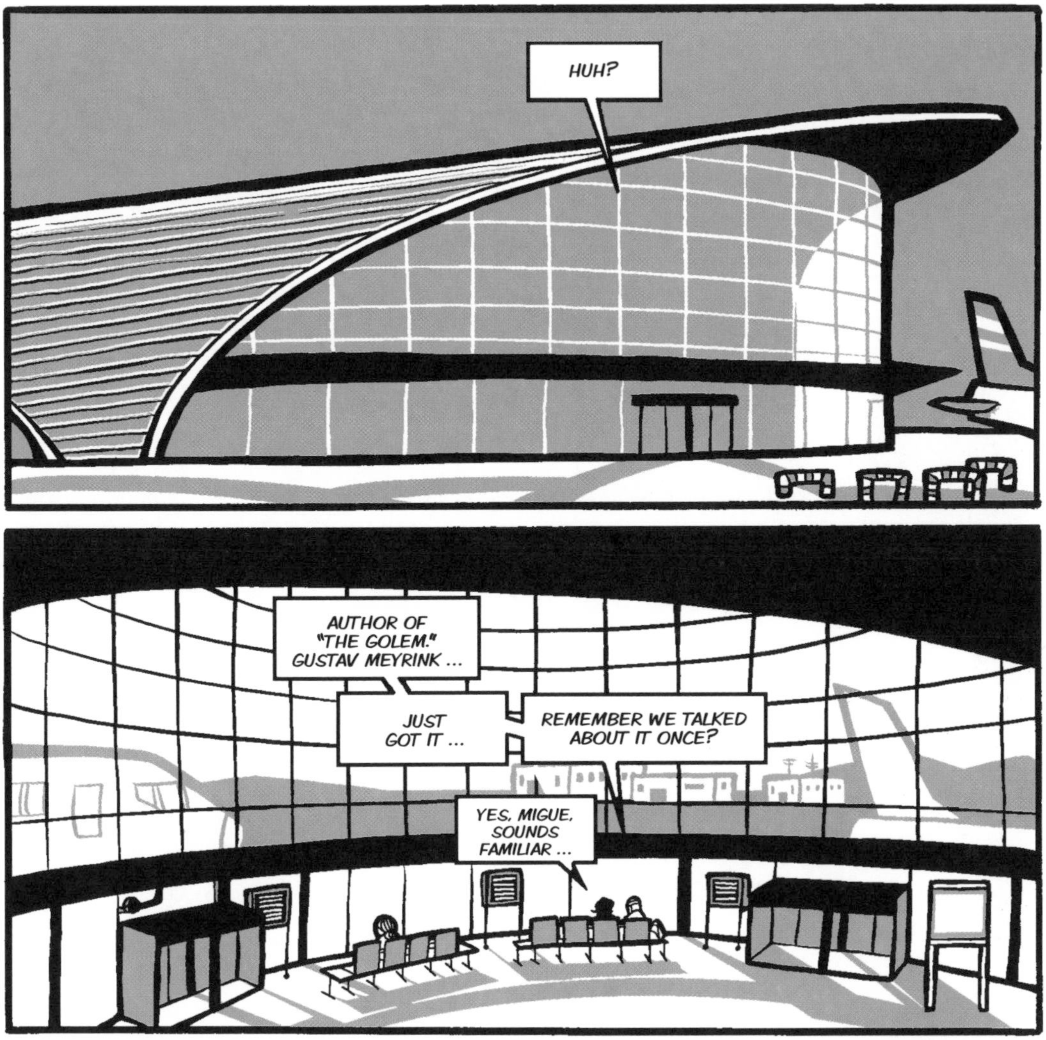
HUH?
AUTHOR OF "THE GOLEM." GUSTAV MEYRINK ...
JUST GOT IT ...
REMEMBER WE TALKED ABOUT IT ONCE?
YES, MIGUE, SOUNDS FAMILIAR ...
THINK LAIA'S OK?

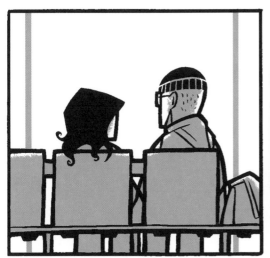

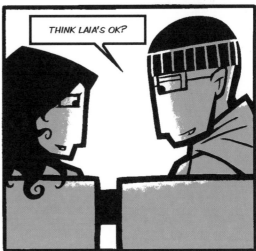

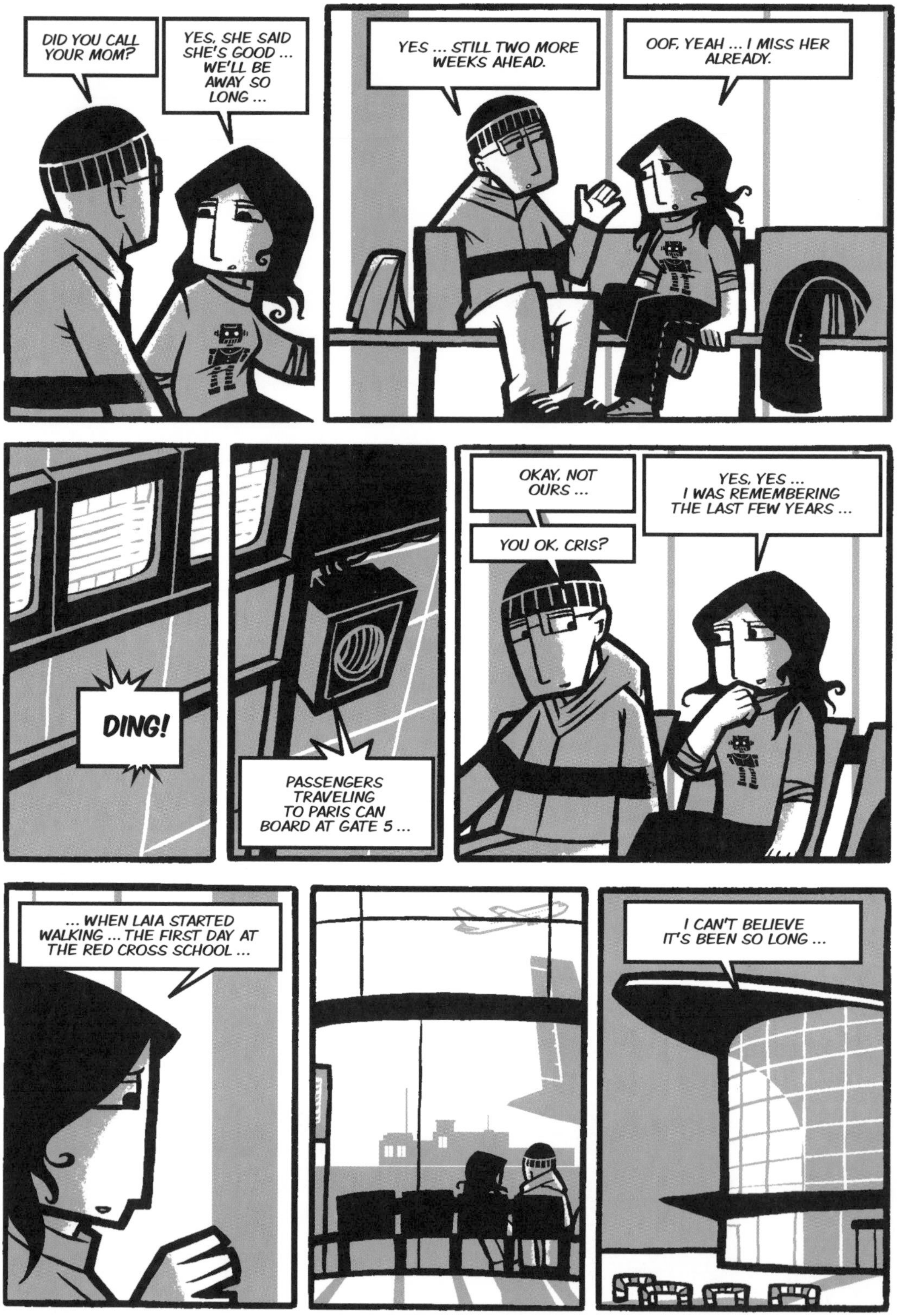
DID YOU CALL YOUR MOM?
YES, SHE SAID SHE'S GOOD ... WE'LL BE AWAY SO LONG ...
YES ... STILL TWO MORE WEEKS AHEAD.
OOF, YEAH ... I MISS HER ALREADY.
DING!
PASSENGERS TRAVELING TO PARIS CAN BOARD AT GATE 5 ...
OKAY, NOT OURS ...
YOU OK, CRIS?
YES, YES ... I WAS REMEMBERING THE LAST FEW YEARS ...
... WHEN LAIA STARTED WALKING ... THE FIRST DAY AT THE RED CROSS SCHOOL ...
I CAN'T BELIEVE IT'S BEEN SO LONG ...

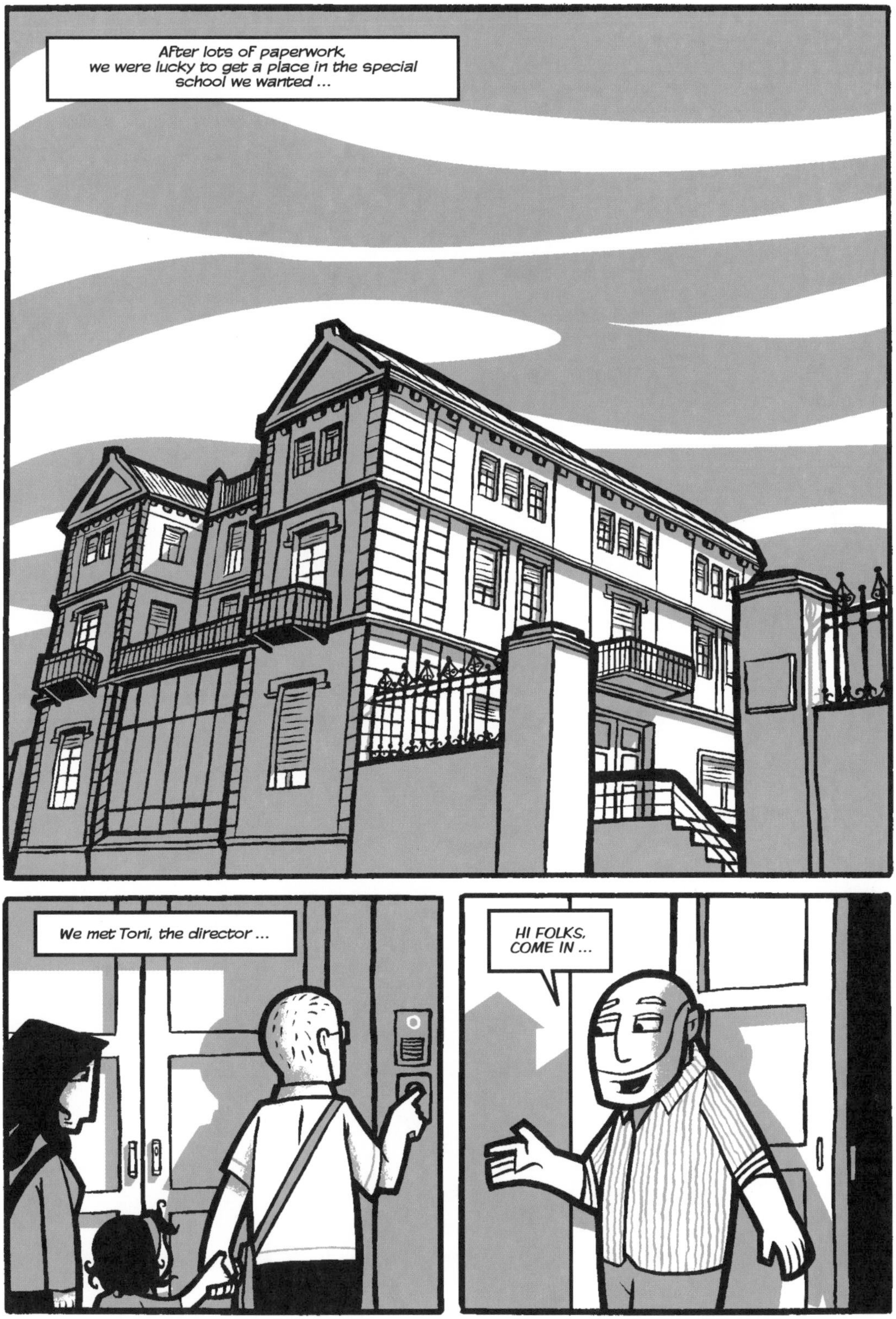
After lots of paperwork,
we were lucky to get a place in the special
school we wanted ...
We met Toni, the director ...
HI FOLKS,
COME IN ...

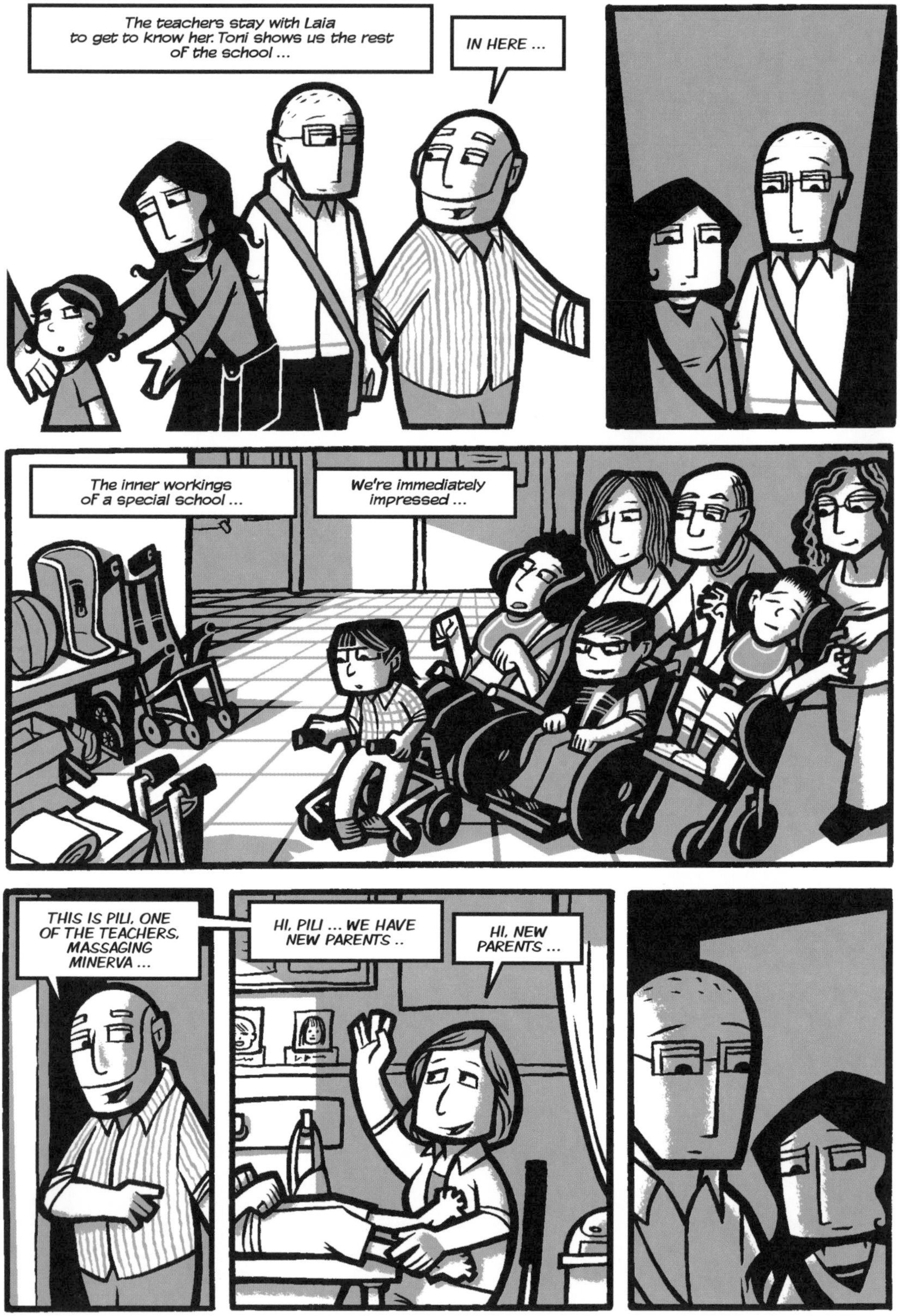
The teachers stay with Laia to get to know her. Toni shows us the rest of the school ...
IN HERE ...
The inner workings of a special school ...
We're immediately impressed ...
THIS IS PILI, ONE OF THE TEACHERS, MASSAGING MINERVA ...
HI, PILI ... WE HAVE NEW PARENTS ..
HI, NEW PARENTS ...

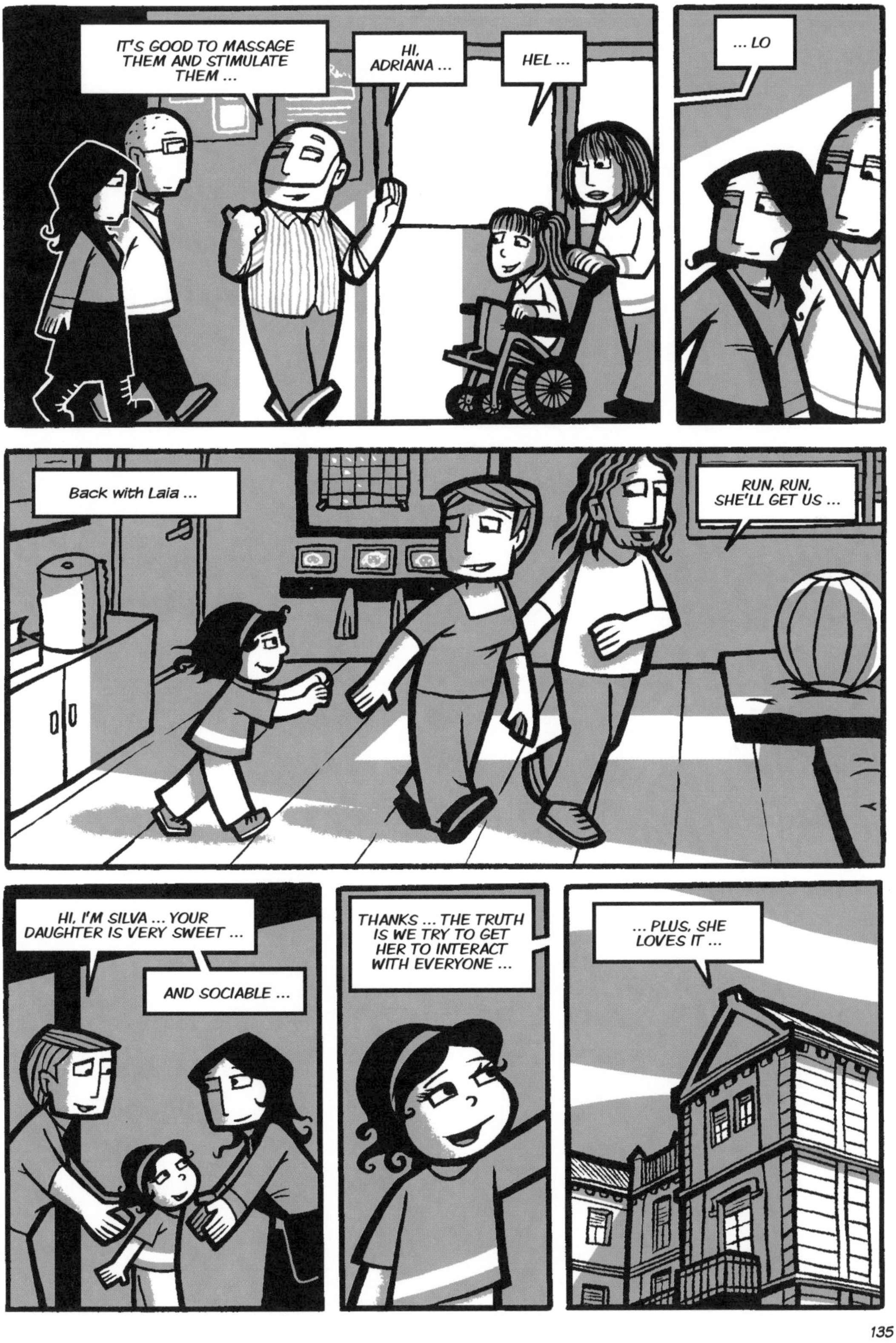
IT'S GOOD TO MASSAGE THEM AND STIMULATE THEM ...
HI, ADRIANA ...
HEL ...
... LO
Back with Laia ...
RUN, RUN, SHE'LL GET US ...
HI, I'M SILVA ... YOUR DAUGHTER IS VERY SWEET ...
AND SOCIABLE ...
THANKS ... THE TRUTH IS WE TRY TO GET HER TO INTERACT WITH EVERYONE ...
... PLUS, SHE LOVES IT ...

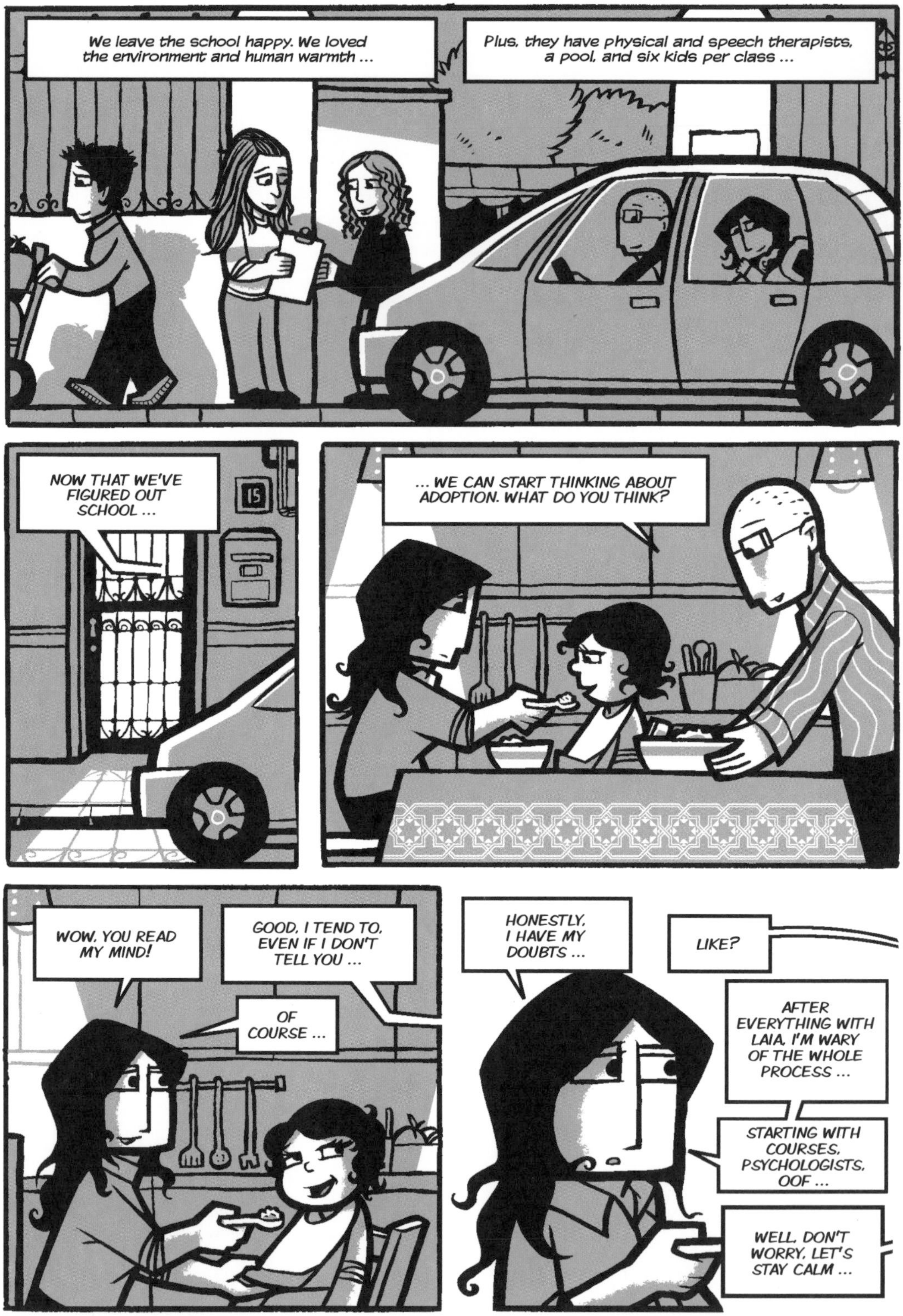
We leave the school happy. We loved the environment and human warmth ...
Plus, they have physical and speech therapists, a pool, and six kids per class ...
NOW THAT WE'VE FIGURED OUT SCHOOL ...
15
... WE CAN START THINKING ABOUT ADOPTION. WHAT DO YOU THINK?
WOW, YOU READ MY MIND!
GOOD, I TEND TO, EVEN IF I DON'T TELL YOU ...
OF COURSE ...
HONESTLY, I HAVE MY DOUBTS ...
LIKE?
AFTER EVERYTHING WITH LAIA, I'M WARY OF THE WHOLE PROCESS ...
STARTING WITH COURSES, PSYCHOLOGISTS, OOF ...
WELL, DON'T WORRY, LET'S STAY CALM ...

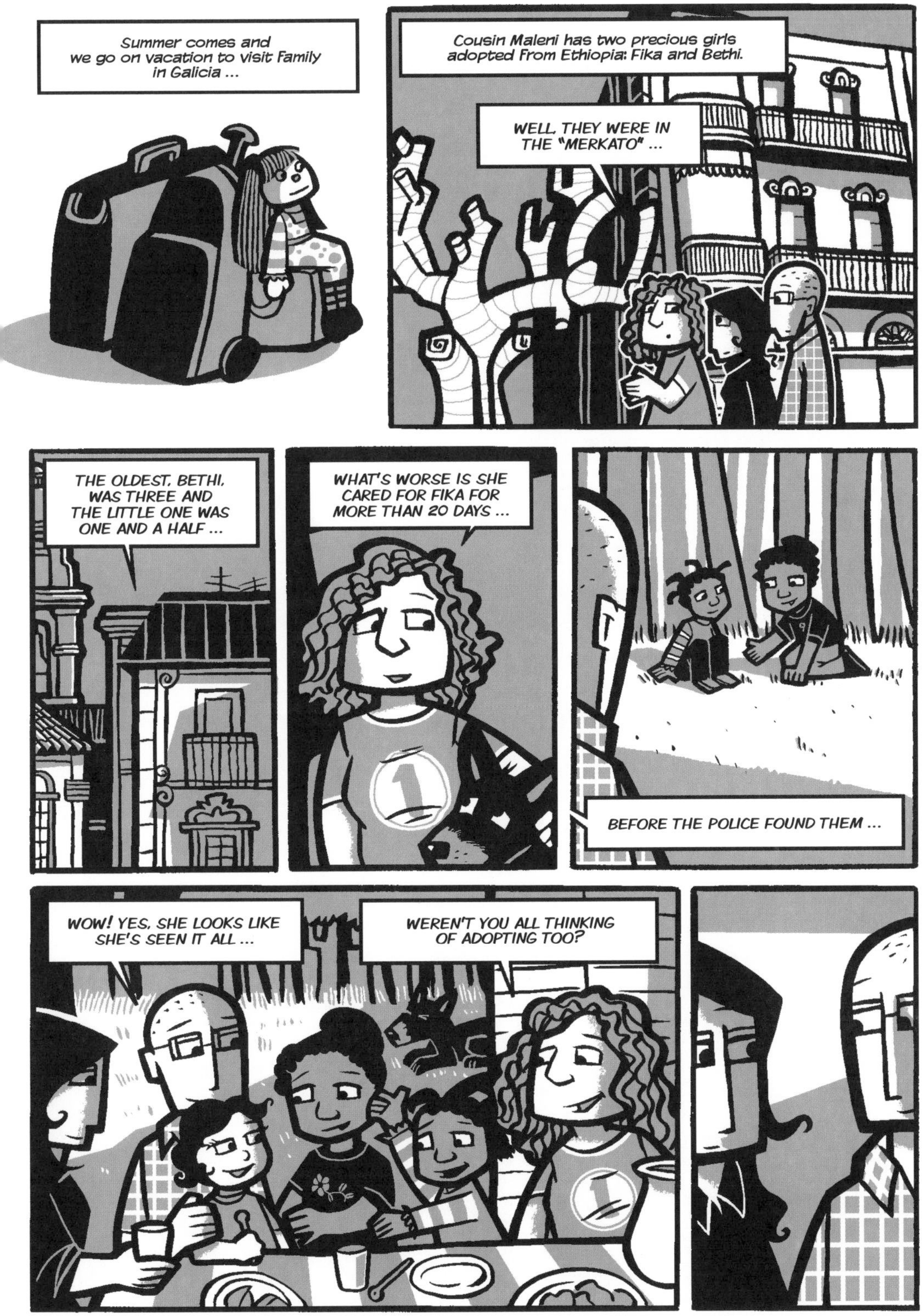
Summer comes and we go on vacation to visit family in Galicia ...
Cousin Maleni has two precious girls adopted from Ethiopia: Fika and Bethi.
WELL, THEY WERE IN THE "MERKATO" ...
THE OLDEST, BETHI, WAS THREE AND THE LITTLE ONE WAS ONE AND A HALF ...
WHAT'S WORSE IS SHE CARED FOR FIKA FOR MORE THAN 20 DAYS ...
BEFORE THE POLICE FOUND THEM ...
WOW! YES, SHE LOOKS LIKE SHE'S SEEN IT ALL ...
WEREN'T YOU ALL THINKING OF ADOPTING TOO?

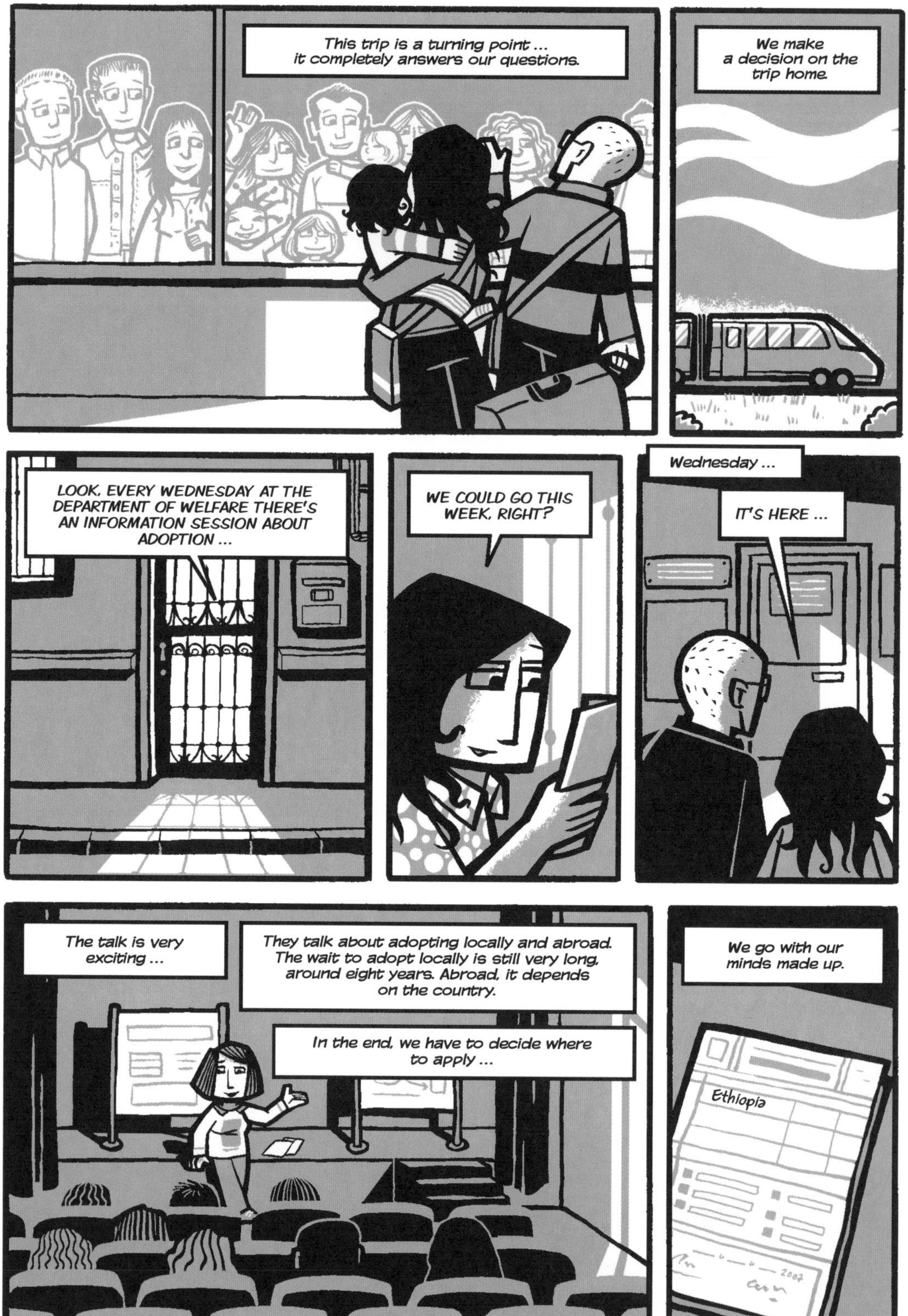
This trip is a turning point ... it completely answers our questions.
We make a decision on the trip home.
LOOK, EVERY WEDNESDAY AT THE DEPARTMENT OF WELFARE THERE'S AN INFORMATION SESSION ABOUT ADOPTION ...
WE COULD GO THIS WEEK, RIGHT?
Wednesday ...
IT'S HERE ...
The talk is very exciting ...
They talk about adopting locally and abroad. The wait to adopt locally is still very long, around eight years. Abroad, it depends on the country.
In the end, we have to decide where to apply ...
We go with our minds made up.
Ethiopia

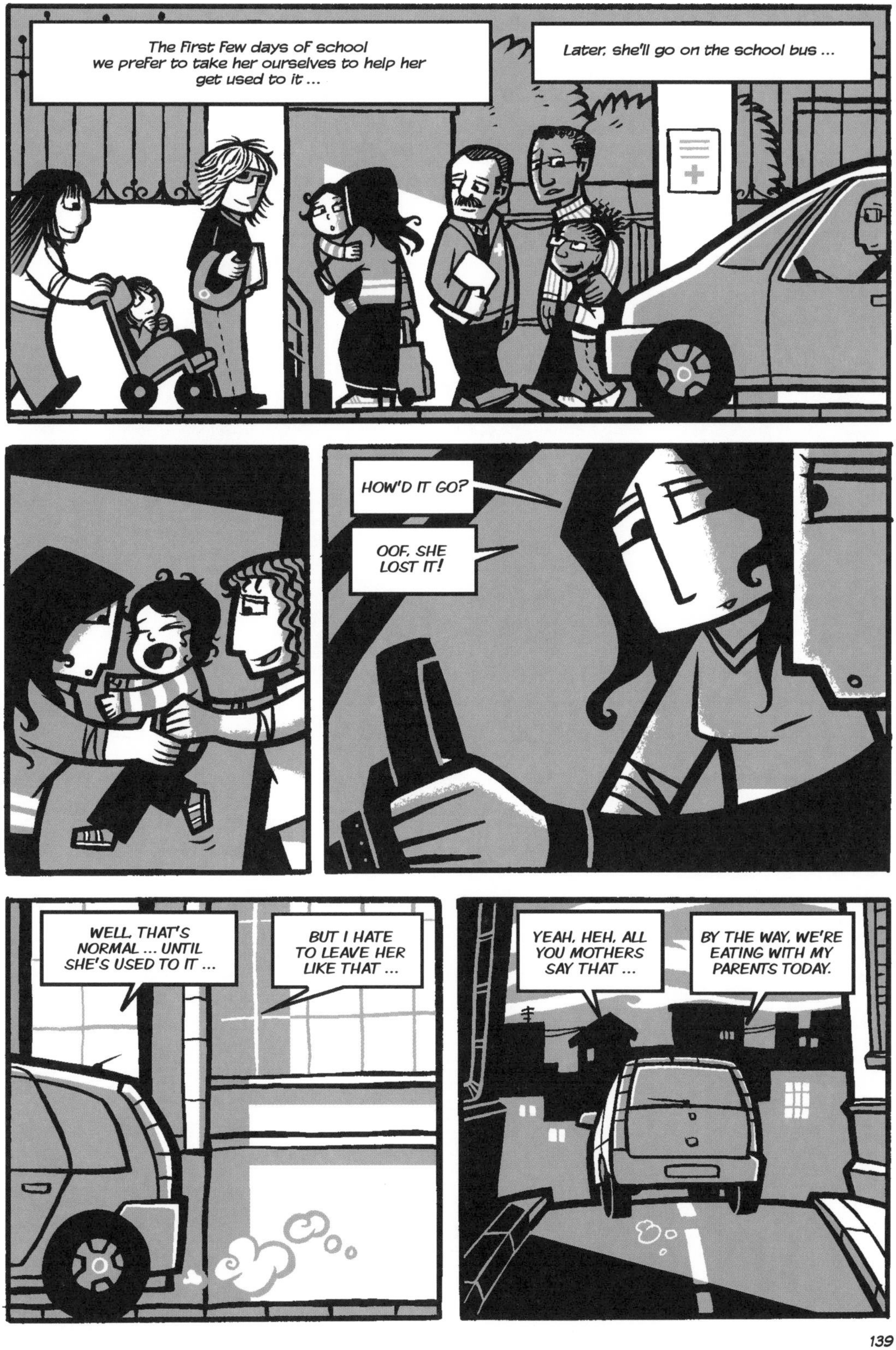
The First few days of school we prefer to take her ourselves to help her get used to it ...
Later, she'll go on the school bus ...
HOW'D IT GO?
OOF, SHE LOST IT!
WELL, THAT'S NORMAL ... UNTIL SHE'S USED TO IT ...
BUT I HATE TO LEAVE HER LIKE THAT ...
YEAH, HEH, ALL YOU MOTHERS SAY THAT ...
BY THE WAY, WE'RE EATING WITH MY PARENTS TODAY.

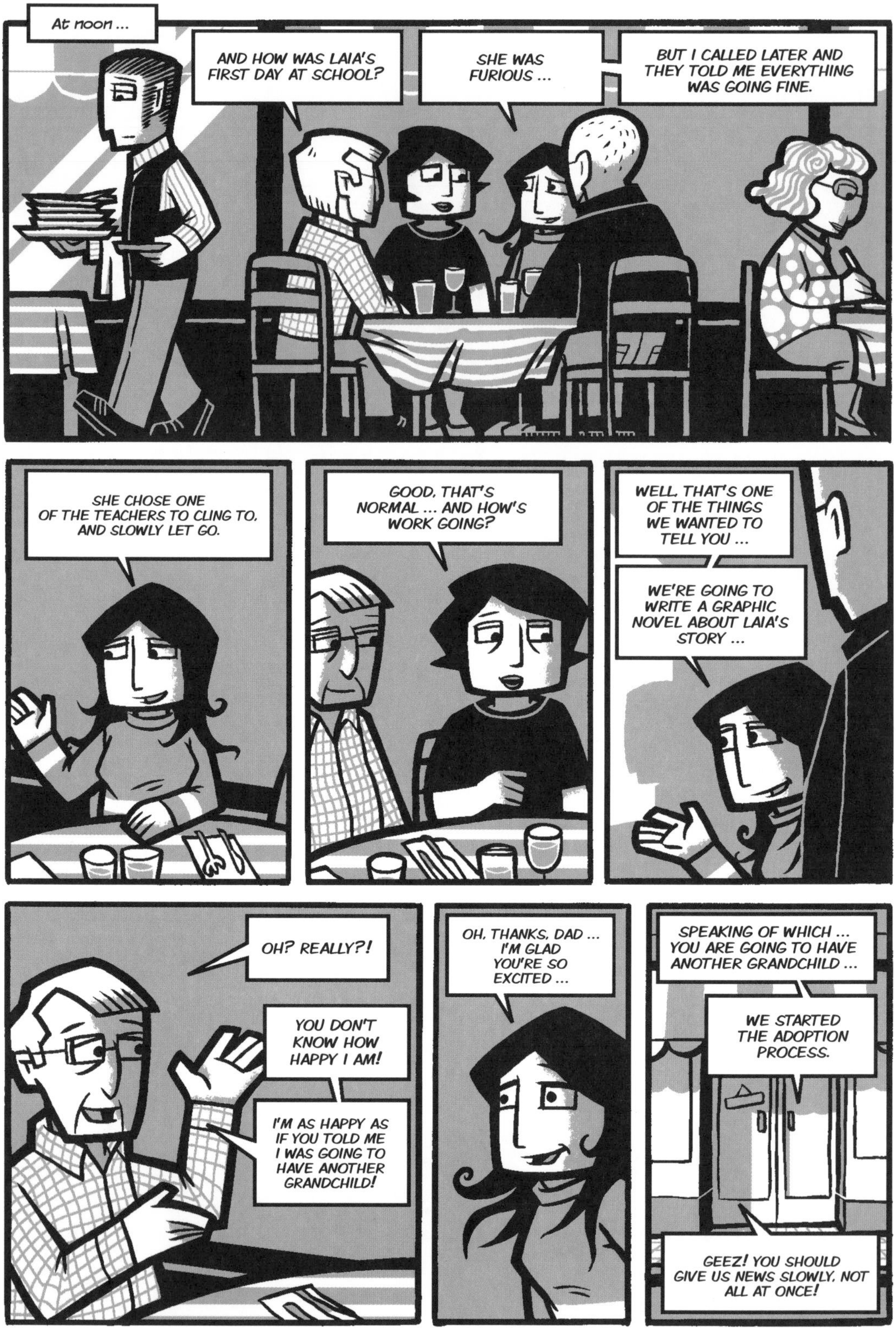
At noon ...
AND HOW WAS LAIA'S FIRST DAY AT SCHOOL?
SHE WAS FURIOUS ...
BUT I CALLED LATER AND THEY TOLD ME EVERYTHING WAS GOING FINE.
SHE CHOSE ONE OF THE TEACHERS TO CLING TO, AND SLOWLY LET GO.
GOOD, THAT'S NORMAL ... AND HOW'S WORK GOING?
WELL, THAT'S ONE OF THE THINGS WE WANTED TO TELL YOU ...
WE'RE GOING TO WRITE A GRAPHIC NOVEL ABOUT LAIA'S STORY ...
OH? REALLY?!
YOU DON'T KNOW HOW HAPPY I AM!
I'M AS HAPPY AS IF YOU TOLD ME I WAS GOING TO HAVE ANOTHER GRANDCHILD!
OH, THANKS, DAD ... I'M GLAD YOU'RE SO EXCITED ...
SPEAKING OF WHICH ... YOU ARE GOING TO HAVE ANOTHER GRANDCHILD ...
WE STARTED THE ADOPTION PROCESS.
GEEZ! YOU SHOULD GIVE US NEWS SLOWLY, NOT ALL AT ONCE!

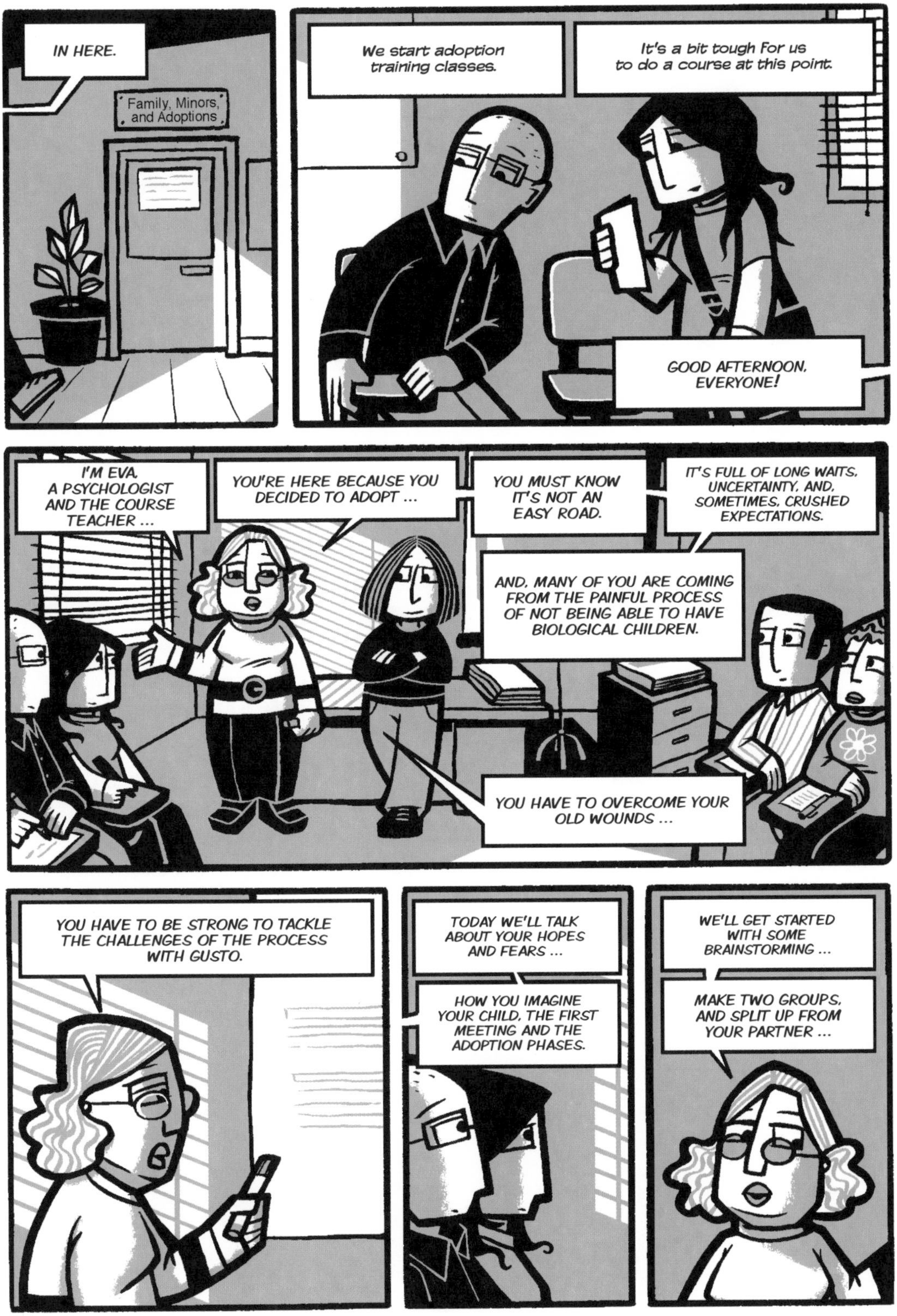
IN HERE.
Family, Minors, and Adoptions
We start adoption training classes.
It's a bit tough for us to do a course at this point.
GOOD AFTERNOON, EVERYONE!
I'M EVA, A PSYCHOLOGIST AND THE COURSE TEACHER ...
YOU'RE HERE BECAUSE YOU DECIDED TO ADOPT ...
YOU MUST KNOW IT'S NOT AN EASY ROAD.
IT'S FULL OF LONG WAITS, UNCERTAINTY, AND, SOMETIMES, CRUSHED EXPECTATIONS.
AND, MANY OF YOU ARE COMING FROM THE PAINFUL PROCESS OF NOT BEING ABLE TO HAVE BIOLOGICAL CHILDREN.
YOU HAVE TO OVERCOME YOUR OLD WOUNDS ...
YOU HAVE TO BE STRONG TO TACKLE THE CHALLENGES OF THE PROCESS WITH GUSTO.
TODAY WE'LL TALK ABOUT YOUR HOPES AND FEARS ...
HOW YOU IMAGINE YOUR CHILD, THE FIRST MEETING AND THE ADOPTION PHASES.
WE'LL GET STARTED WITH SOME BRAINSTORMING ...
MAKE TWO GROUPS, AND SPLIT UP FROM YOUR PARTNER ...

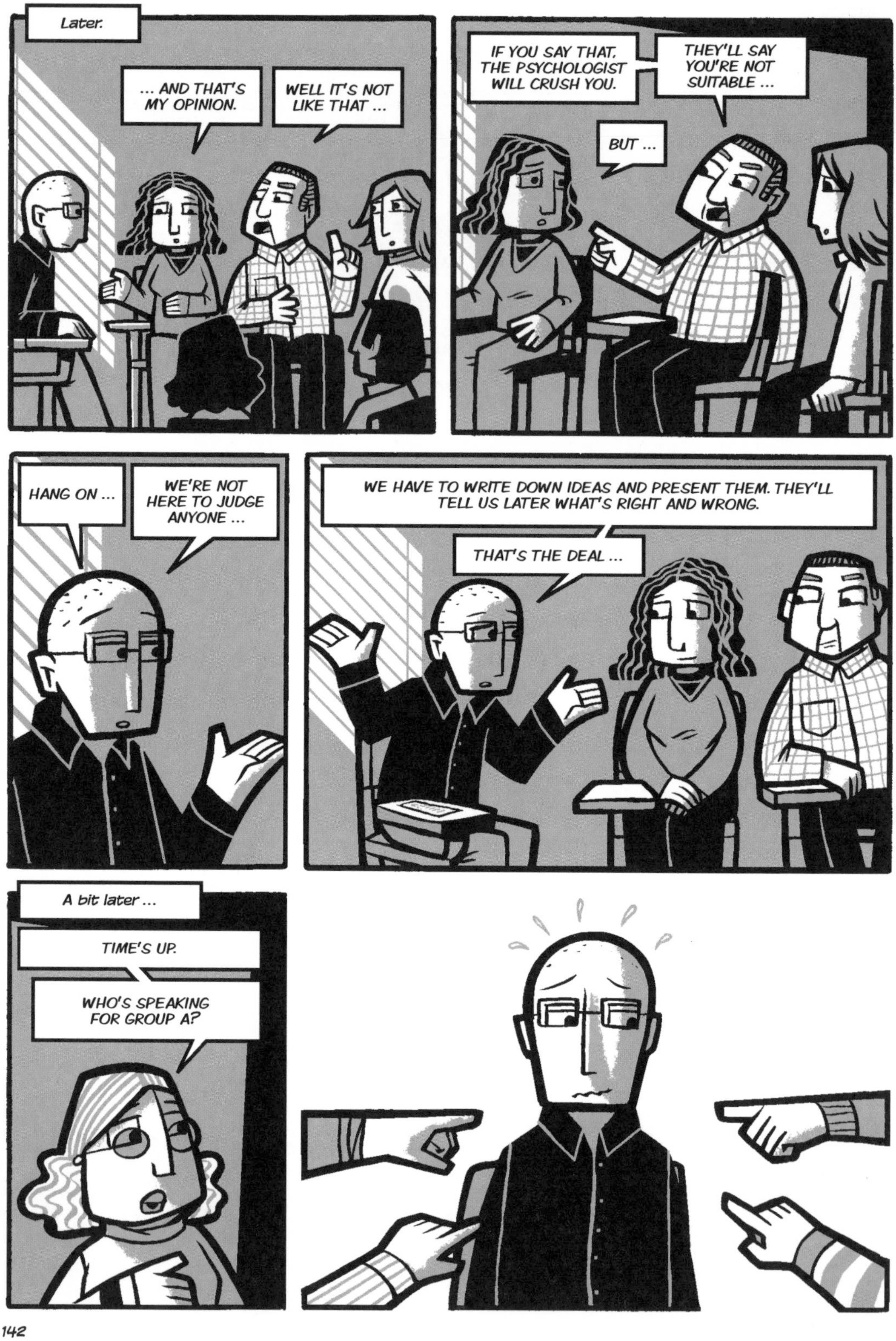
Later.
... AND THAT'S MY OPINION.
WELL IT'S NOT LIKE THAT ...
IF YOU SAY THAT, THE PSYCHOLOGIST WILL CRUSH YOU.
THEY'LL SAY YOU'RE NOT SUITABLE ...
BUT ...
HANG ON ...
WE'RE NOT HERE TO JUDGE ANYONE ...
WE HAVE TO WRITE DOWN IDEAS AND PRESENT THEM. THEY'LL TELL US LATER WHAT'S RIGHT AND WRONG.
THAT'S THE DEAL ...
A bit later ...
TIME'S UP.
WHO'S SPEAKING FOR GROUP A?

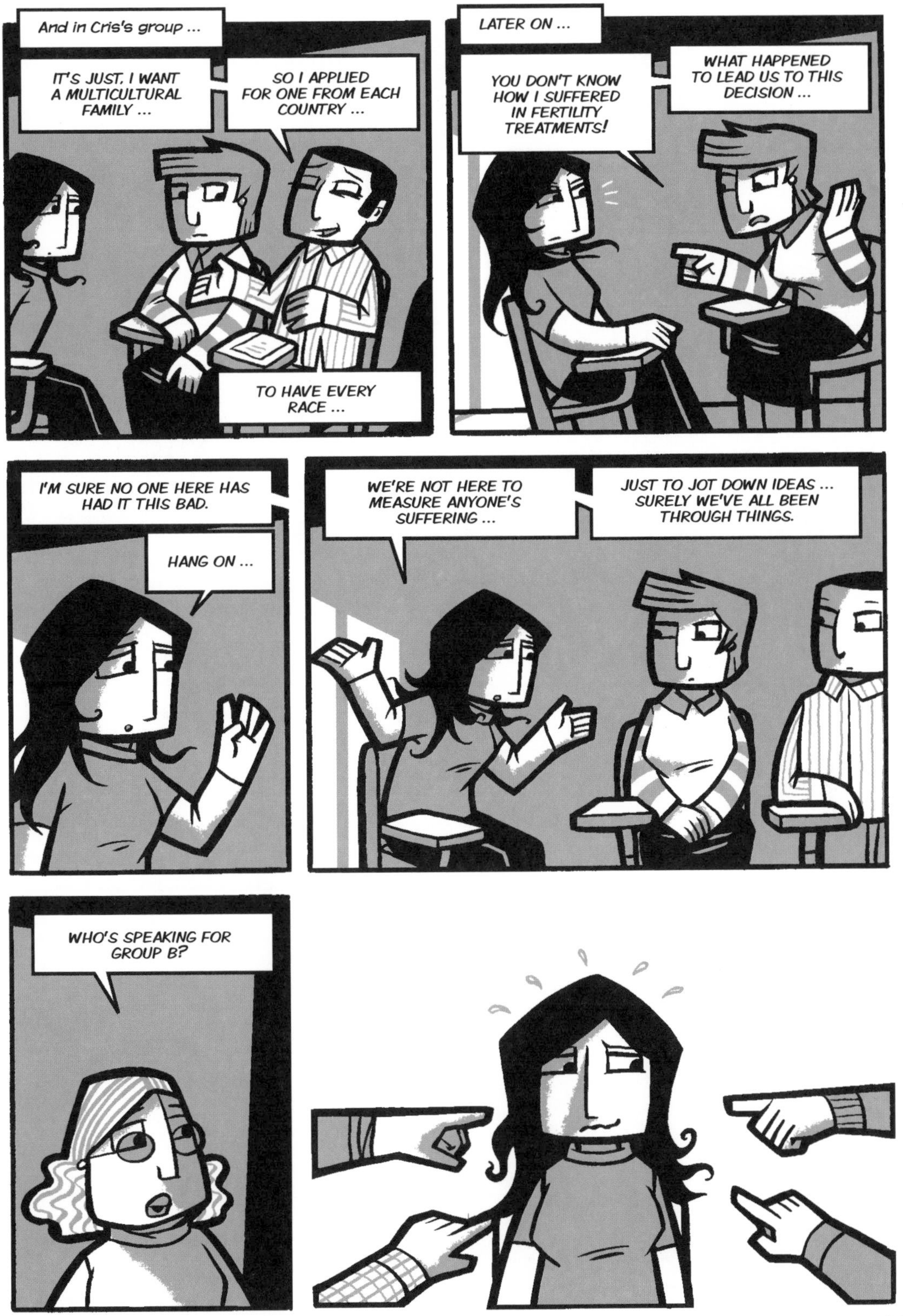
And in Cris's group ...
IT'S JUST, I WANT A MULTICULTURAL FAMILY ...
SO I APPLIED FOR ONE FROM EACH COUNTRY ...
TO HAVE EVERY RACE ...
LATER ON ...
YOU DON'T KNOW HOW I SUFFERED IN FERTILITY TREATMENTS!
WHAT HAPPENED TO LEAD US TO THIS DECISION ...
I'M SURE NO ONE HERE HAS HAD IT THIS BAD.
HANG ON ...
WE'RE NOT HERE TO MEASURE ANYONE'S SUFFERING ...
JUST TO JOT DOWN IDEAS ... SURELY WE'VE ALL BEEN THROUGH THINGS.
WHO'S SPEAKING FOR GROUP B?

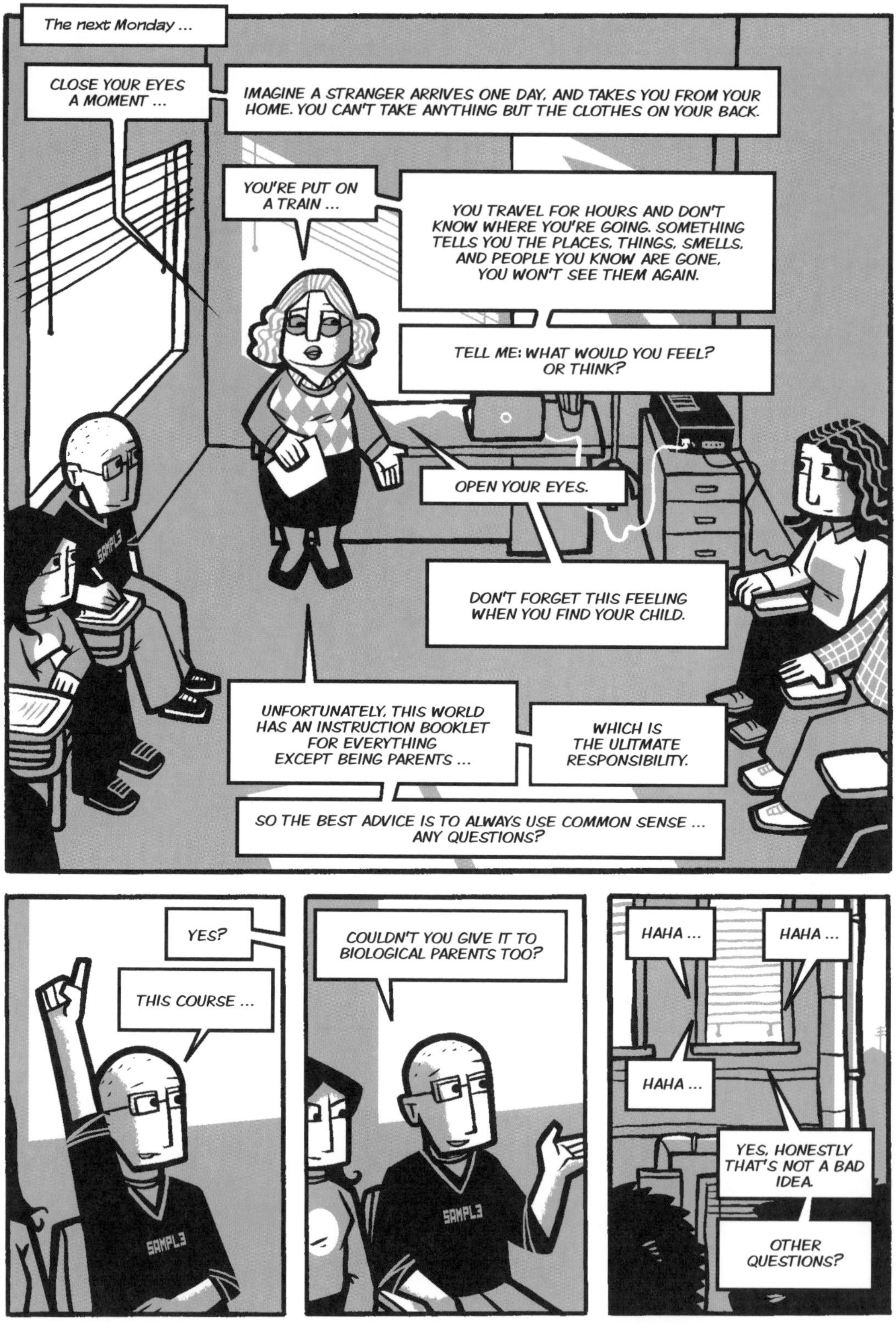
The next Monday ...
CLOSE YOUR EYES A MOMENT ...
IMAGINE A STRANGER ARRIVES ONE DAY, AND TAKES YOU FROM YOUR HOME. YOU CAN'T TAKE ANYTHING BUT THE CLOTHES ON YOUR BACK.
YOU'RE PUT ON A TRAIN ...
YOU TRAVEL FOR HOURS AND DON'T KNOW WHERE YOU'RE GOING. SOMETHING TELLS YOU THE PLACES, THINGS, SMELLS, AND PEOPLE YOU KNOW ARE GONE, YOU WON'T SEE THEM AGAIN.
TELL ME: WHAT WOULD YOU FEEL? OR THINK?
OPEN YOUR EYES.
DON'T FORGET THIS FEELING WHEN YOU FIND YOUR CHILD.
UNFORTUNATELY, THIS WORLD HAS AN INSTRUCTION BOOKLET FOR EVERYTHING EXCEPT BEING PARENTS ...
WHICH IS THE ULTIMATE RESPONSIBILITY.
SO THE BEST ADVICE IS TO ALWAYS USE COMMON SENSE ... ANY QUESTIONS?
YES?
THIS COURSE ...
SAMPL3
COULDN'T YOU GIVE IT TO BIOLOGICAL PARENTS TOO?
SAMPL3
HAHA ...
HAHA ...
HAHA ...
YES, HONESTLY THAT'S NOT A BAD IDEA.
OTHER QUESTIONS?

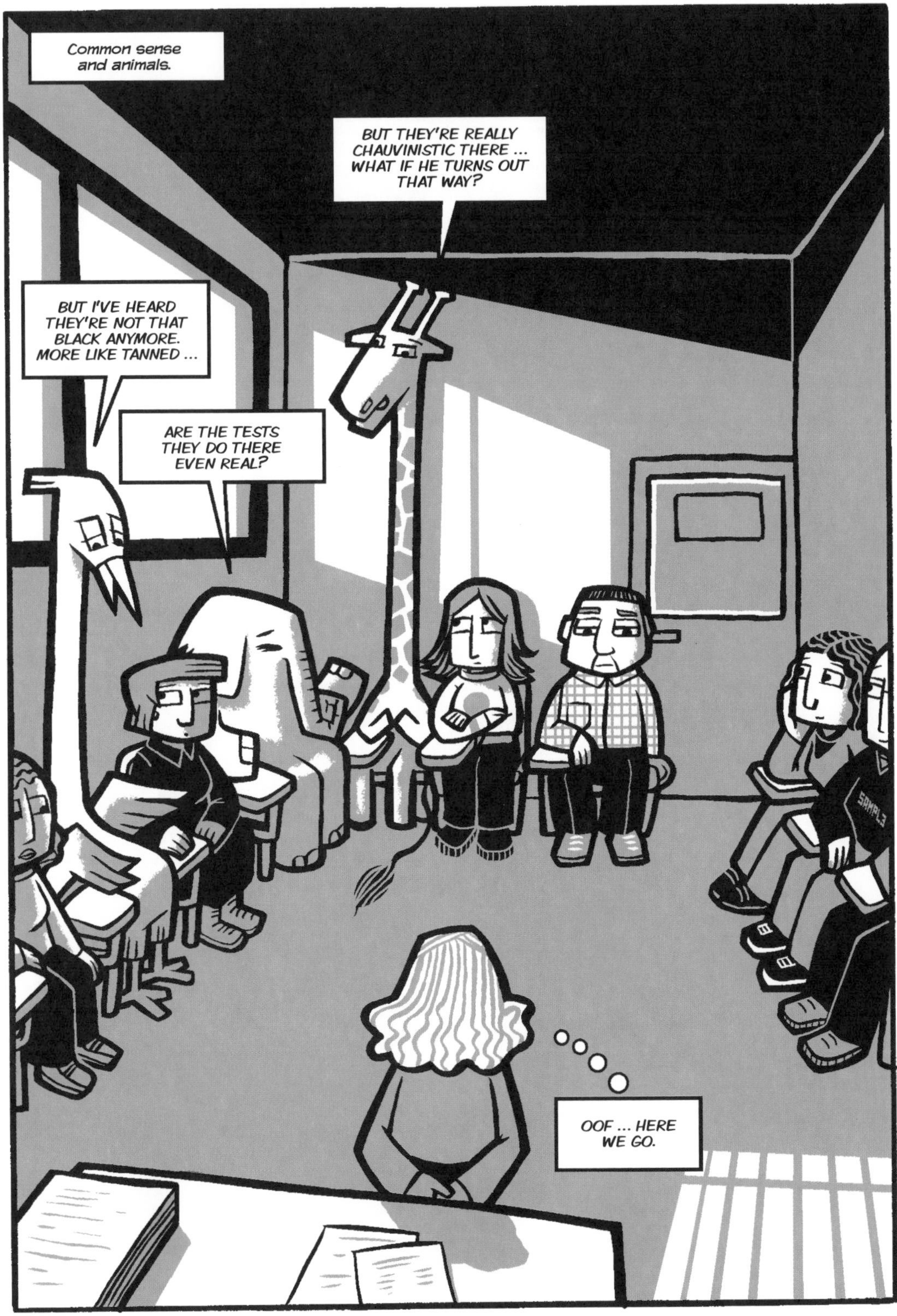
Common sense and animals.
BUT THEY'RE REALLY CHAUVINISTIC THERE ... WHAT IF HE TURNS OUT THAT WAY?
BUT I'VE HEARD THEY'RE NOT THAT BLACK ANYMORE. MORE LIKE TANNED ...
ARE THE TESTS THEY DO THERE EVEN REAL?
OOF ... HERE WE GO.

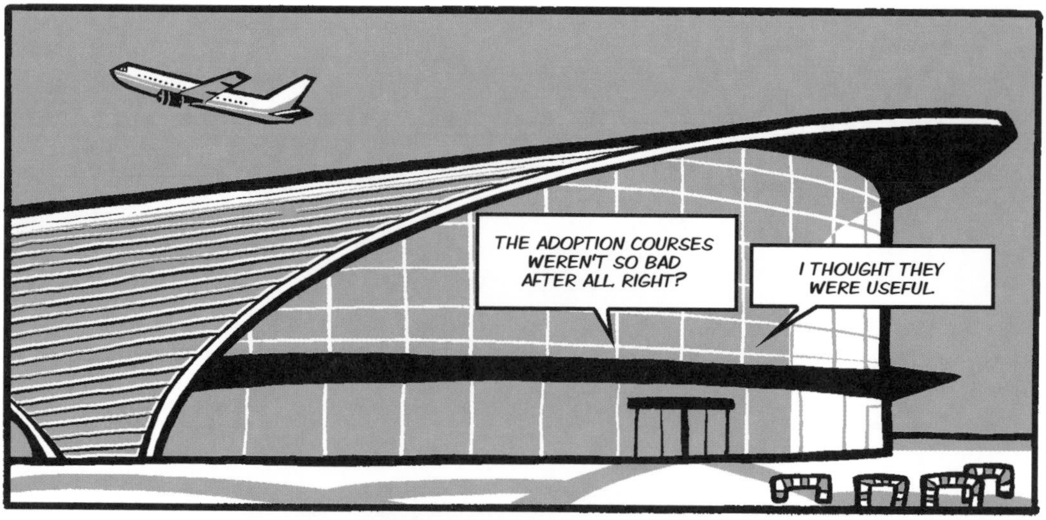
THE ADOPTION COURSES WEREN'T SO BAD AFTER ALL, RIGHT?
I THOUGHT THEY WERE USEFUL.

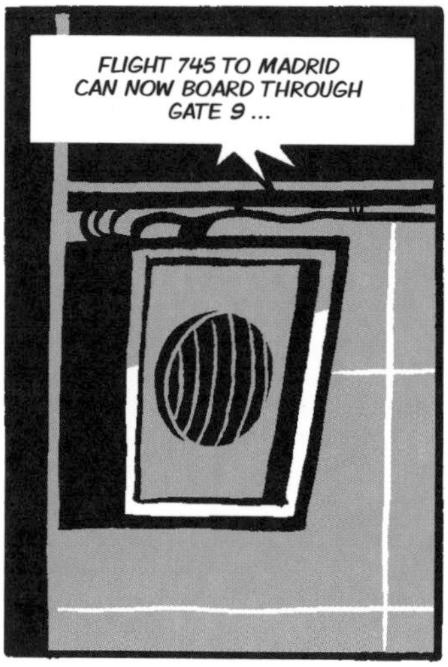
FLIGHT 745 TO MADRID CAN NOW BOARD THROUGH GATE 9 ...

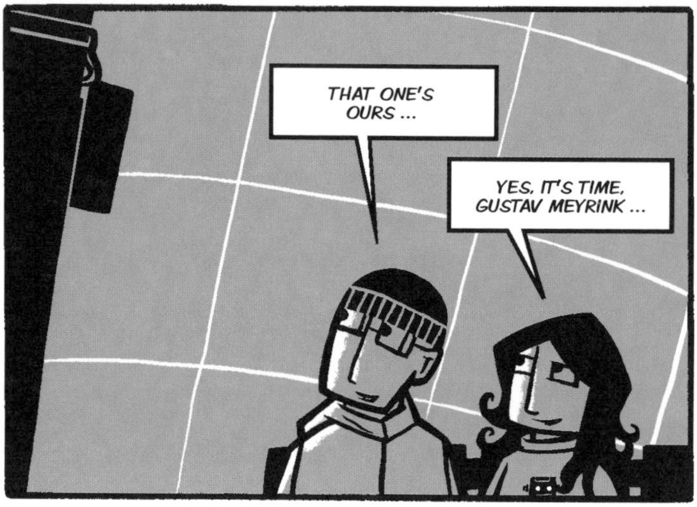
THAT ONE'S OURS ...
YES, IT'S TIME, GUSTAV MEYRINK ...

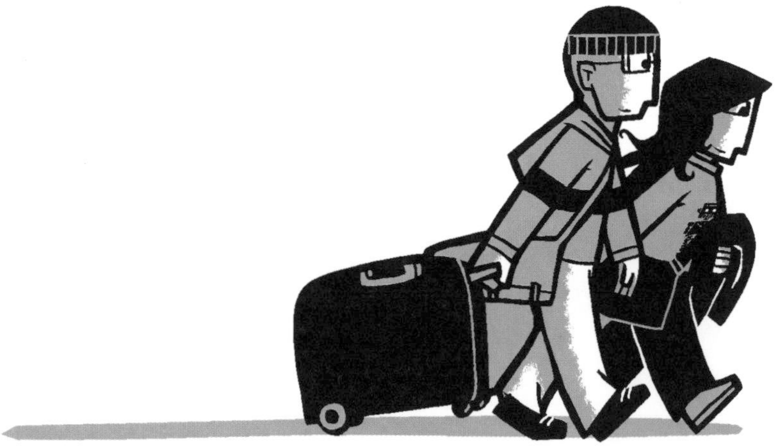

Chapter 2
INTEGRATION

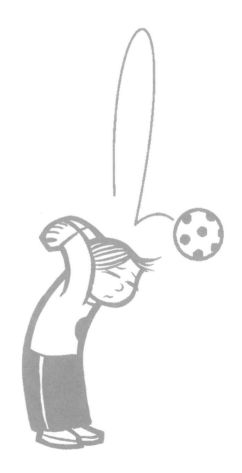

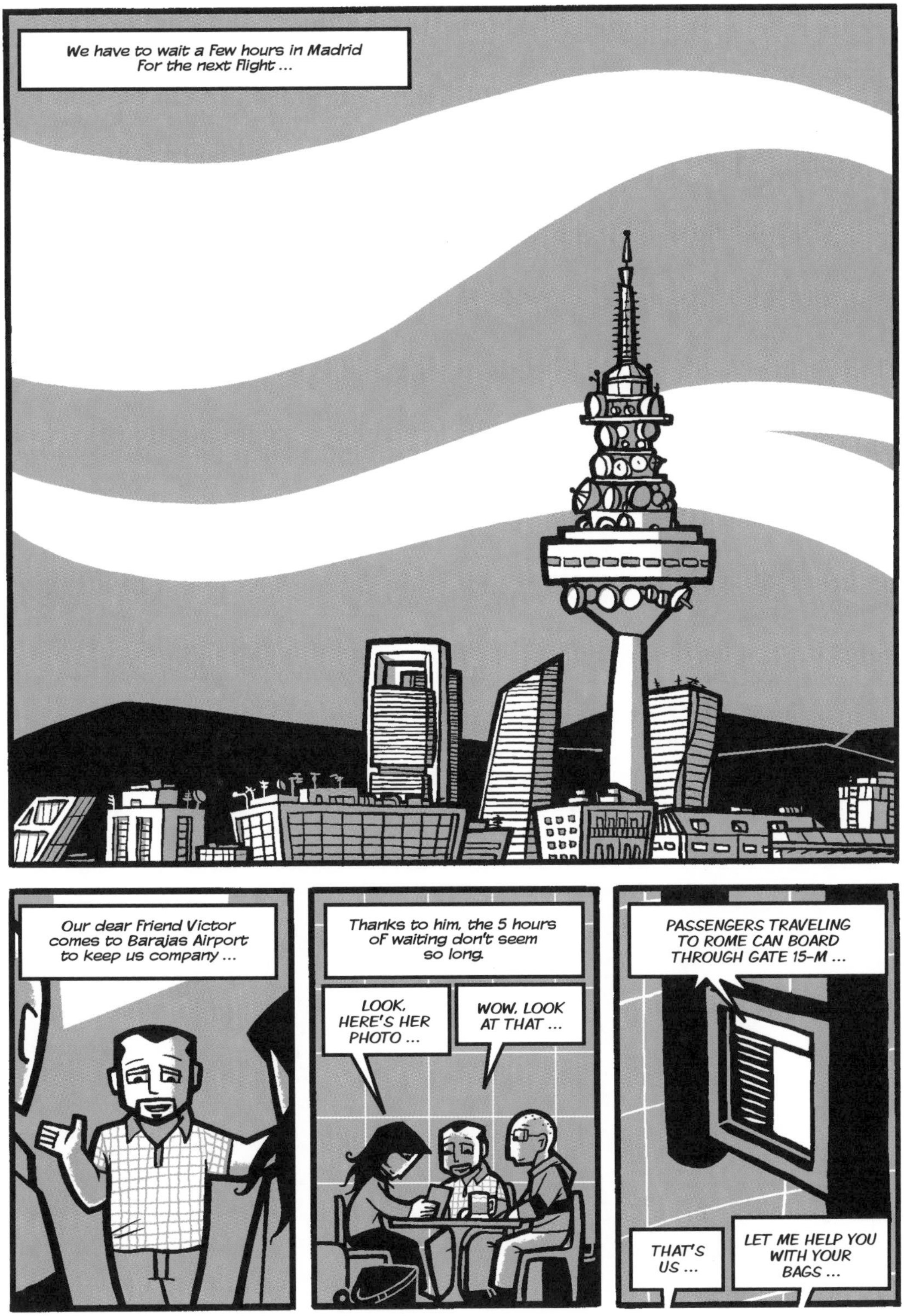
We have to wait a Few hours in Madrid For the next Flight ...
Our dear Friend Victor comes to Barajas Airport to keep us company ...
Thanks to him, the 5 hours of waiting don't seem so long.
LOOK, HERE'S HER PHOTO ...
WOW, LOOK AT THAT ...
PASSENGERS TRAVELING TO ROME CAN BOARD THROUGH GATE 15-M ...
THAT'S US ...
LET ME HELP YOU WITH YOUR BAGS ...

BUT, VICTOR ... LEAVE US SOMETHING ...
NO, NO, I WANT A SPOT IN YOUR NEXT COMIC, HEHE ...
BYE, FRIENDS! SAFE TRAVELS!
WHAT'S SO FUNNY?
EH ... I WAS REMEMBERING AFTERNOONS IN THE PLAZA ...

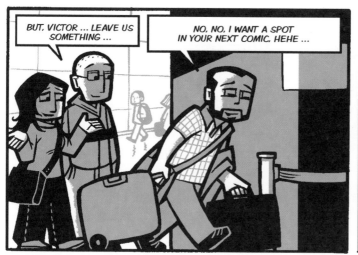

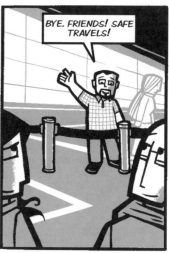

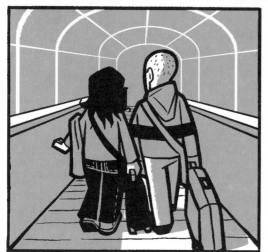

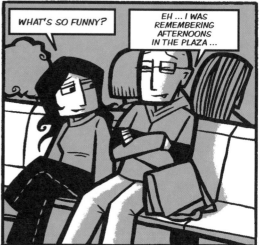

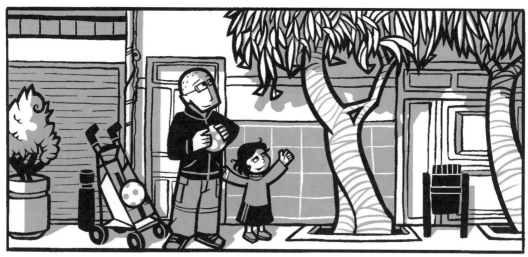

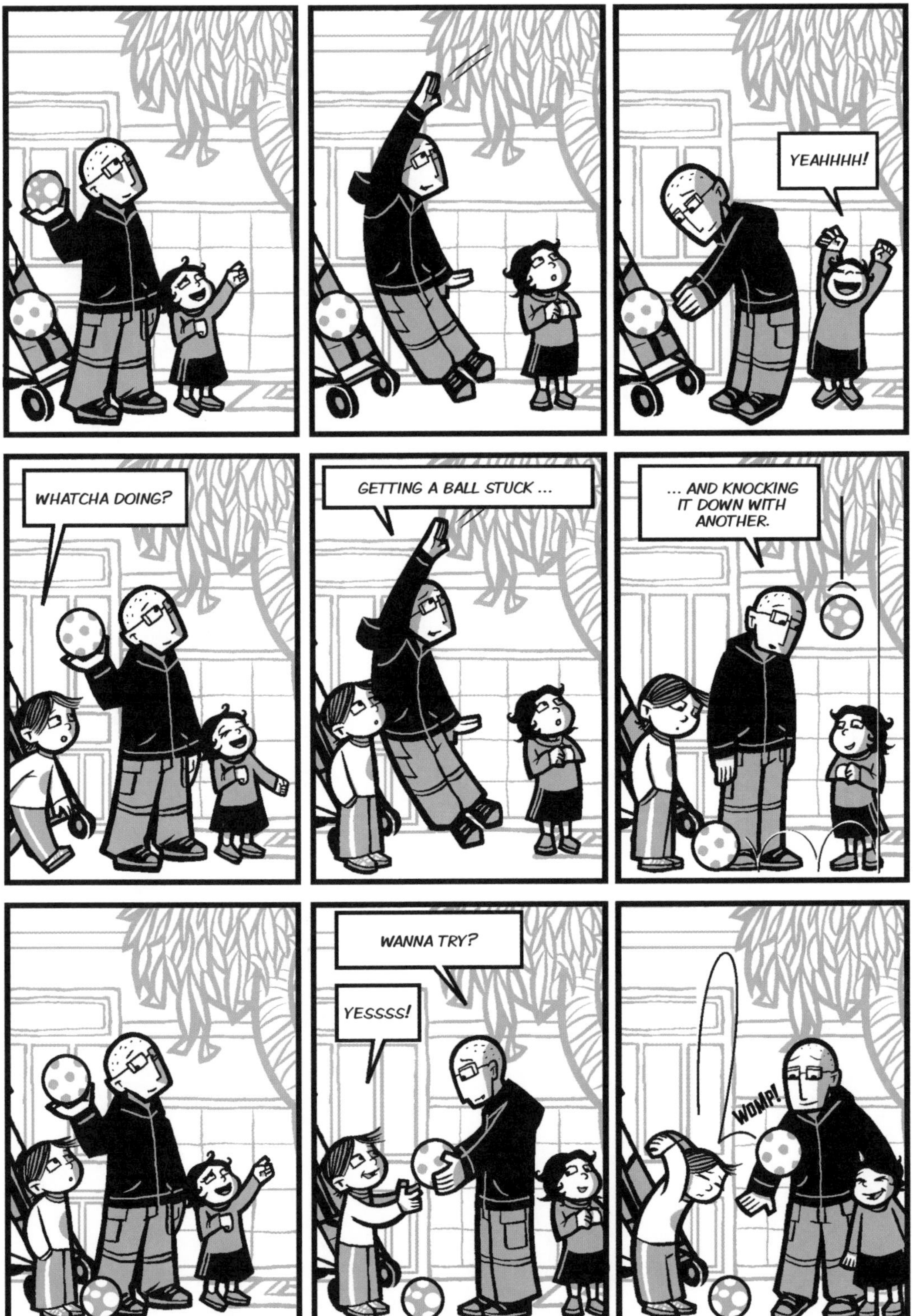
YEAHHHH!
WHATCHA DOING?
GETTING A BALL STUCK ...
... AND KNOCKING IT DOWN WITH ANOTHER.
WANNA TRY?
YESSSS!
WOMP!

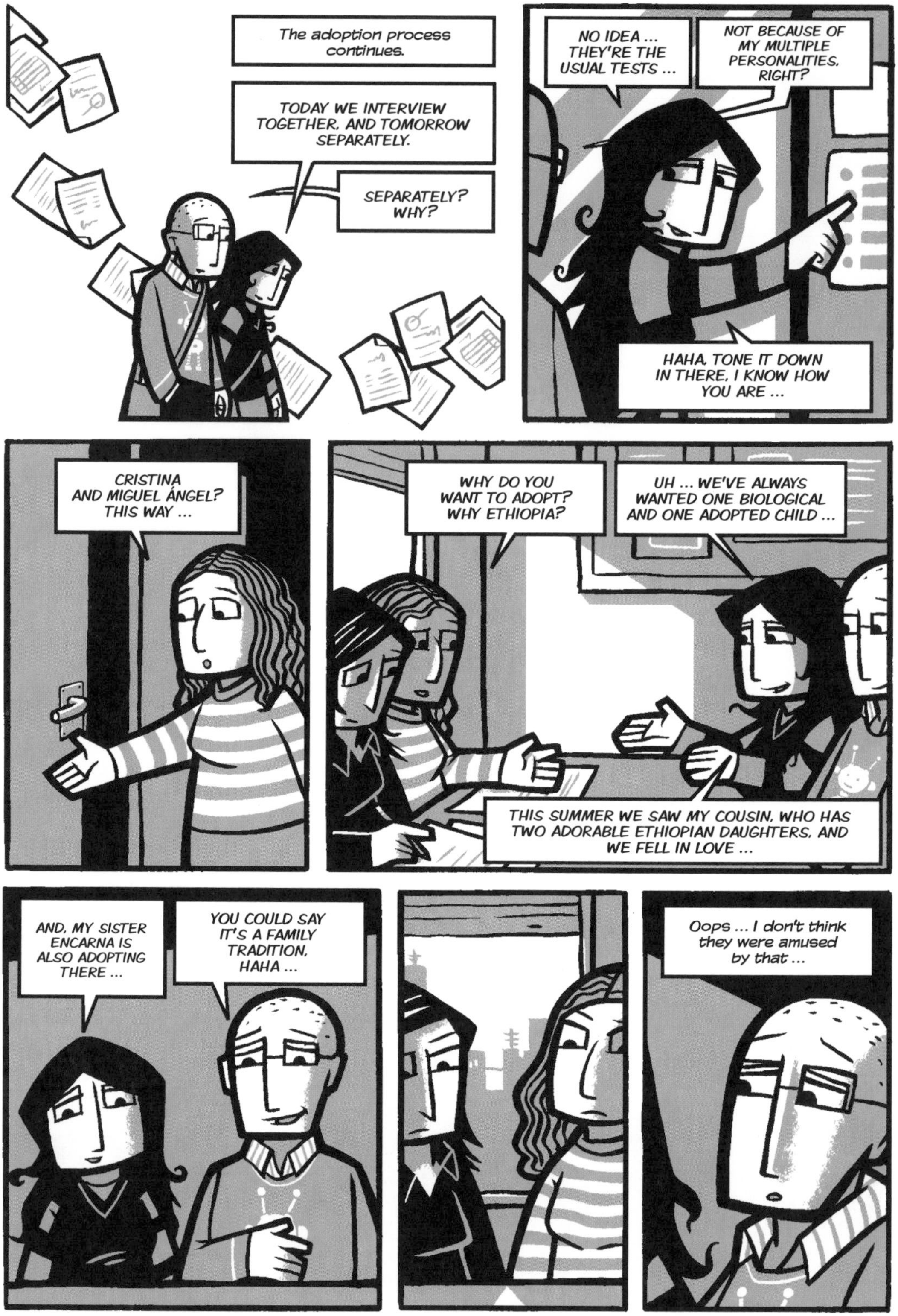
The adoption process continues.
TODAY WE INTERVIEW TOGETHER, AND TOMORROW SEPARATELY.
SEPARATELY? WHY?
NO IDEA ... THEY'RE THE USUAL TESTS ...
NOT BECAUSE OF MY MULTIPLE PERSONALITIES, RIGHT?
HAHA, TONE IT DOWN IN THERE, I KNOW HOW YOU ARE ...
CRISTINA AND MIGUEL ÁNGEL? THIS WAY ...
WHY DO YOU WANT TO ADOPT? WHY ETHIOPIA?
UH ... WE'VE ALWAYS WANTED ONE BIOLOGICAL AND ONE ADOPTED CHILD ...
THIS SUMMER WE SAW MY COUSIN, WHO HAS TWO ADORABLE ETHIOPIAN DAUGHTERS, AND WE FELL IN LOVE ...
AND, MY SISTER ENCARNA IS ALSO ADOPTING THERE ...
YOU COULD SAY IT'S A FAMILY TRADITION, HAHA ...
Oops ... I don't think they were amused by that ...

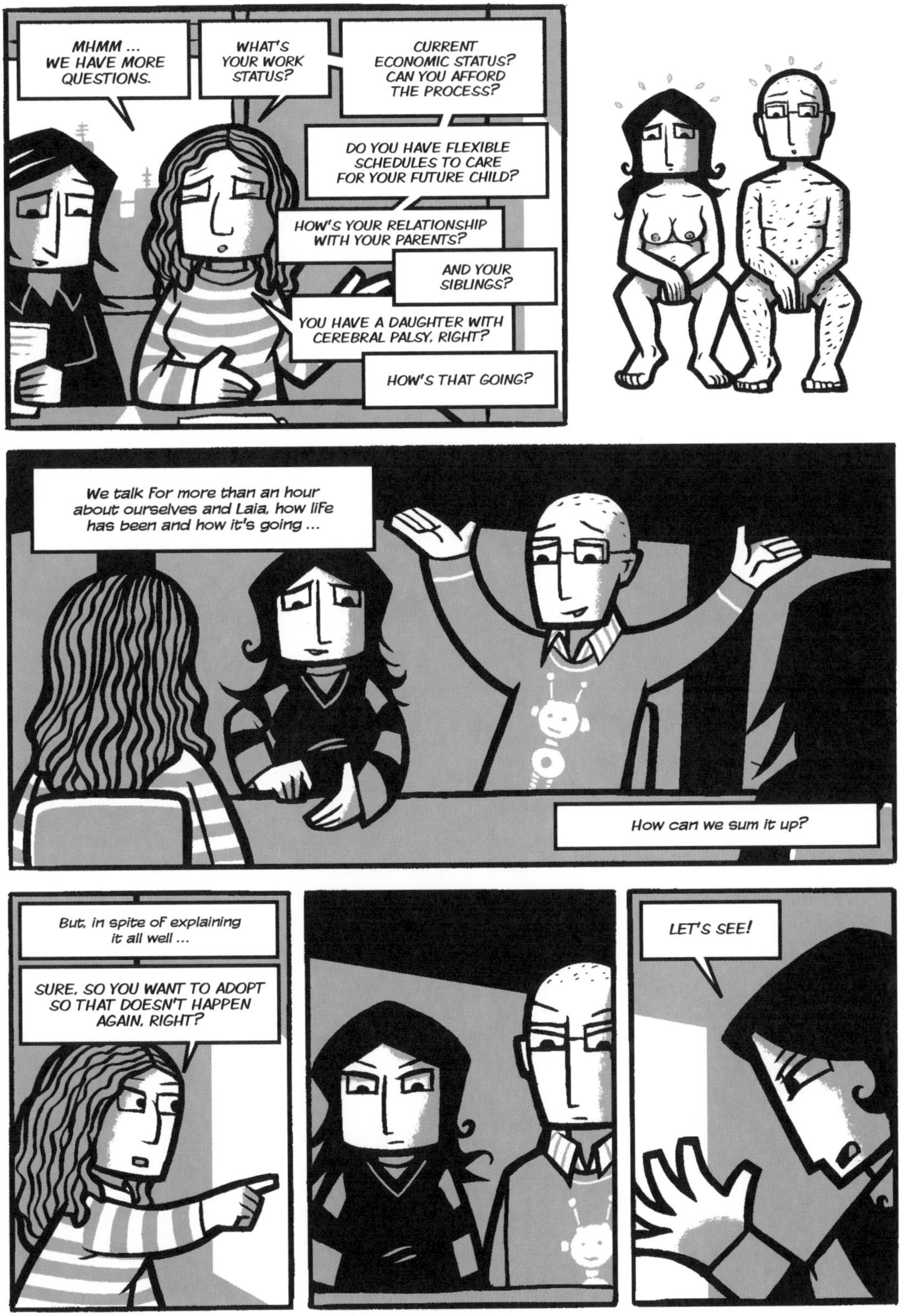
MHMM ... WE HAVE MORE QUESTIONS.
WHAT'S YOUR WORK STATUS?
CURRENT ECONOMIC STATUS? CAN YOU AFFORD THE PROCESS?
DO YOU HAVE FLEXIBLE SCHEDULES TO CARE FOR YOUR FUTURE CHILD?
HOW'S YOUR RELATIONSHIP WITH YOUR PARENTS?
AND YOUR SIBLINGS?
YOU HAVE A DAUGHTER WITH CEREBRAL PALSY, RIGHT?
HOW'S THAT GOING?
We talk for more than an hour about ourselves and Laia, how life has been and how it's going ...
How can we sum it up?
But, in spite of explaining it all well ...
SURE, SO YOU WANT TO ADOPT SO THAT DOESN'T HAPPEN AGAIN, RIGHT?
LET'S SEE!

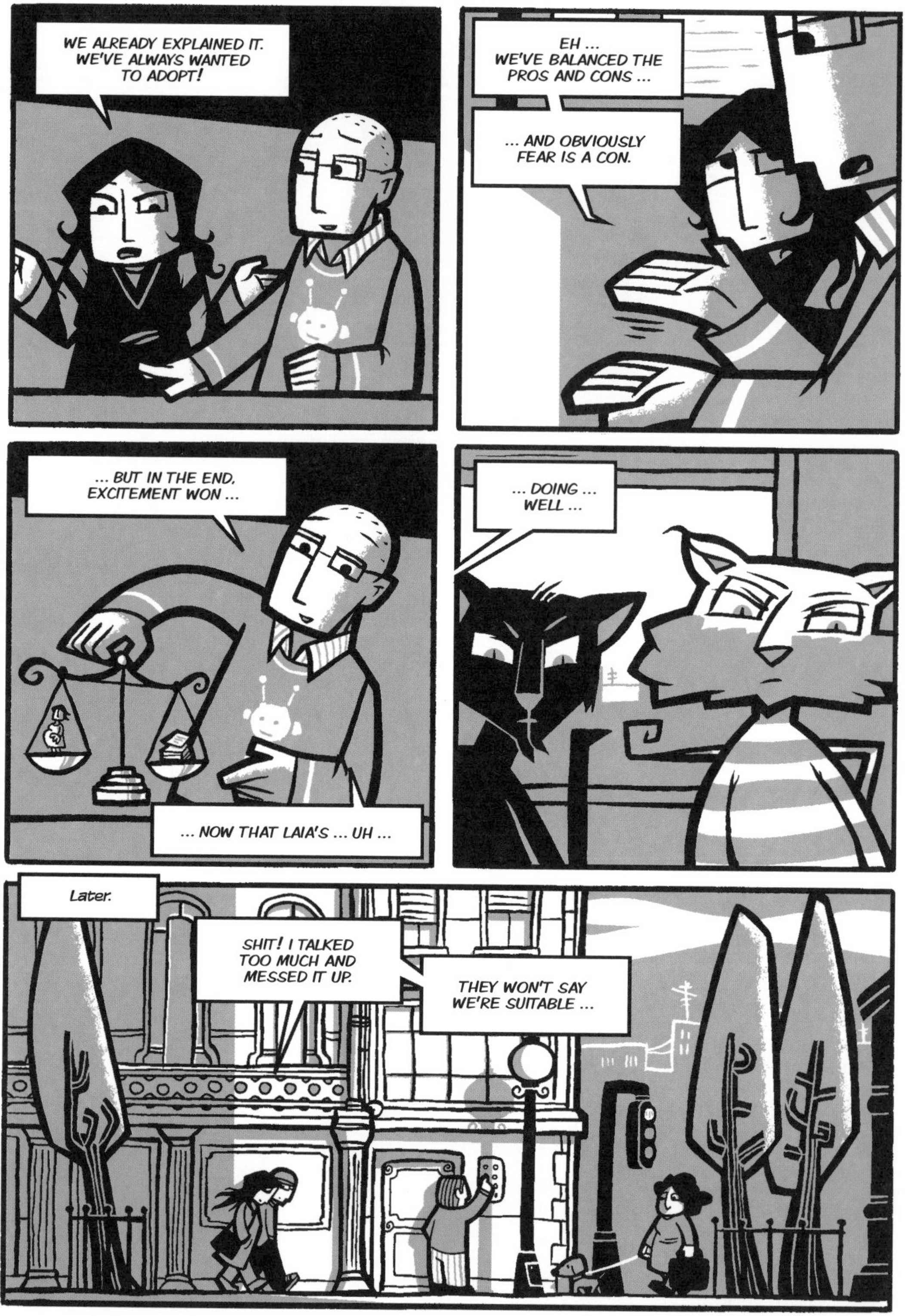
WE ALREADY EXPLAINED IT. WE'VE ALWAYS WANTED TO ADOPT!
EH ... WE'VE BALANCED THE PROS AND CONS ...
... AND OBVIOUSLY FEAR IS A CON.
... BUT IN THE END, EXCITEMENT WON ...
... NOW THAT LAIA'S ... UH ...
... DOING ... WELL ...
Later.
SHIT! I TALKED TOO MUCH AND MESSED IT UP.
THEY WON'T SAY WE'RE SUITABLE ...

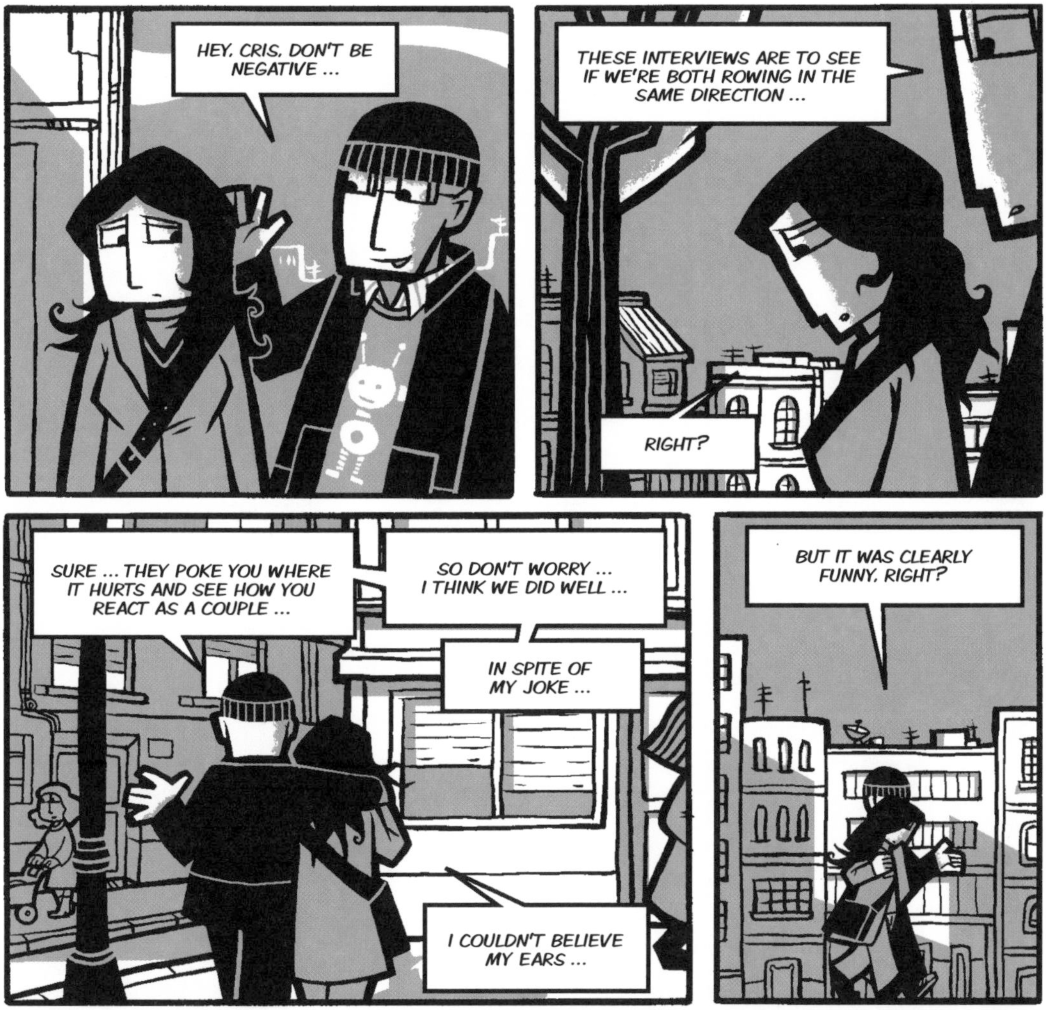
HEY, CRIS, DON'T BE NEGATIVE ...
THESE INTERVIEWS ARE TO SEE IF WE'RE BOTH ROWING IN THE SAME DIRECTION ...
RIGHT?
SURE ... THEY POKE YOU WHERE IT HURTS AND SEE HOW YOU REACT AS A COUPLE ...
SO DON'T WORRY ... I THINK WE DID WELL ...
IN SPITE OF MY JOKE ...
I COULDN'T BELIEVE MY EARS ...
BUT IT WAS CLEARLY FUNNY, RIGHT?

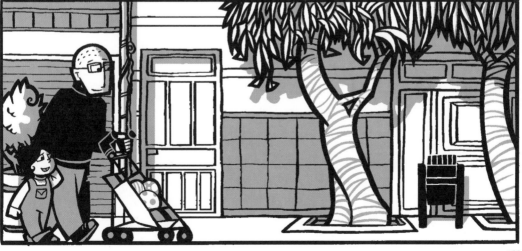

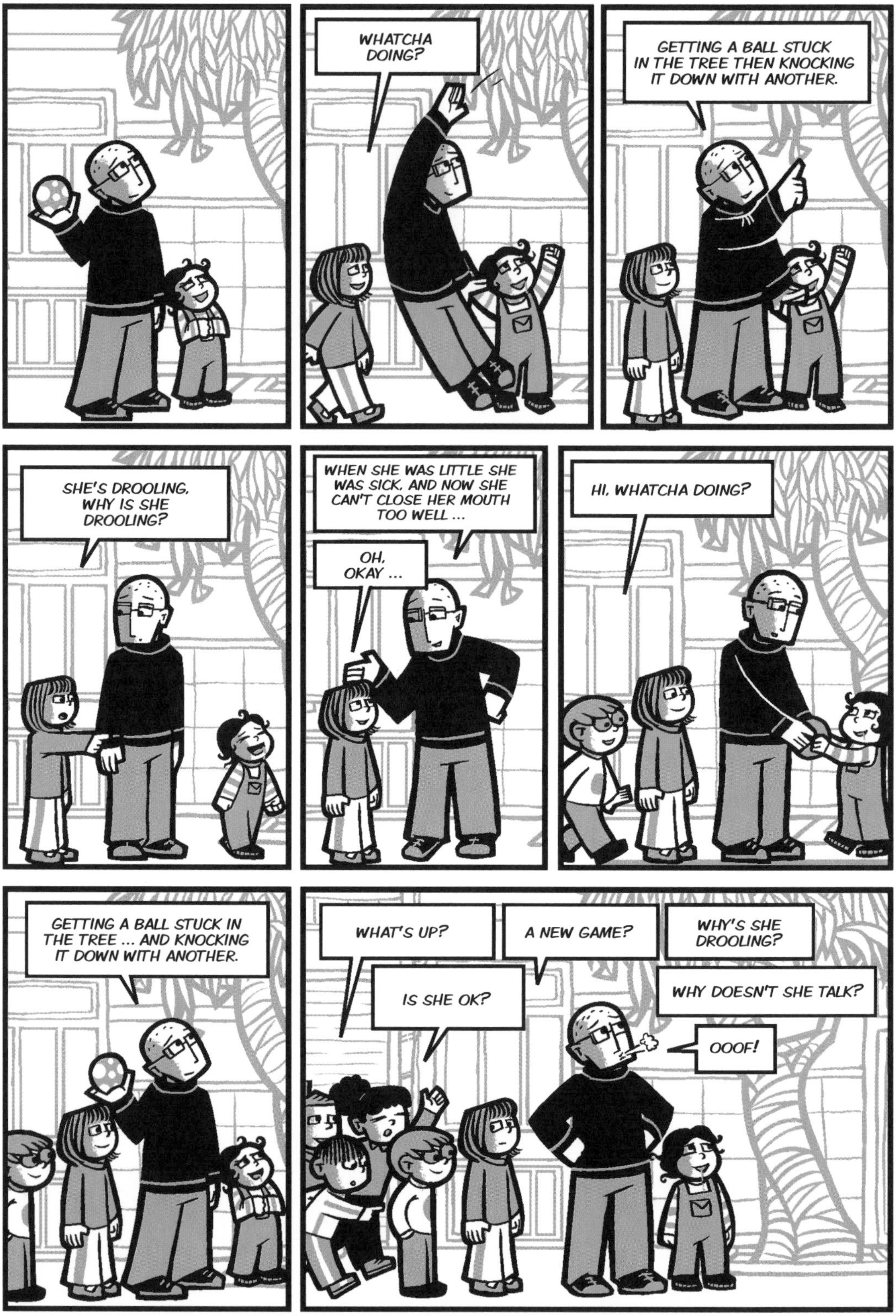
WHATCHA DOING?
GETTING A BALL STUCK IN THE TREE THEN KNOCKING IT DOWN WITH ANOTHER.
SHE'S DROOLING, WHY IS SHE DROOLING?
WHEN SHE WAS LITTLE SHE WAS SICK, AND NOW SHE CAN'T CLOSE HER MOUTH TOO WELL ...
OH, OKAY ...
HI, WHATCHA DOING?
GETTING A BALL STUCK IN THE TREE ... AND KNOCKING IT DOWN WITH ANOTHER.
WHAT'S UP?
IS SHE OK?
A NEW GAME?
WHY'S SHE DROOLING?
WHY DOESN'T SHE TALK?
OOOF!

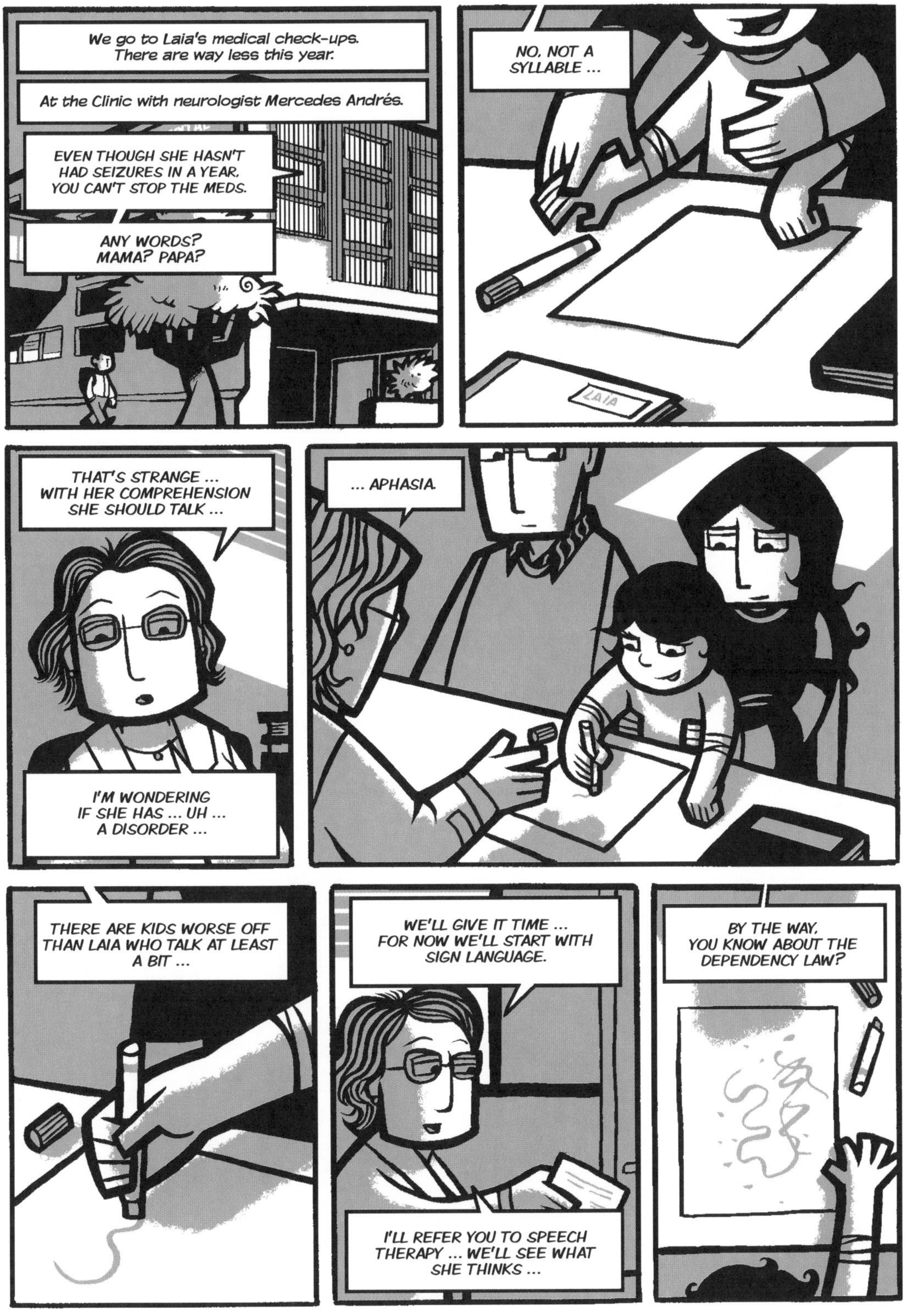
We go to Laia's medical check-ups. There are way less this year.
At the Clinic with neurologist Mercedes Andrés.
EVEN THOUGH SHE HASN'T HAD SEIZURES IN A YEAR, YOU CAN'T STOP THE MEDS.
ANY WORDS? MAMA? PAPA?
NO, NOT A SYLLABLE ...
LAIA
THAT'S STRANGE ... WITH HER COMPREHENSION SHE SHOULD TALK ...
I'M WONDERING IF SHE HAS ... UH ... A DISORDER ...
... APHASIA.
THERE ARE KIDS WORSE OFF THAN LAIA WHO TALK AT LEAST A BIT ...
WE'LL GIVE IT TIME ... FOR NOW WE'LL START WITH SIGN LANGUAGE.
I'LL REFER YOU TO SPEECH THERAPY ... WE'LL SEE WHAT SHE THINKS ...
BY THE WAY, YOU KNOW ABOUT THE DEPENDENCY LAW?

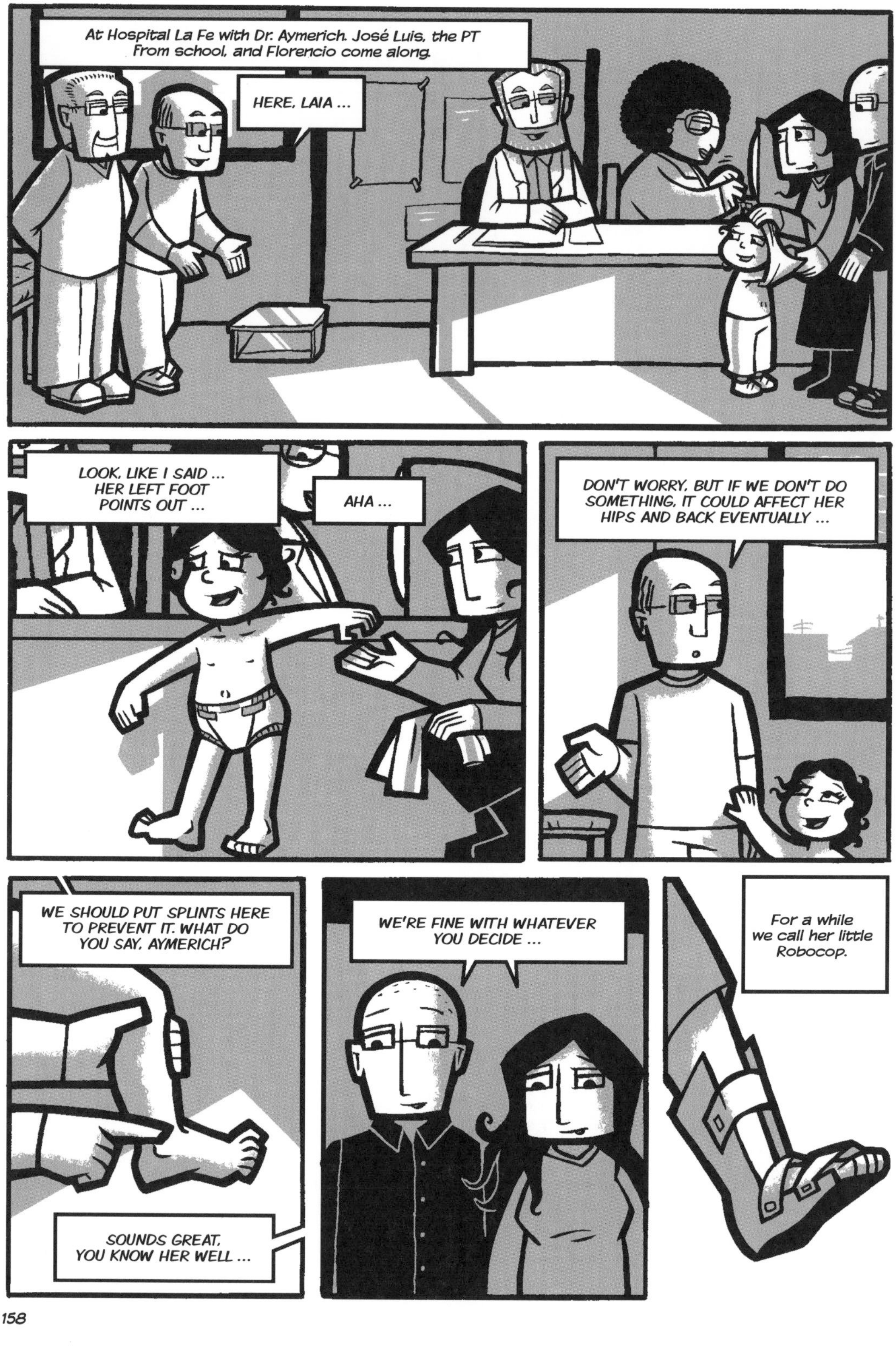
At Hospital La Fe with Dr. Aymerich. José Luis, the PT from school, and Florencio come along.
HERE, LAIA ...
LOOK, LIKE I SAID ... HER LEFT FOOT POINTS OUT ...
AHA ...
DON'T WORRY, BUT IF WE DON'T DO SOMETHING, IT COULD AFFECT HER HIPS AND BACK EVENTUALLY ...
WE SHOULD PUT SPLINTS HERE TO PREVENT IT. WHAT DO YOU SAY, AYMERICH?
SOUNDS GREAT, YOU KNOW HER WELL ...
WE'RE FINE WITH WHATEVER YOU DECIDE ...
For a while we call her little Robocop.

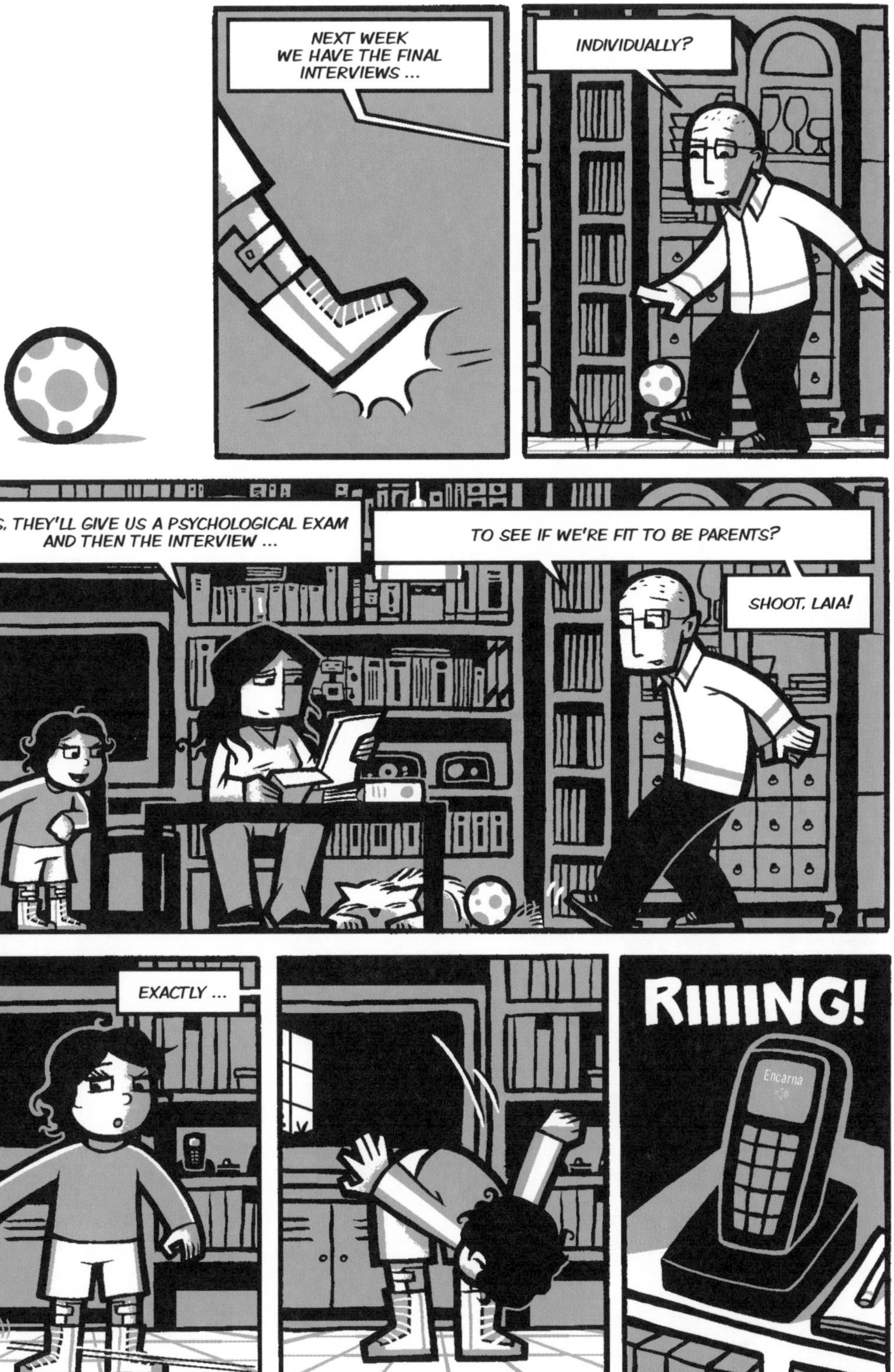
NEXT WEEK WE HAVE THE FINAL INTERVIEWS ...
INDIVIDUALLY?
YES, THEY'LL GIVE US A PSYCHOLOGICAL EXAM AND THEN THE INTERVIEW ...
TO SEE IF WE'RE FIT TO BE PARENTS?
SHOOT, LAIA!
EXACTLY ...
RIIIING!
Encarna

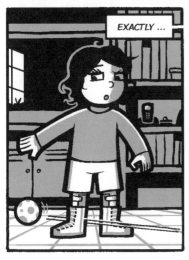

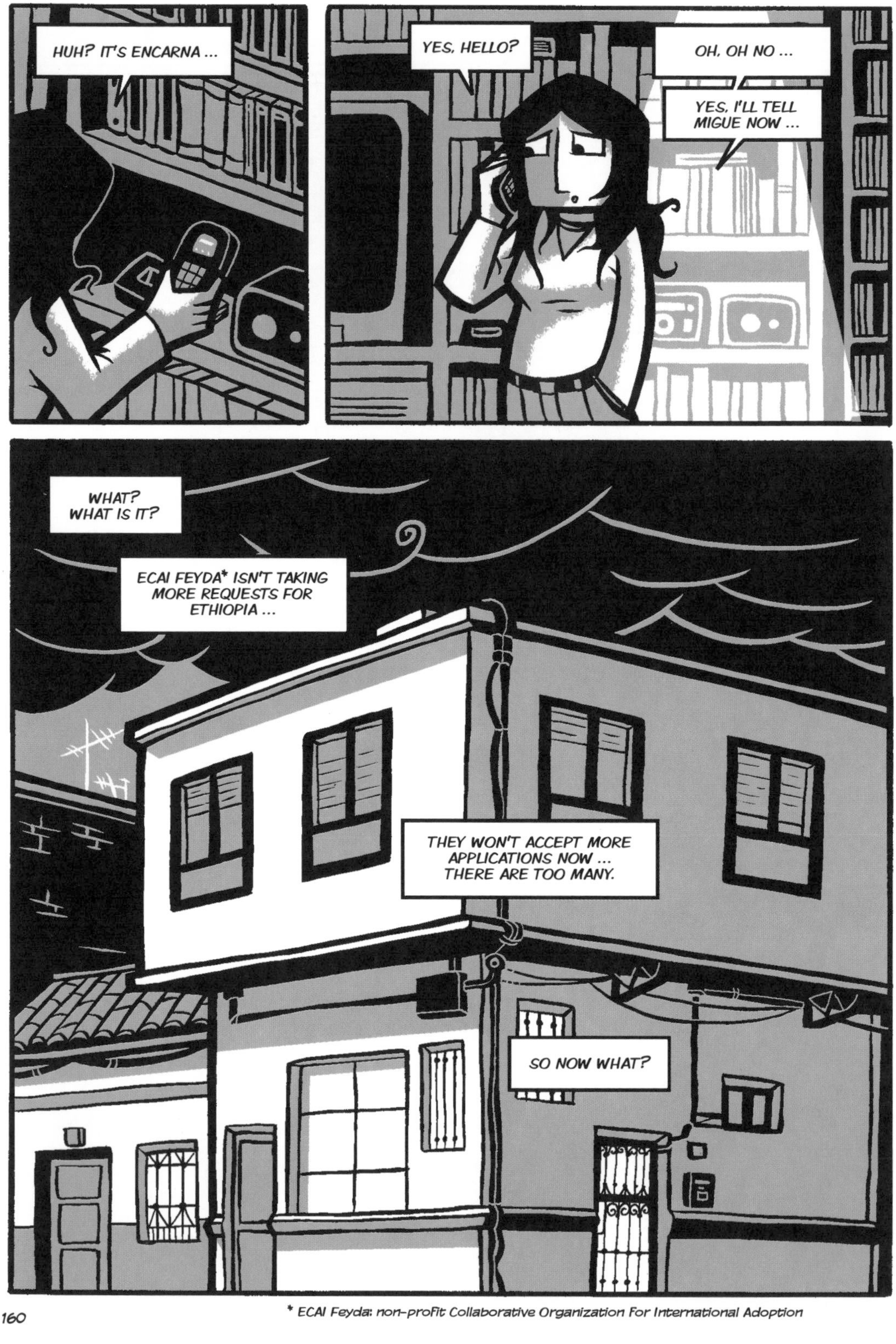
HUH? IT'S ENCARNA ...
YES, HELLO?
OH, OH NO ...
YES, I'LL TELL MIGUE NOW ...
WHAT? WHAT IS IT?
ECAI FEYDA* ISN'T TAKING MORE REQUESTS FOR ETHIOPIA ...
THEY WON'T ACCEPT MORE APPLICATIONS NOW ... THERE ARE TOO MANY.
SO NOW WHAT?

* ECAI Feyda: non-profit Collaborative Organization For International Adoption

Chapter 3
SUITABILITY

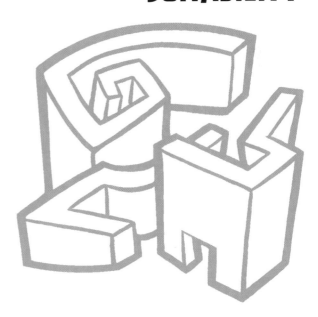

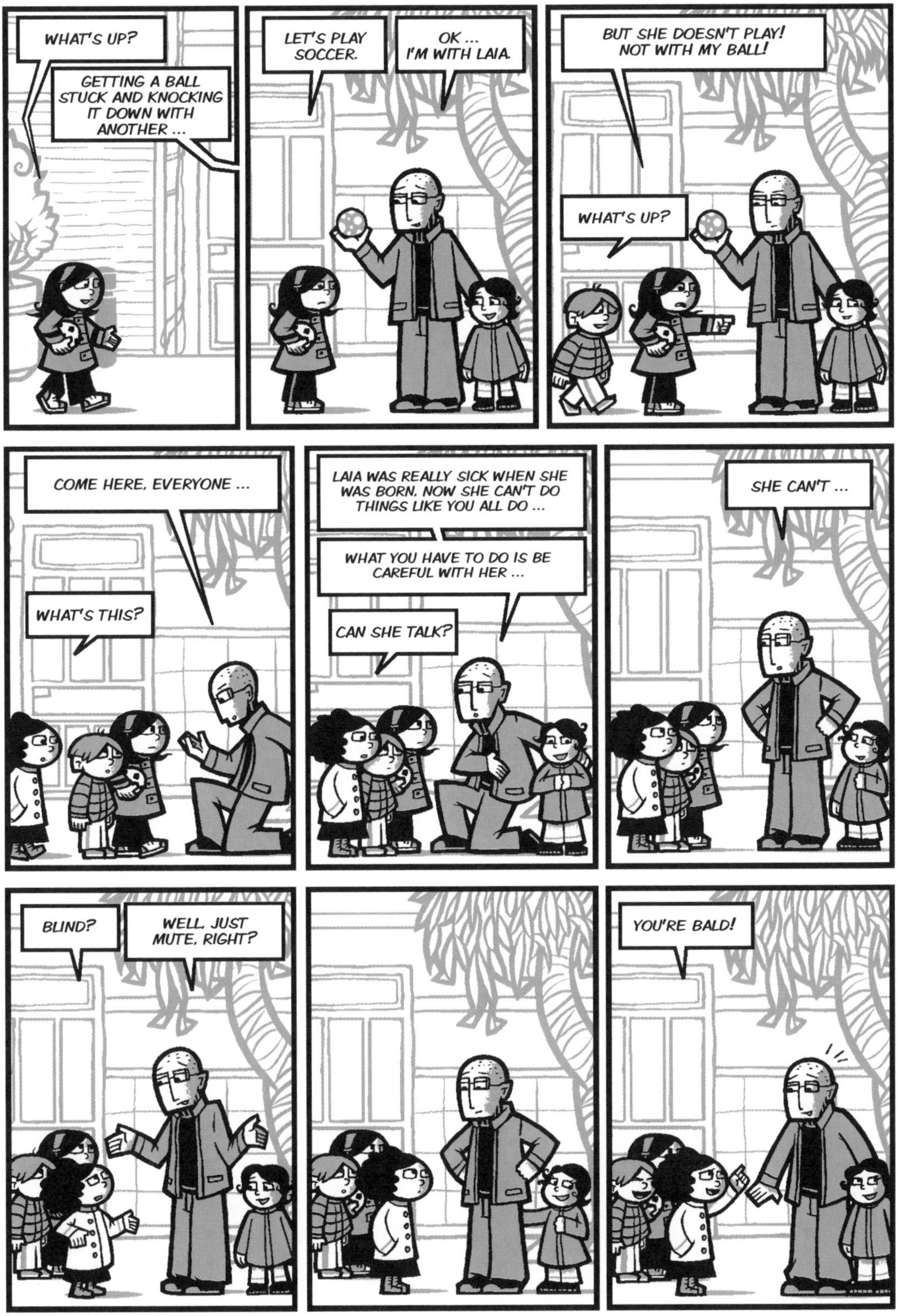
WHAT'S UP?
GETTING A BALL STUCK AND KNOCKING IT DOWN WITH ANOTHER ...
LET'S PLAY SOCCER.
OK ... I'M WITH LAIA.
BUT SHE DOESN'T PLAY! NOT WITH MY BALL!
WHAT'S UP?
COME HERE, EVERYONE ...
WHAT'S THIS?
LAIA WAS REALLY SICK WHEN SHE WAS BORN, NOW SHE CAN'T DO THINGS LIKE YOU ALL DO ...
WHAT YOU HAVE TO DO IS BE CAREFUL WITH HER ...
CAN SHE TALK?
SHE CAN'T ...
BLIND?
WELL, JUST MUTE, RIGHT?
YOU'RE BALD!

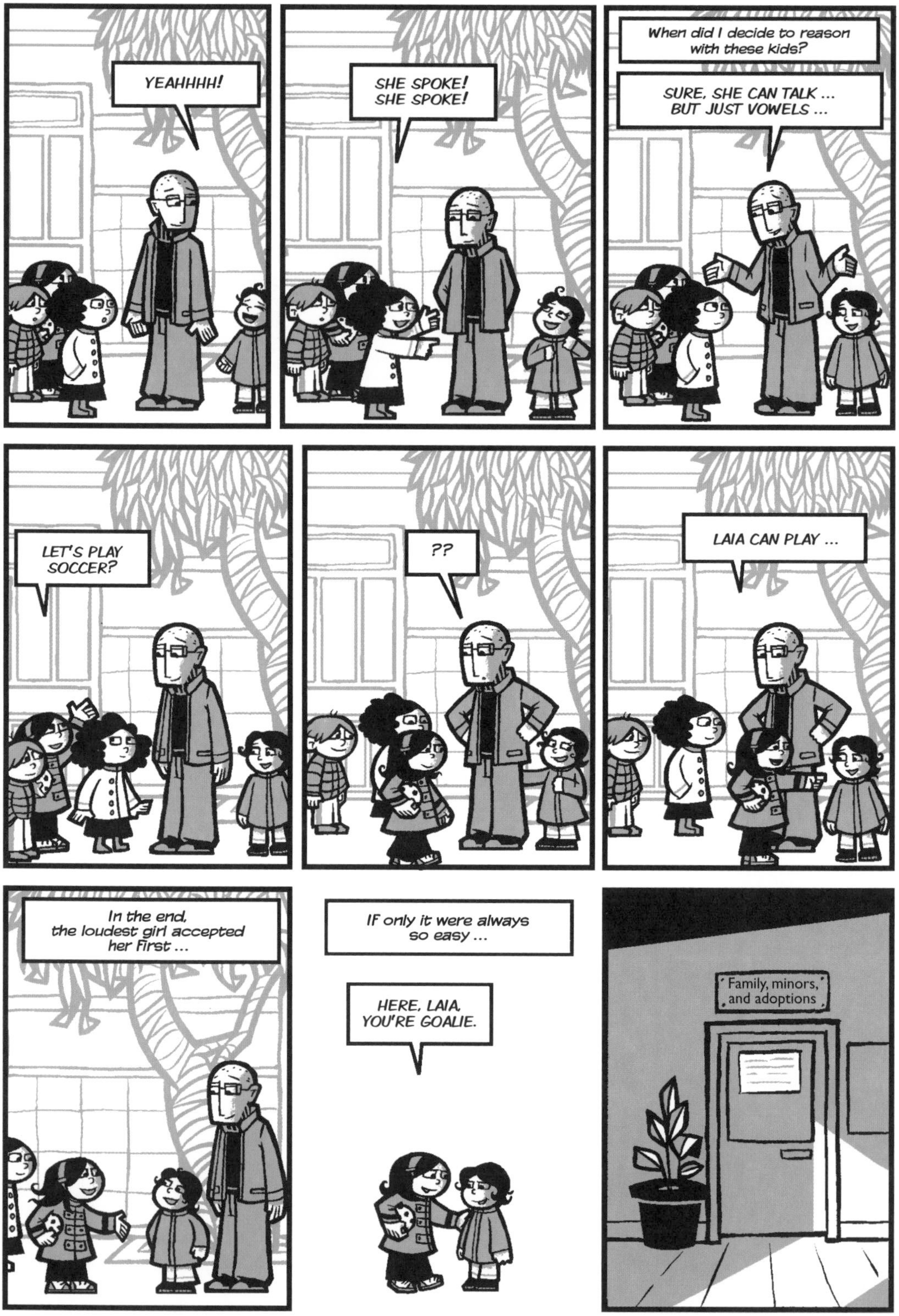
YEAHHHH!
SHE SPOKE! SHE SPOKE!
When did I decide to reason with these kids?
SURE, SHE CAN TALK ... BUT JUST VOWELS ...
LET'S PLAY SOCCER?
??
LAIA CAN PLAY ...
In the end, the loudest girl accepted her first ...
IF only it were always so easy ...
HERE, LAIA. YOU'RE GOALIE.
Family, minors, and adoptions

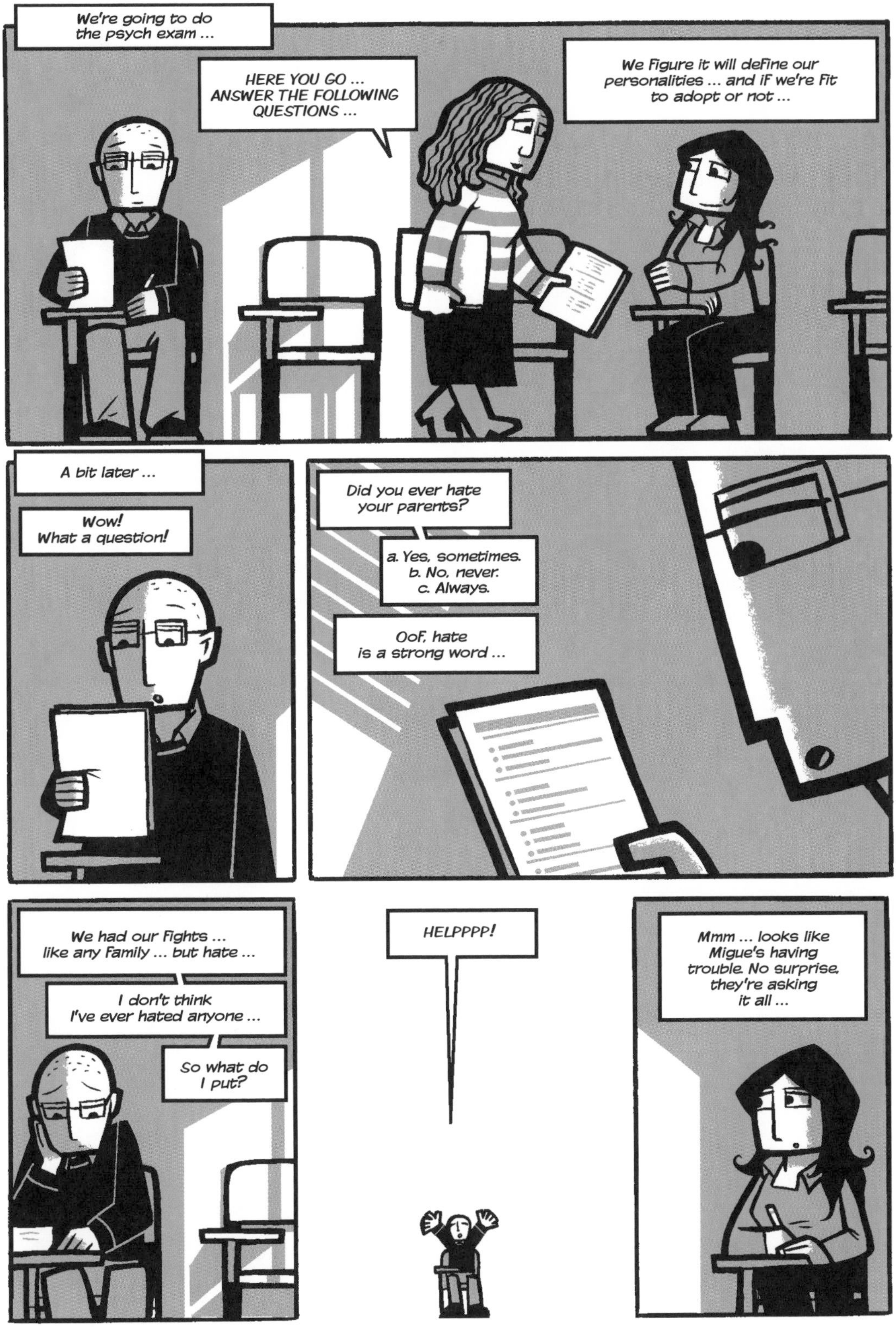
We're going to do the psych exam ...
HERE YOU GO ... ANSWER THE FOLLOWING QUESTIONS ...
We figure it will define our personalities ... and if we're fit to adopt or not ...
A bit later ...
Wow! What a question!
Did you ever hate your parents?
a. Yes, sometimes. b. No, never. c. Always.
Oof, hate is a strong word ...
We had our fights ... like any family ... but hate ...
I don't think I've ever hated anyone ...
So what do I put?
HELPPPP!
Mmm ... looks like Migue's having trouble. No surprise, they're asking it all ...

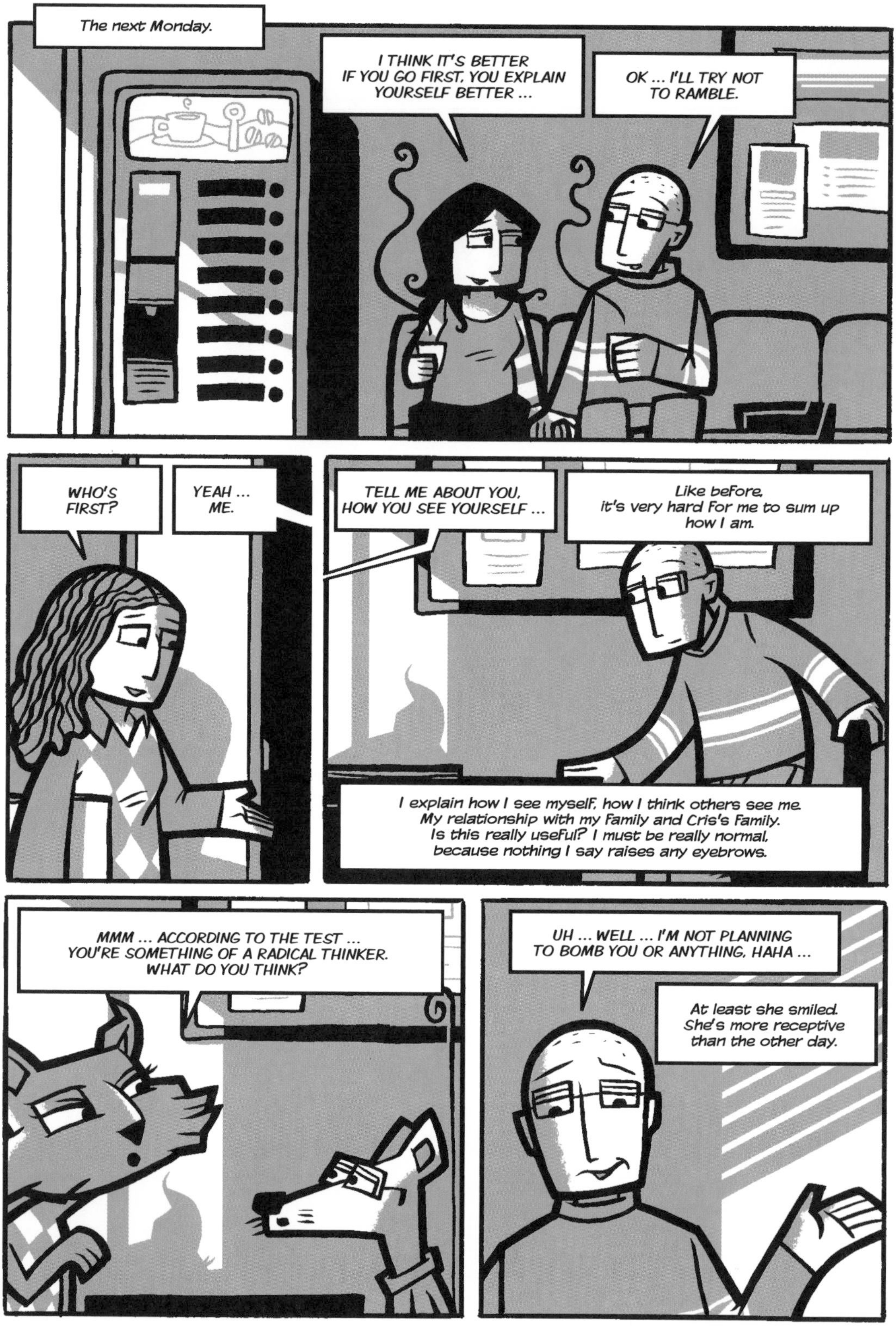
The next Monday.
I THINK IT'S BETTER IF YOU GO FIRST. YOU EXPLAIN YOURSELF BETTER ...
OK ... I'LL TRY NOT TO RAMBLE.
WHO'S FIRST?
YEAH ... ME.
TELL ME ABOUT YOU, HOW YOU SEE YOURSELF ...
Like before, it's very hard for me to sum up how I am.
I explain how I see myself, how I think others see me. My relationship with my family and Cris's family. Is this really useful? I must be really normal, because nothing I say raises any eyebrows.
MMM ... ACCORDING TO THE TEST ... YOU'RE SOMETHING OF A RADICAL THINKER. WHAT DO YOU THINK?
UH ... WELL ... I'M NOT PLANNING TO BOMB YOU OR ANYTHING, HAHA ...
At least she smiled. She's more receptive than the other day.

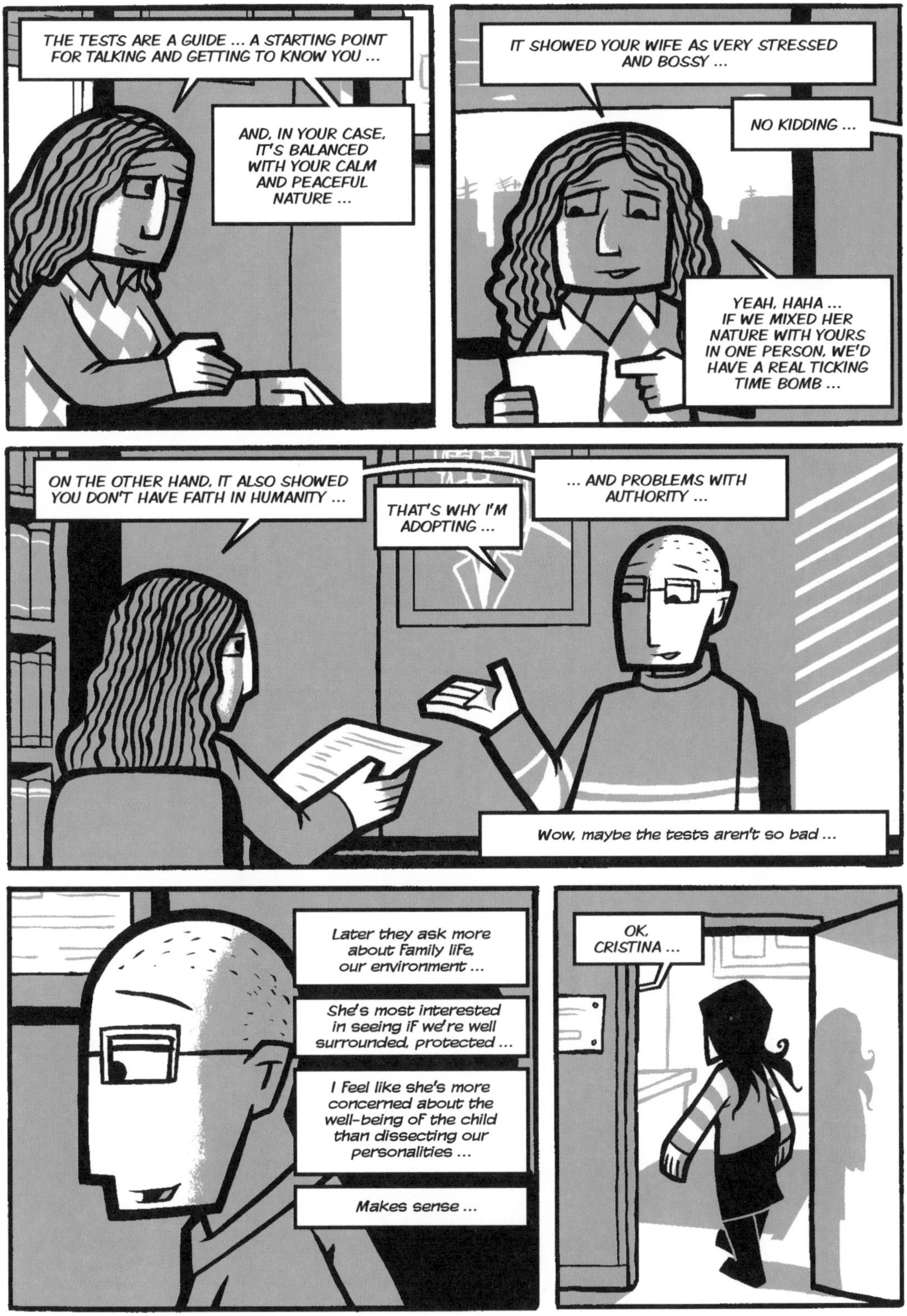
THE TESTS ARE A GUIDE ... A STARTING POINT FOR TALKING AND GETTING TO KNOW YOU ...
AND, IN YOUR CASE, IT'S BALANCED WITH YOUR CALM AND PEACEFUL NATURE ...
IT SHOWED YOUR WIFE AS VERY STRESSED AND BOSSY ...
NO KIDDING ...
YEAH, HAHA ... IF WE MIXED HER NATURE WITH YOURS IN ONE PERSON, WE'D HAVE A REAL TICKING TIME BOMB ...
ON THE OTHER HAND, IT ALSO SHOWED YOU DON'T HAVE FAITH IN HUMANITY ...
THAT'S WHY I'M ADOPTING ...
... AND PROBLEMS WITH AUTHORITY ...
Wow, maybe the tests aren't so bad ...
Later they ask more about family life, our environment ...
She's most interested in seeing if we're well surrounded, protected ...
I feel like she's more concerned about the well-being of the child than dissecting our personalities ...
Makes sense ...
OK, CRISTINA ...

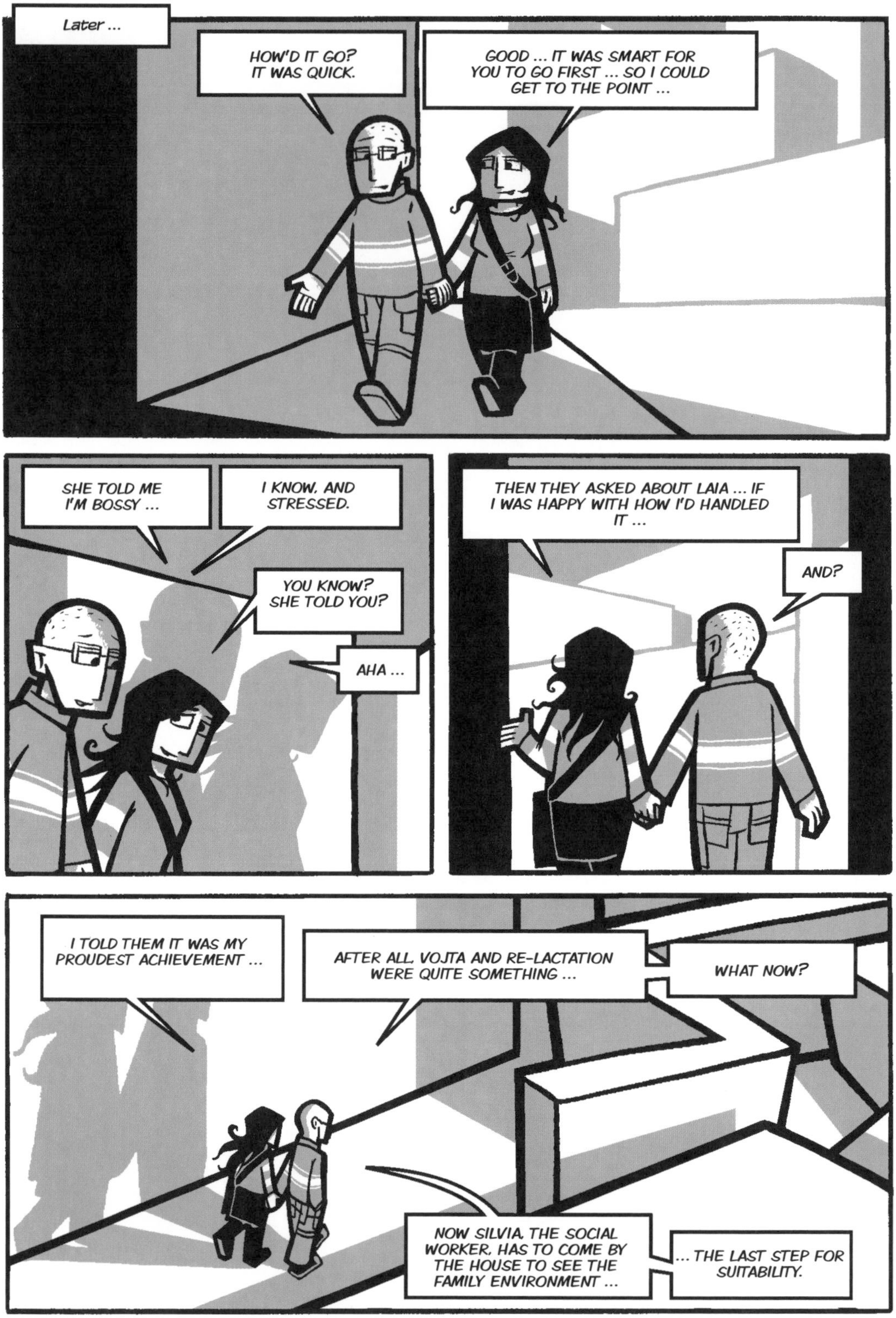
Later ...
HOW'D IT GO? IT WAS QUICK.
GOOD ... IT WAS SMART FOR YOU TO GO FIRST ... SO I COULD GET TO THE POINT ...
SHE TOLD ME I'M BOSSY ...
I KNOW, AND STRESSED.
YOU KNOW? SHE TOLD YOU?
AHA ...
THEN THEY ASKED ABOUT LAIA ... IF I WAS HAPPY WITH HOW I'D HANDLED IT ...
AND?
I TOLD THEM IT WAS MY PROUDEST ACHIEVEMENT ...
AFTER ALL, VOJTA AND RE-LACTATION WERE QUITE SOMETHING ...
WHAT NOW?
NOW SILVIA, THE SOCIAL WORKER, HAS TO COME BY THE HOUSE TO SEE THE FAMILY ENVIRONMENT ...
... THE LAST STEP FOR SUITABILITY.

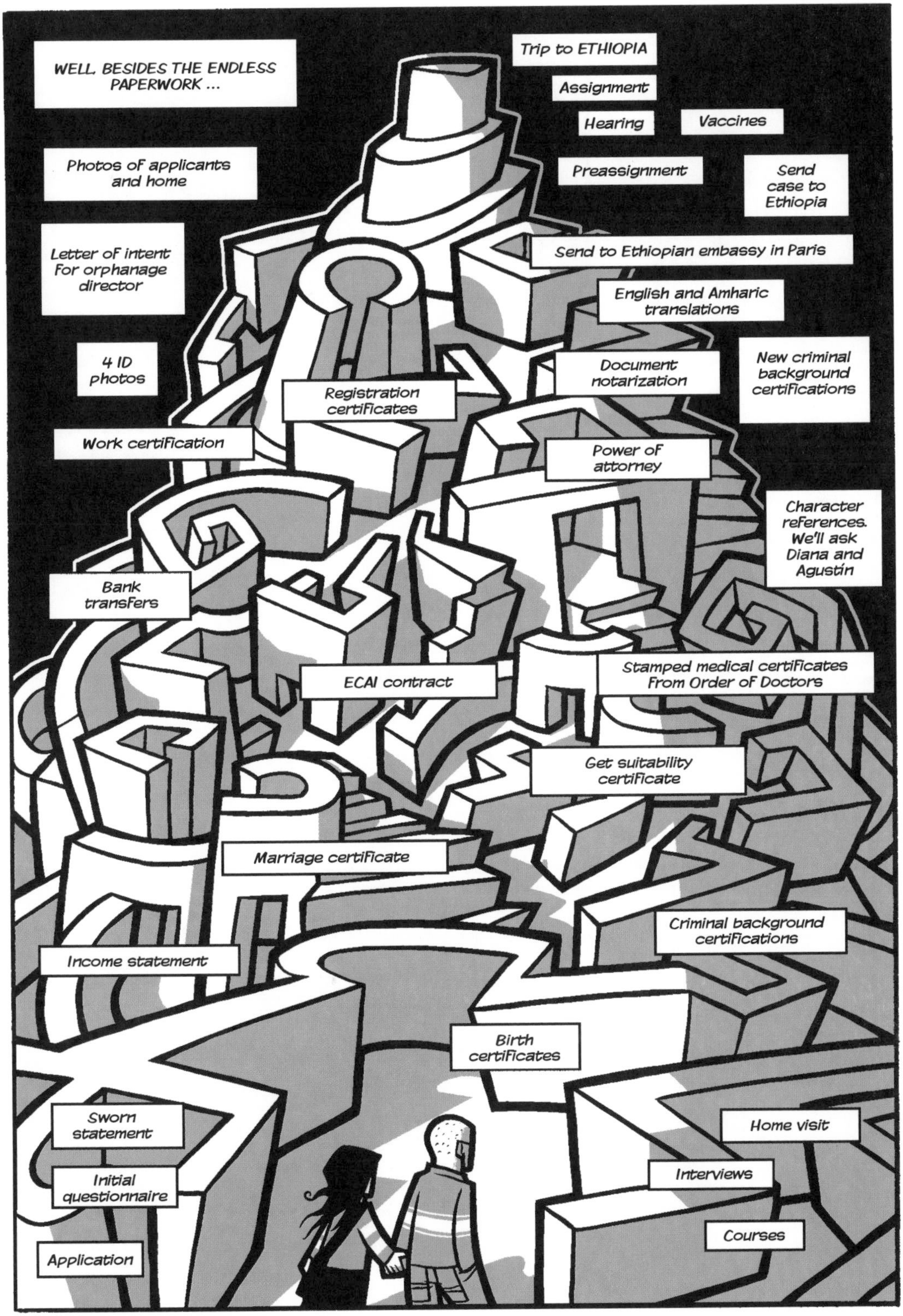
WELL, BESIDES THE ENDLESS PAPERWORK ...
Trip to ETHIOPIA
Assignment
Hearing
Vaccines
Photos of applicants and home
Preassignment
Send case to Ethiopia
Letter of intent for orphanage director
Send to Ethiopian embassy in Paris
English and Amharic translations
4 ID photos
Registration certificates
Document notarization
New criminal background certifications
Work certification
Power of attorney
Character references. We'll ask Diana and Agustín
Bank transfers
ECAI contract
Stamped medical certificates from Order of Doctors
Get suitability certificate
Marriage certificate
Criminal background certifications
Income statement
Birth certificates
Sworn statement
Home visit
Initial questionnaire
Interviews
Courses
Application

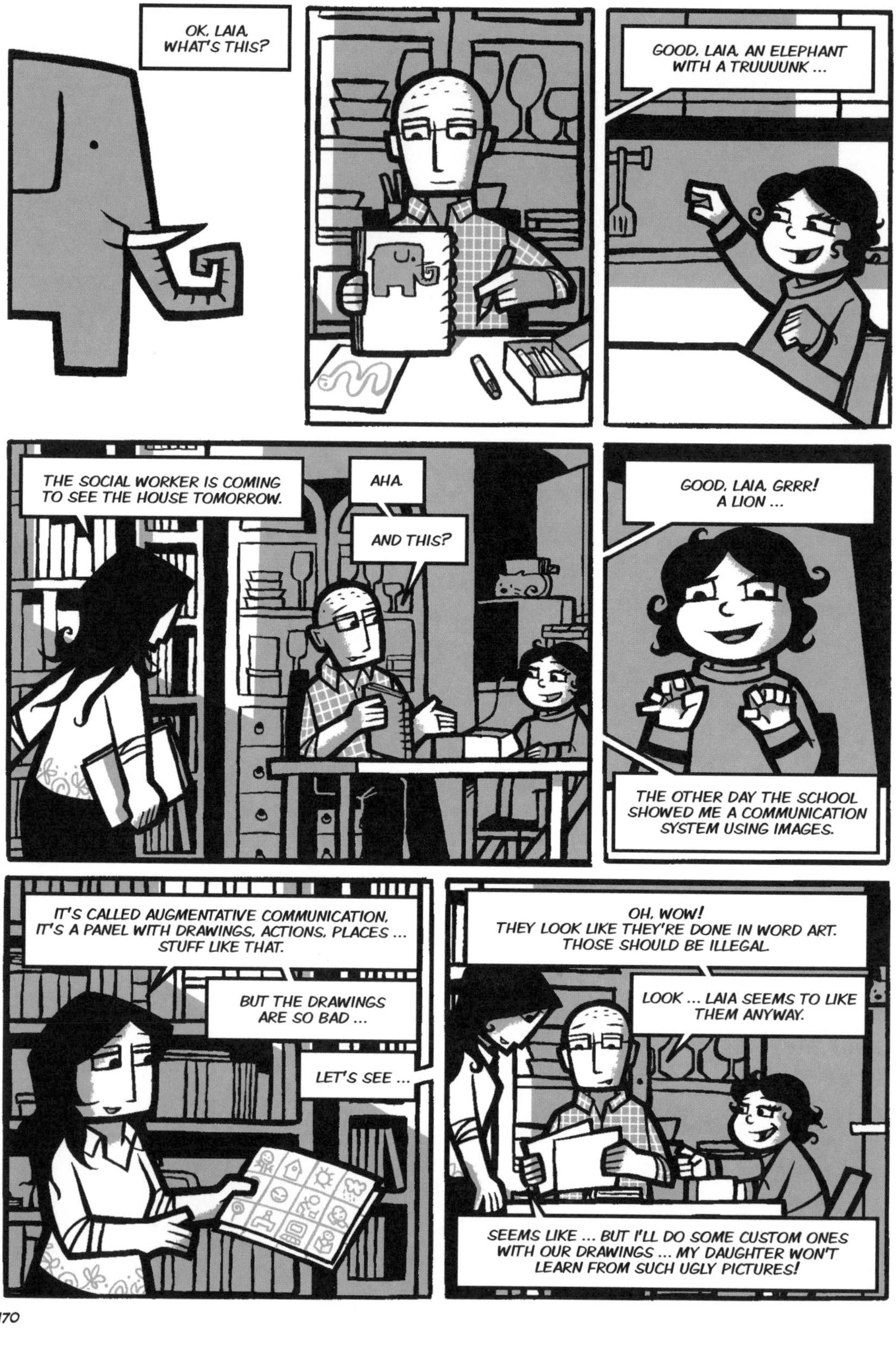
OK, LAIA, WHAT'S THIS?
GOOD, LAIA, AN ELEPHANT WITH A TRUUUUNK ...
THE SOCIAL WORKER IS COMING TO SEE THE HOUSE TOMORROW.
AHA.
AND THIS?
GOOD, LAIA, GRRR! A LION ...
THE OTHER DAY THE SCHOOL SHOWED ME A COMMUNICATION SYSTEM USING IMAGES.
IT'S CALLED AUGMENTATIVE COMMUNICATION. IT'S A PANEL WITH DRAWINGS, ACTIONS, PLACES ... STUFF LIKE THAT.
BUT THE DRAWINGS ARE SO BAD ...
LET'S SEE ...
OH, WOW! THEY LOOK LIKE THEY'RE DONE IN WORD ART. THOSE SHOULD BE ILLEGAL.
LOOK ... LAIA SEEMS TO LIKE THEM ANYWAY.
SEEMS LIKE ... BUT I'LL DO SOME CUSTOM ONES WITH OUR DRAWINGS ... MY DAUGHTER WON'T LEARN FROM SUCH UGLY PICTURES!

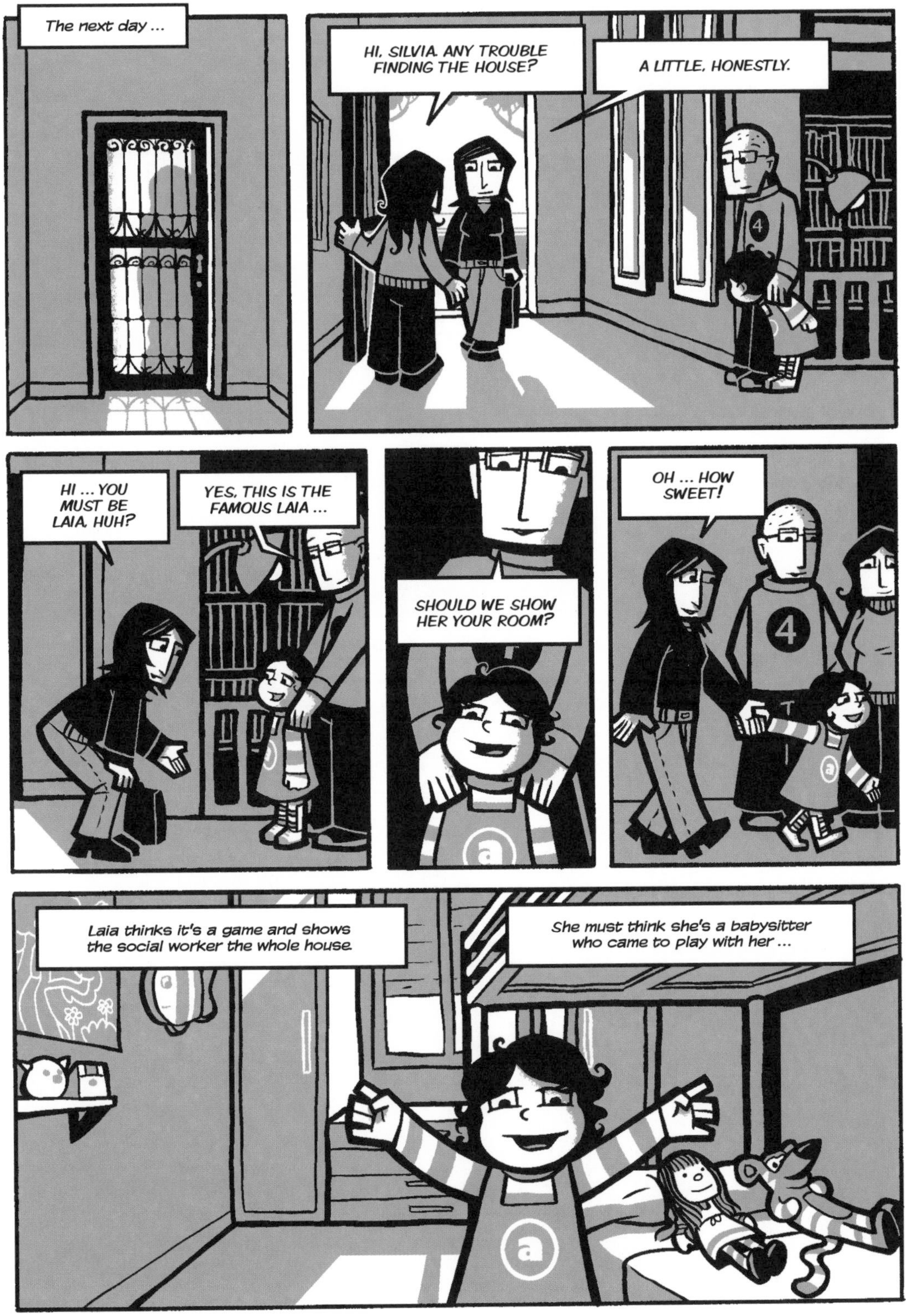
The next day ...
HI, SILVIA. ANY TROUBLE FINDING THE HOUSE?
A LITTLE, HONESTLY.
HI ... YOU MUST BE LAIA, HUH?
YES, THIS IS THE FAMOUS LAIA ...
SHOULD WE SHOW HER YOUR ROOM?
OH ... HOW SWEET!
Laia thinks it's a game and shows the social worker the whole house.
She must think she's a babysitter who came to play with her ...

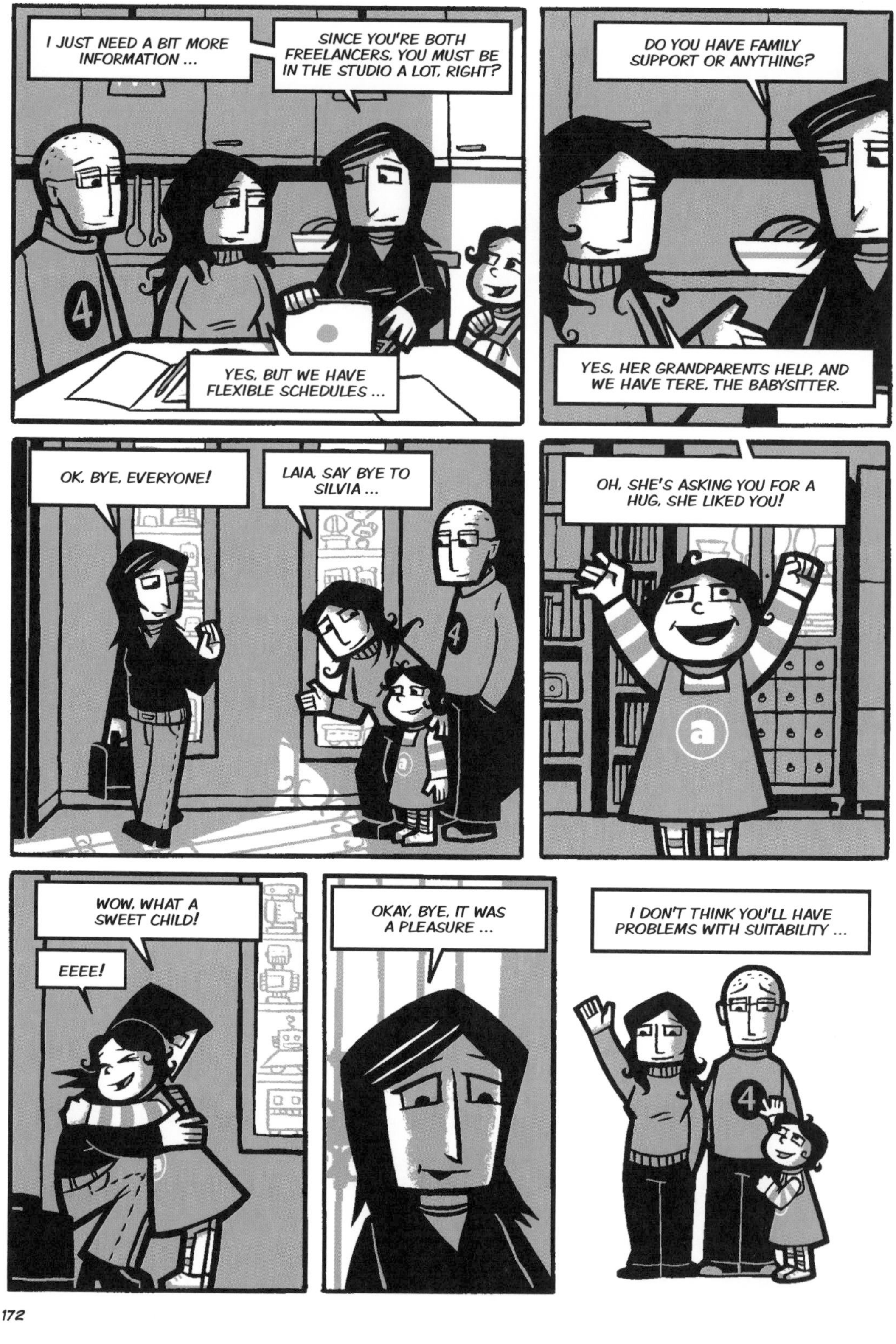
I JUST NEED A BIT MORE INFORMATION ...
SINCE YOU'RE BOTH FREELANCERS, YOU MUST BE IN THE STUDIO A LOT, RIGHT?
YES, BUT WE HAVE FLEXIBLE SCHEDULES ...
DO YOU HAVE FAMILY SUPPORT OR ANYTHING?
YES, HER GRANDPARENTS HELP, AND WE HAVE TERE, THE BABYSITTER.
OK, BYE, EVERYONE!
LAIA, SAY BYE TO SILVIA ...
OH, SHE'S ASKING YOU FOR A HUG, SHE LIKED YOU!
WOW, WHAT A SWEET CHILD!
EEEE!
OKAY, BYE, IT WAS A PLEASURE ...
I DON'T THINK YOU'LL HAVE PROBLEMS WITH SUITABILITY ...

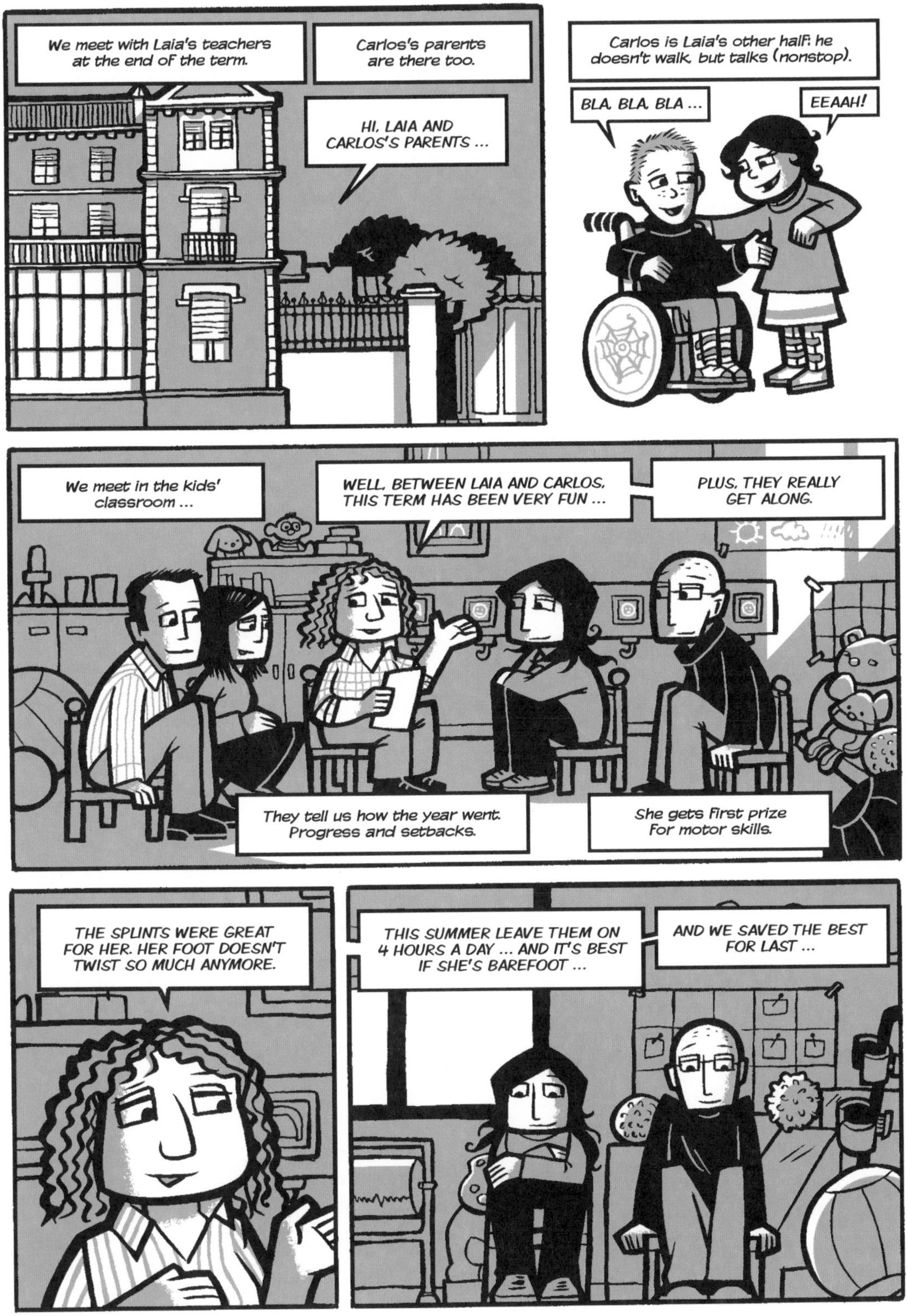
We meet with Laia's teachers at the end of the term.
Carlos's parents are there too.
HI, LAIA AND CARLOS'S PARENTS ...
Carlos is Laia's other half: he doesn't walk, but talks (nonstop).
BLA, BLA, BLA ...
EEAAH!
We meet in the kids' classroom ...
WELL, BETWEEN LAIA AND CARLOS, THIS TERM HAS BEEN VERY FUN ...
PLUS, THEY REALLY GET ALONG.
They tell us how the year went. Progress and setbacks.
She gets first prize for motor skills.
THE SPLINTS WERE GREAT FOR HER. HER FOOT DOESN'T TWIST SO MUCH ANYMORE.
THIS SUMMER LEAVE THEM ON 4 HOURS A DAY ... AND IT'S BEST IF SHE'S BAREFOOT ...
AND WE SAVED THE BEST FOR LAST ...

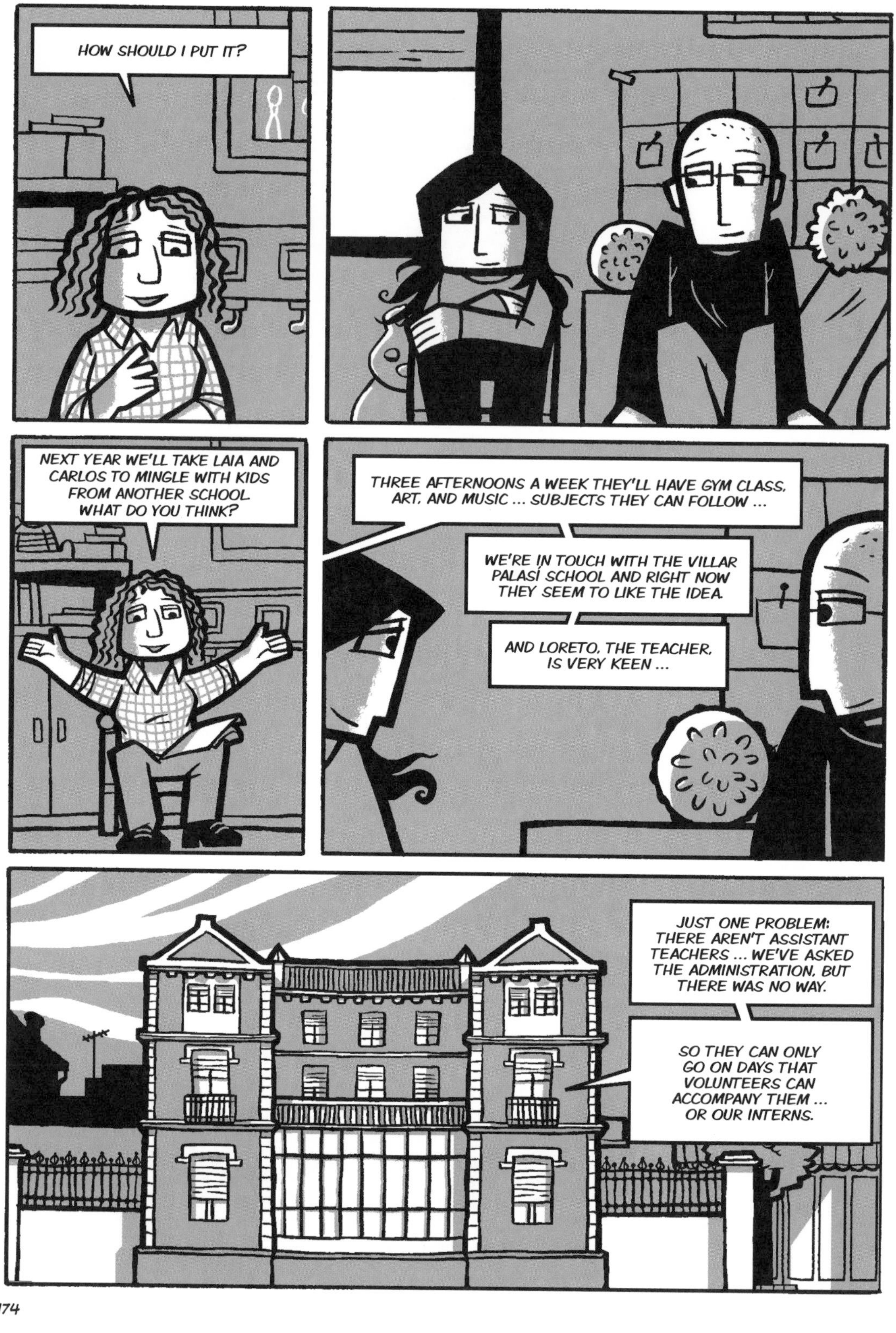
HOW SHOULD I PUT IT?
NEXT YEAR WE'LL TAKE LAIA AND CARLOS TO MINGLE WITH KIDS FROM ANOTHER SCHOOL. WHAT DO YOU THINK?
THREE AFTERNOONS A WEEK THEY'LL HAVE GYM CLASS, ART, AND MUSIC ... SUBJECTS THEY CAN FOLLOW ...
WE'RE IN TOUCH WITH THE VILLAR PALASÍ SCHOOL AND RIGHT NOW THEY SEEM TO LIKE THE IDEA.
AND LORETO, THE TEACHER, IS VERY KEEN ...
JUST ONE PROBLEM: THERE AREN'T ASSISTANT TEACHERS ... WE'VE ASKED THE ADMINISTRATION, BUT THERE WAS NO WAY.
SO THEY CAN ONLY GO ON DAYS THAT VOLUNTEERS CAN ACCOMPANY THEM ... OR OUR INTERNS.

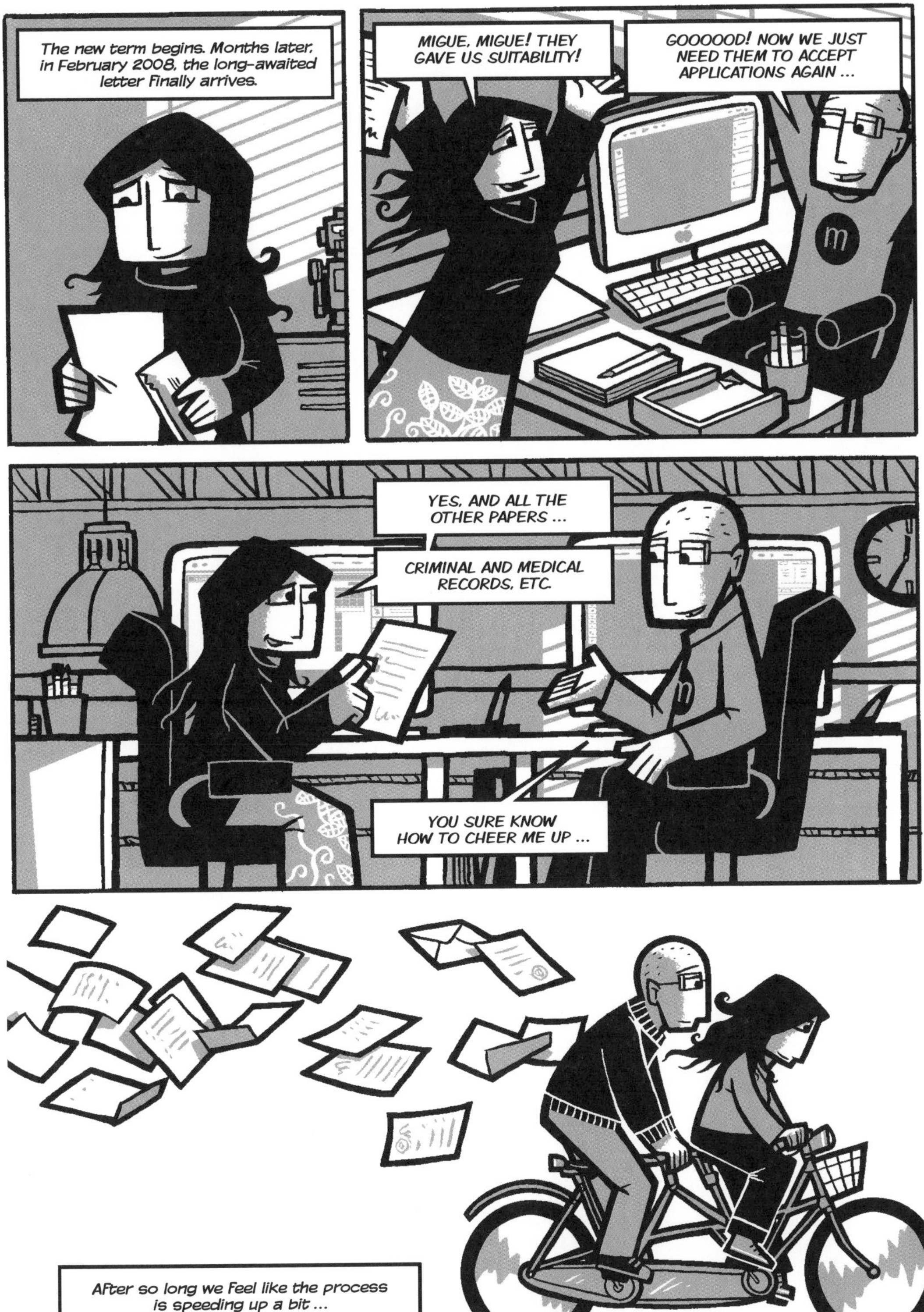
The new term begins. Months later, in February 2008, the long-awaited letter finally arrives.
MIGUE, MIGUE! THEY GAVE US SUITABILITY!
GOOOOOD! NOW WE JUST NEED THEM TO ACCEPT APPLICATIONS AGAIN ...
YES, AND ALL THE OTHER PAPERS ...
CRIMINAL AND MEDICAL RECORDS, ETC.
YOU SURE KNOW HOW TO CHEER ME UP ...
After so long we feel like the process is speeding up a bit ...

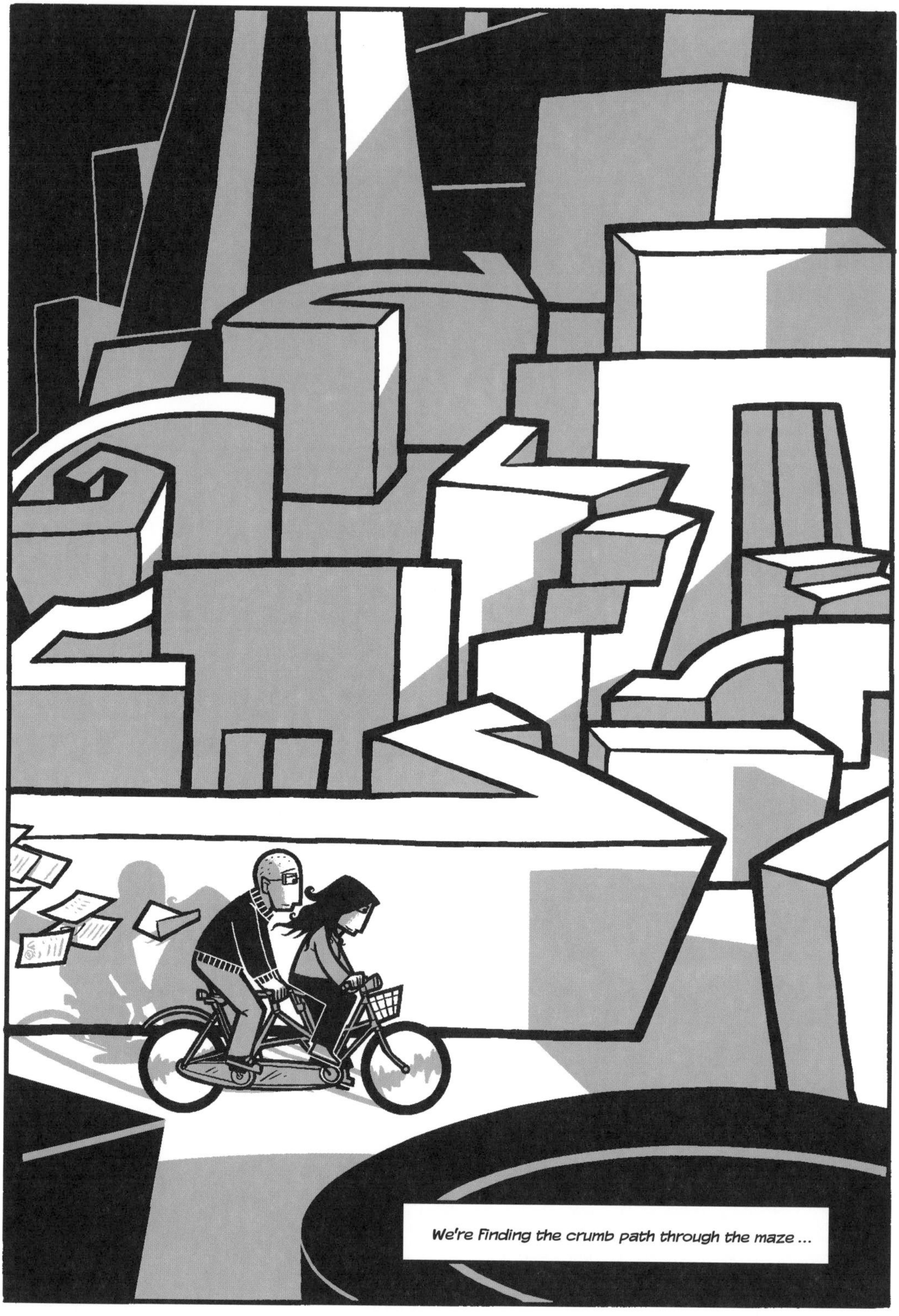
We're finding the crumb path through the maze ...

Chapter 4
THE DISABILITY LAW

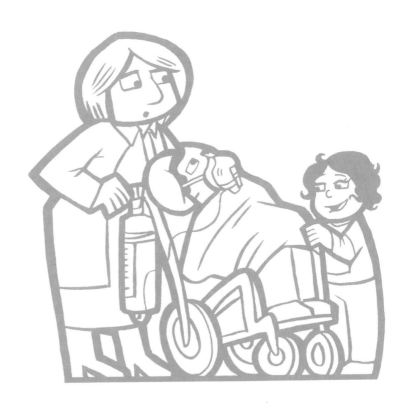

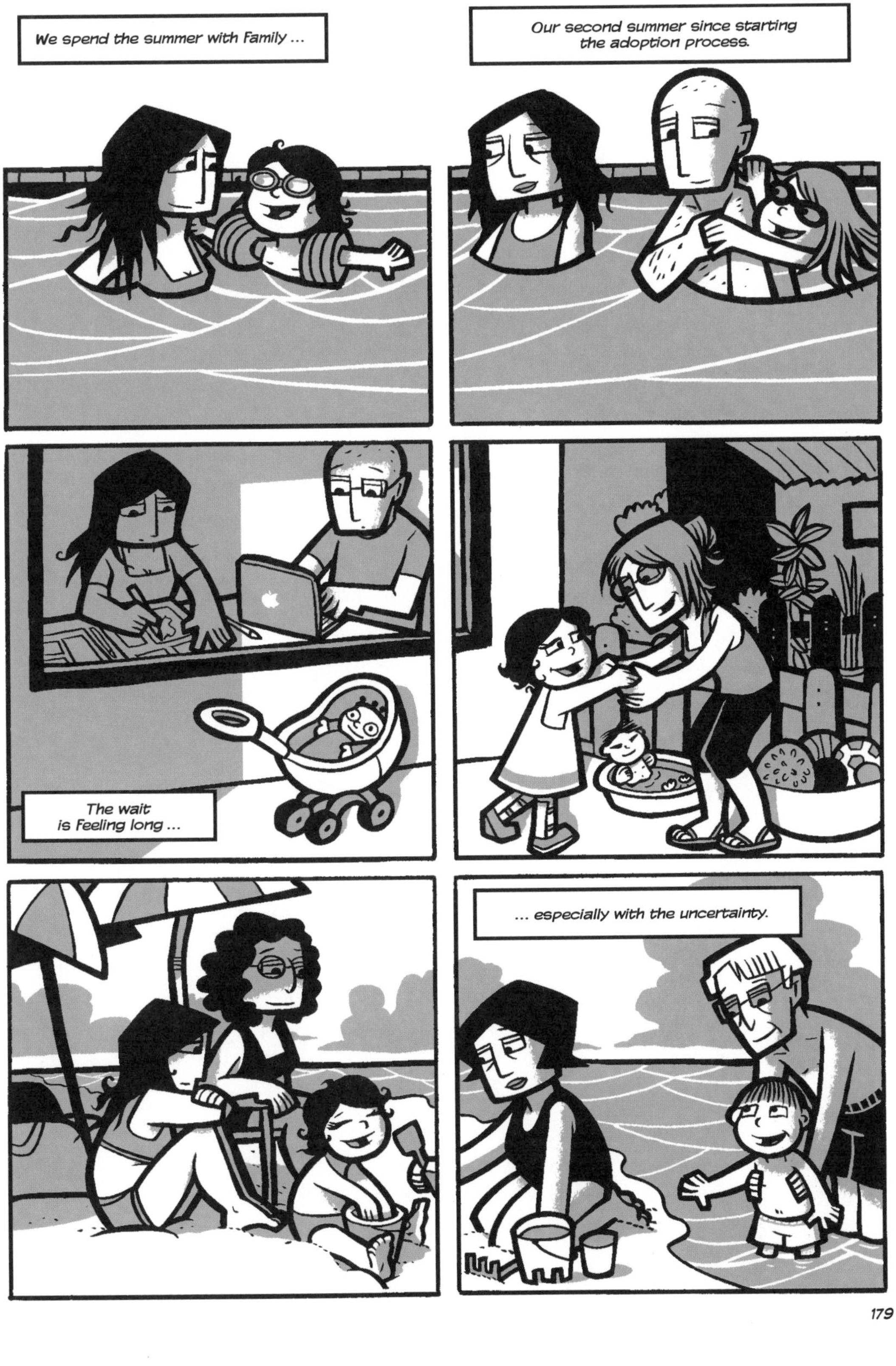
We spend the summer with family ...
Our second summer since starting the adoption process.
The wait is feeling long ...
... especially with the uncertainty.

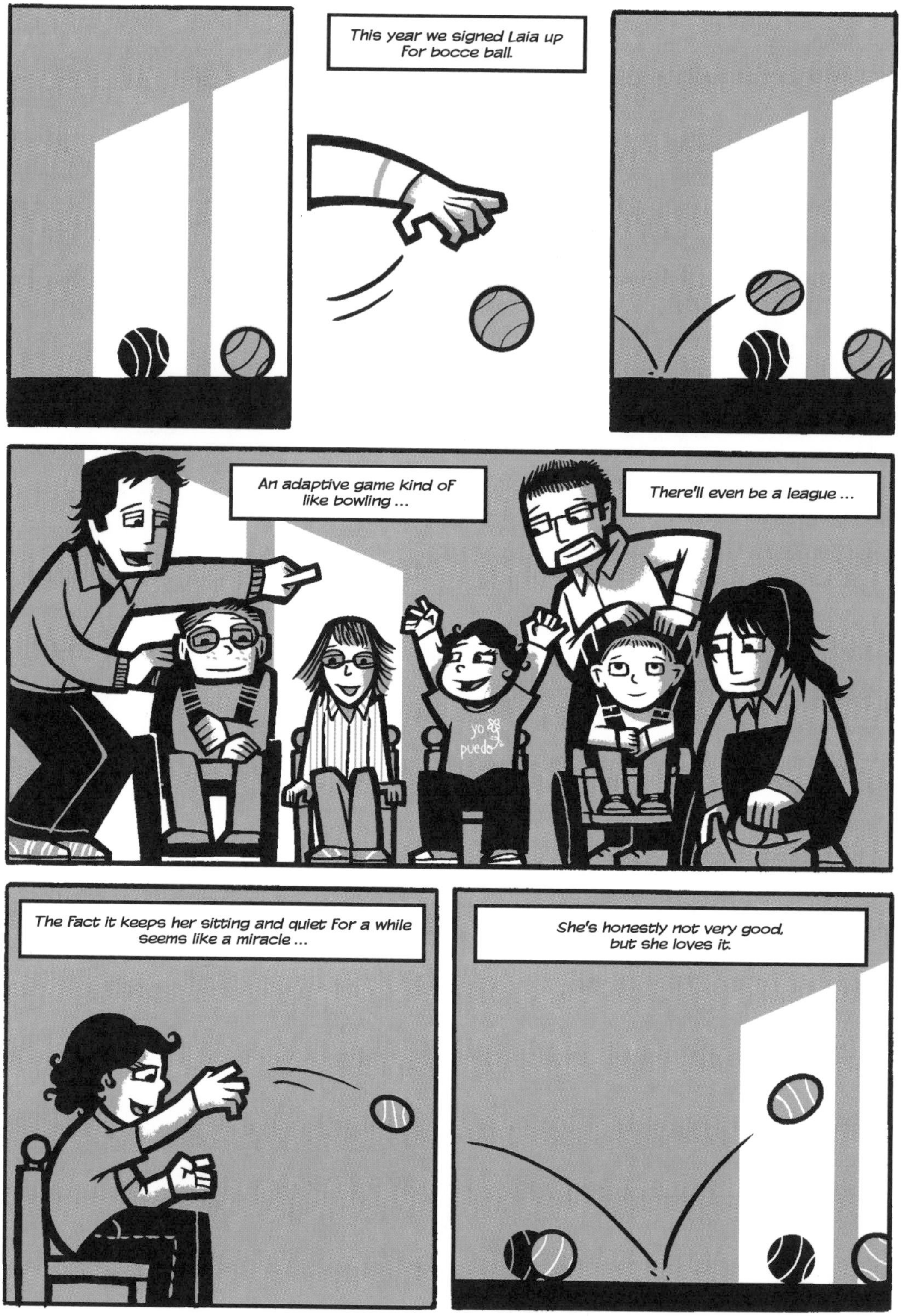
This year we signed Laia up for bocce ball.
An adaptive game kind of like bowling ...
There'll even be a league ...
yo puedo
The fact it keeps her sitting and quiet for a while seems like a miracle ...
She's honestly not very good, but she loves it.

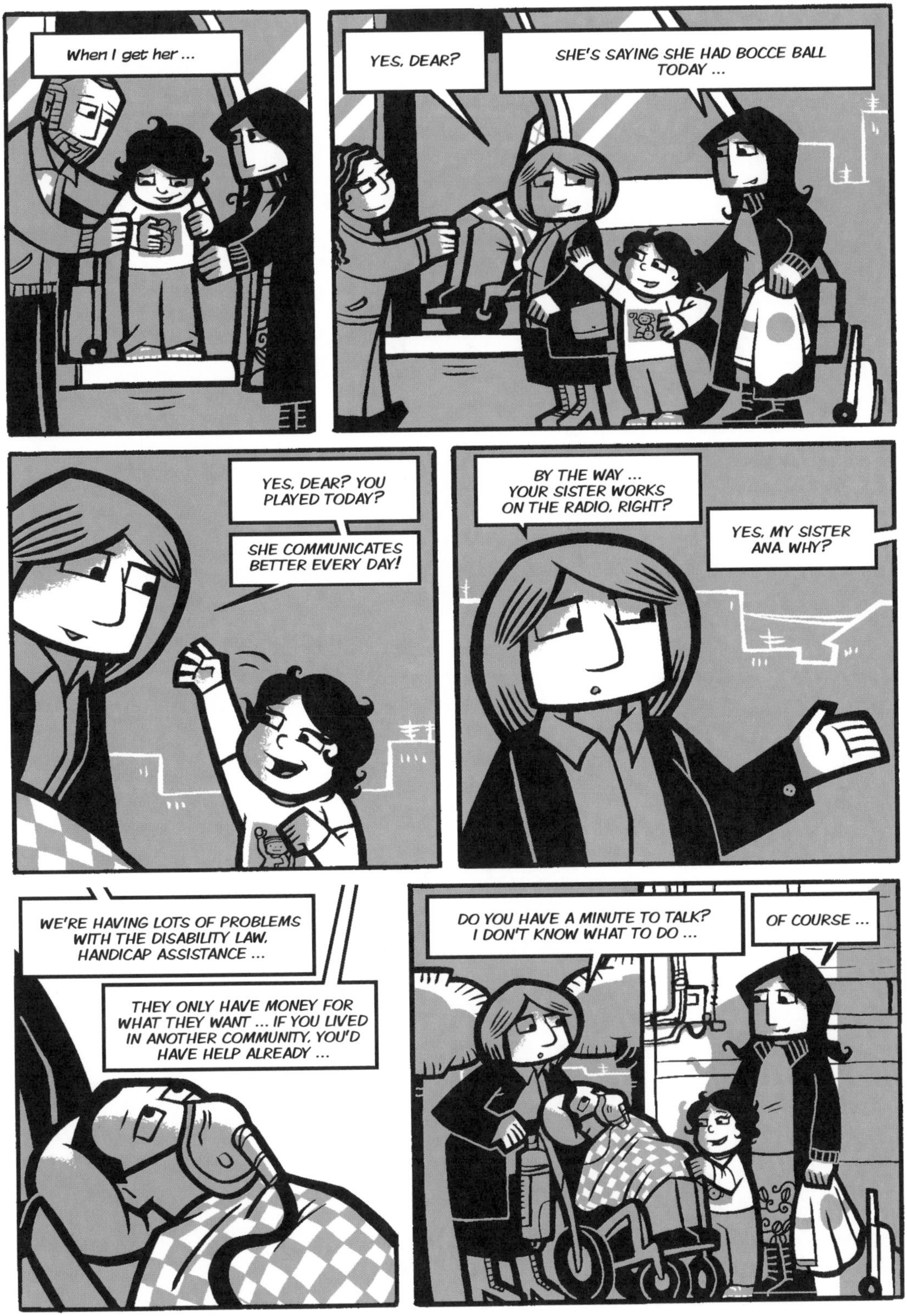
When I get her ...
YES, DEAR?
SHE'S SAYING SHE HAD BOCCE BALL TODAY ...
YES, DEAR? YOU PLAYED TODAY?
SHE COMMUNICATES BETTER EVERY DAY!
BY THE WAY ... YOUR SISTER WORKS ON THE RADIO, RIGHT?
YES, MY SISTER ANA. WHY?
WE'RE HAVING LOTS OF PROBLEMS WITH THE DISABILITY LAW, HANDICAP ASSISTANCE ...
THEY ONLY HAVE MONEY FOR WHAT THEY WANT ... IF YOU LIVED IN ANOTHER COMMUNITY, YOU'D HAVE HELP ALREADY ...
DO YOU HAVE A MINUTE TO TALK? I DON'T KNOW WHAT TO DO ...
OF COURSE ...

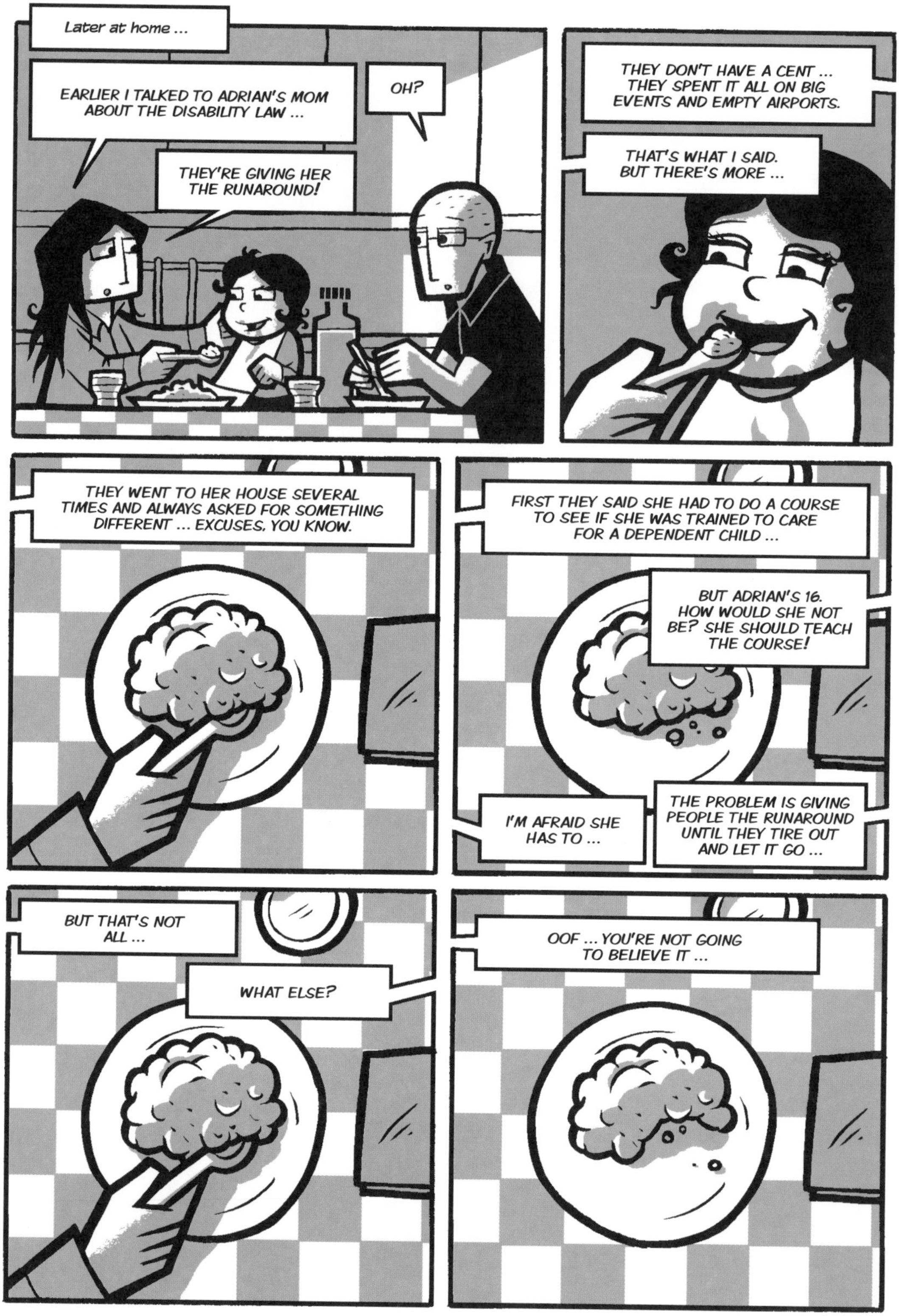

Later at home ...
EARLIER I TALKED TO ADRIAN'S MOM ABOUT THE DISABILITY LAW ...
THEY'RE GIVING HER THE RUNAROUND!
OH?
THEY DON'T HAVE A CENT ... THEY SPENT IT ALL ON BIG EVENTS AND EMPTY AIRPORTS.
THAT'S WHAT I SAID. BUT THERE'S MORE ...
THEY WENT TO HER HOUSE SEVERAL TIMES AND ALWAYS ASKED FOR SOMETHING DIFFERENT ... EXCUSES, YOU KNOW.
FIRST THEY SAID SHE HAD TO DO A COURSE TO SEE IF SHE WAS TRAINED TO CARE FOR A DEPENDENT CHILD ...
BUT ADRIAN'S 16. HOW WOULD SHE NOT BE? SHE SHOULD TEACH THE COURSE!
I'M AFRAID SHE HAS TO ...
THE PROBLEM IS GIVING PEOPLE THE RUNAROUND UNTIL THEY TIRE OUT AND LET IT GO ...
BUT THAT'S NOT ALL ...
WHAT ELSE?
OOF ... YOU'RE NOT GOING TO BELIEVE IT ...

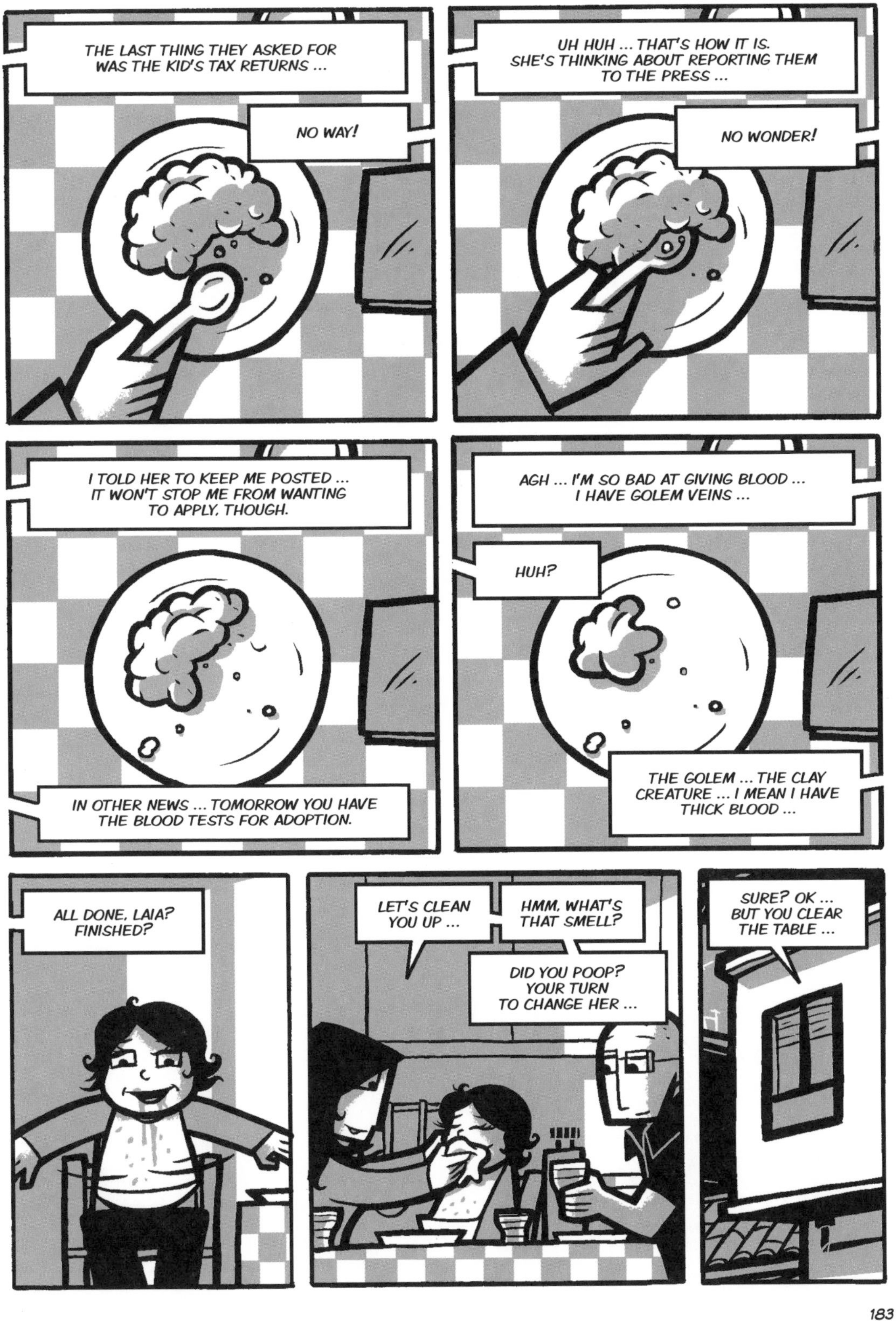
THE LAST THING THEY ASKED FOR WAS THE KID'S TAX RETURNS ...
NO WAY!
UH HUH ... THAT'S HOW IT IS. SHE'S THINKING ABOUT REPORTING THEM TO THE PRESS ...
NO WONDER!
I TOLD HER TO KEEP ME POSTED ... IT WON'T STOP ME FROM WANTING TO APPLY, THOUGH.
IN OTHER NEWS ... TOMORROW YOU HAVE THE BLOOD TESTS FOR ADOPTION.
AGH ... I'M SO BAD AT GIVING BLOOD ... I HAVE GOLEM VEINS ...
HUH?
THE GOLEM ... THE CLAY CREATURE ... I MEAN I HAVE THICK BLOOD ...
ALL DONE, LAIA? FINISHED?
LET'S CLEAN YOU UP ...
HMM, WHAT'S THAT SMELL?
DID YOU POOP? YOUR TURN TO CHANGE HER ...
SURE? OK ... BUT YOU CLEAR THE TABLE ...

Medical certificate, part 1.

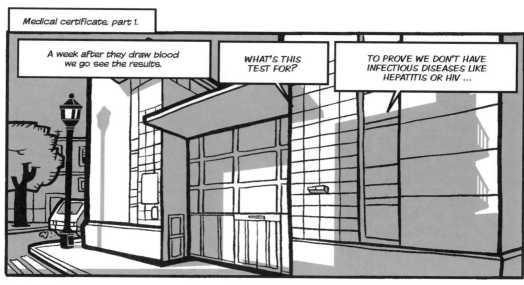

A week after they draw blood we go see the results.

WHAT'S THIS TEST FOR?

TO PROVE WE DON'T HAVE INFECTIOUS DISEASES LIKE HEPATITIS OR HIV ...

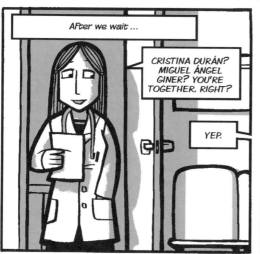

After we wait ...

CRISTINA DURÁN? MIGUEL ÁNGEL GINER? YOU'RE TOGETHER, RIGHT?

YEP.

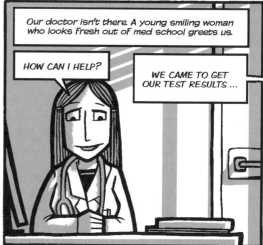

Our doctor isn't there. A young smiling woman who looks fresh out of med school greets us.

HOW CAN I HELP?

WE CAME TO GET OUR TEST RESULTS ...

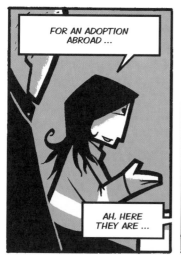

FOR AN ADOPTION ABROAD ...

AH, HERE THEY ARE ...

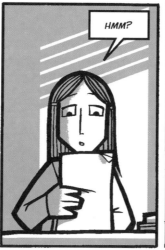

HMM?

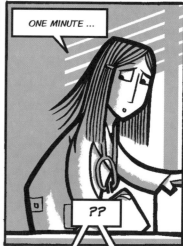

ONE MINUTE ...

??

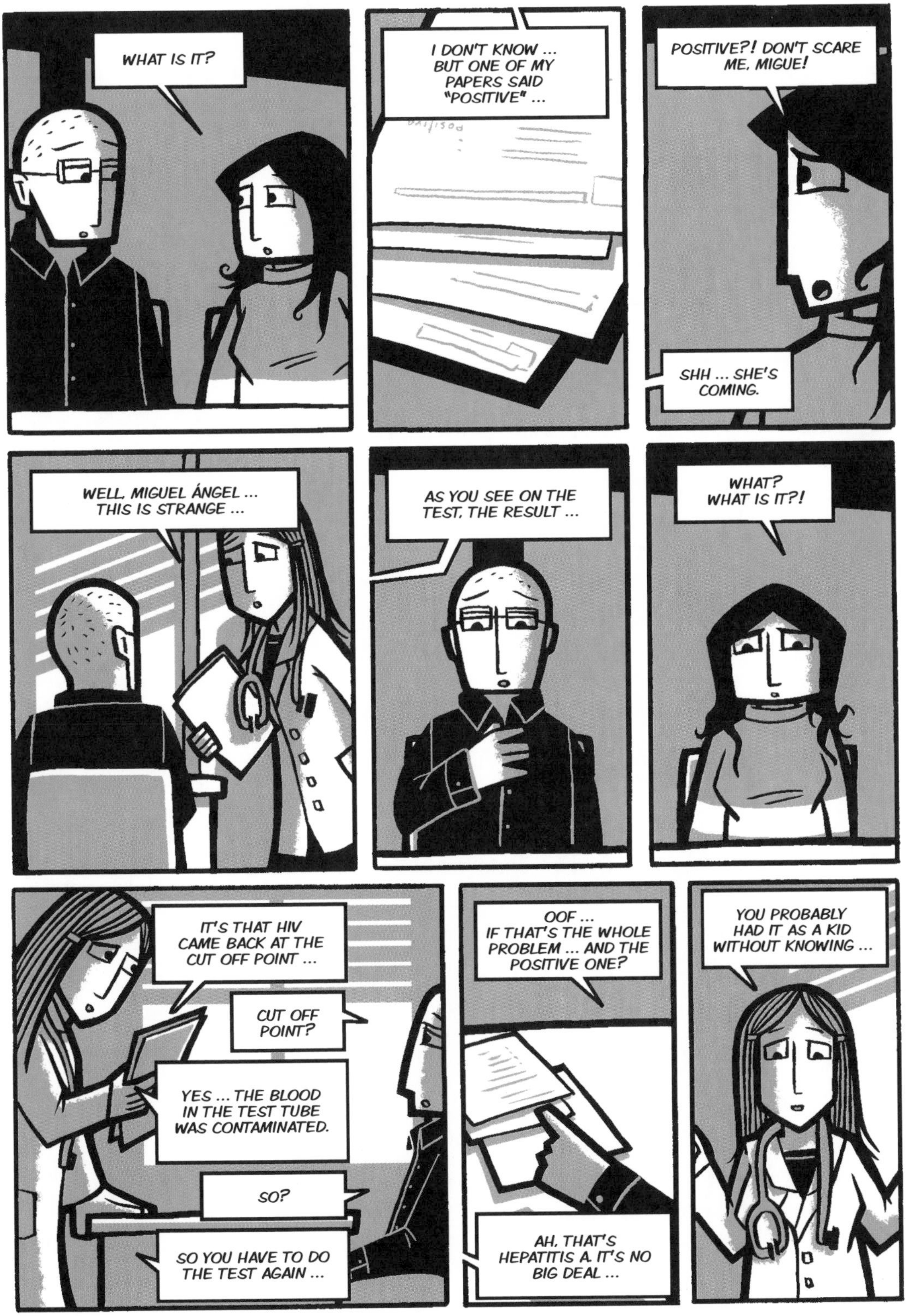
WHAT IS IT?
I DON'T KNOW ... BUT ONE OF MY PAPERS SAID "POSITIVE" ...
POSITIVE?! DON'T SCARE ME, MIGUE!
SHH ... SHE'S COMING.
WELL, MIGUEL ÁNGEL ... THIS IS STRANGE ...
AS YOU SEE ON THE TEST, THE RESULT ...
WHAT? WHAT IS IT?!
IT'S THAT HIV CAME BACK AT THE CUT OFF POINT ...
CUT OFF POINT?
YES ... THE BLOOD IN THE TEST TUBE WAS CONTAMINATED.
SO?
SO YOU HAVE TO DO THE TEST AGAIN ...
OOF ... IF THAT'S THE WHOLE PROBLEM ... AND THE POSITIVE ONE?
AH, THAT'S HEPATITIS A. IT'S NO BIG DEAL ...
YOU PROBABLY HAD IT AS A KID WITHOUT KNOWING ...

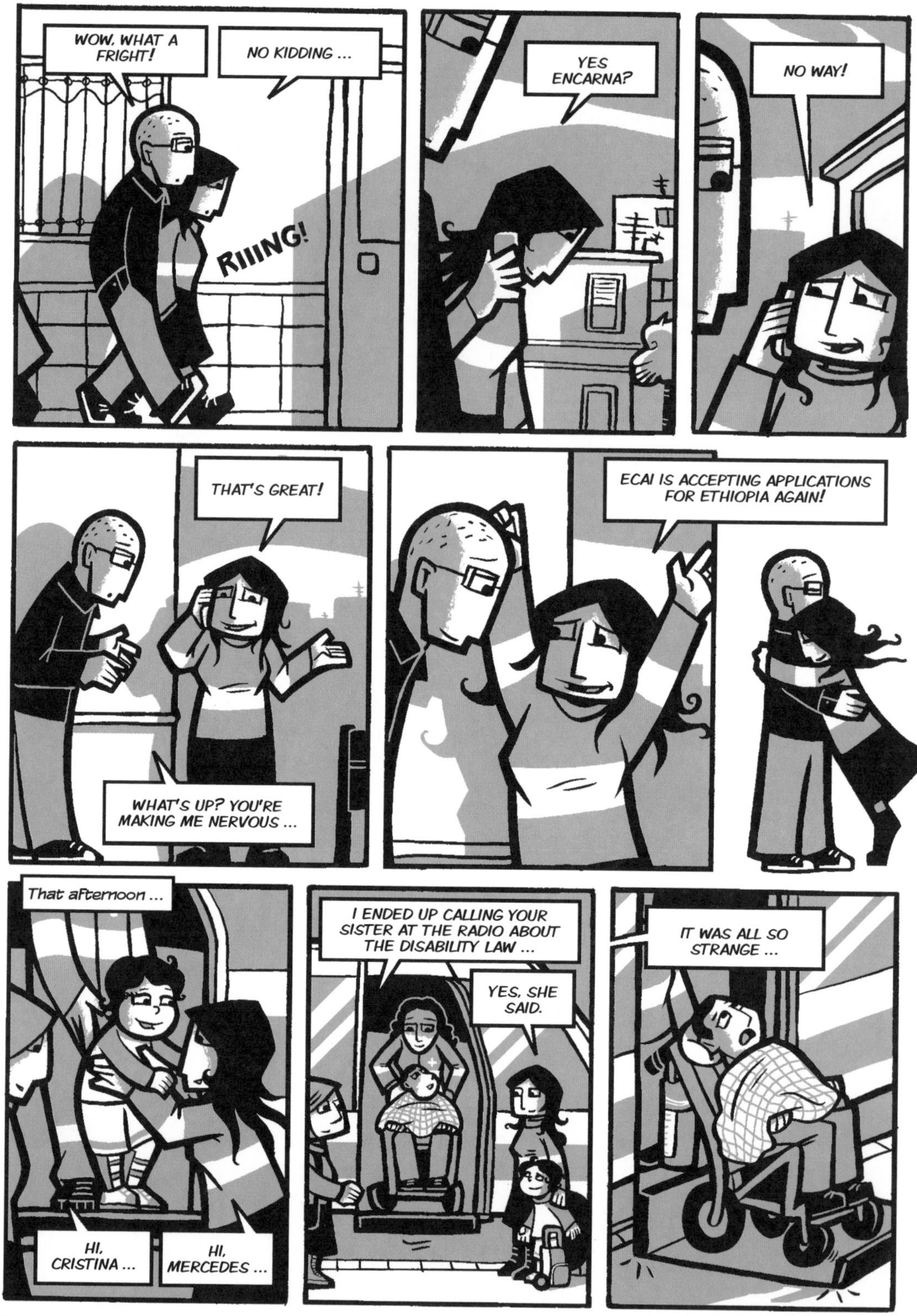

WOW, WHAT A FRIGHT!
NO KIDDING ...
RIIING!
YES ENCARNA?
NO WAY!
THAT'S GREAT!
WHAT'S UP? YOU'RE MAKING ME NERVOUS ...
ECAI IS ACCEPTING APPLICATIONS FOR ETHIOPIA AGAIN!
That afternoon ...
HI, CRISTINA ...
HI, MERCEDES ...
I ENDED UP CALLING YOUR SISTER AT THE RADIO ABOUT THE DISABILITY LAW ...
YES, SHE SAID.
IT WAS ALL SO STRANGE ...

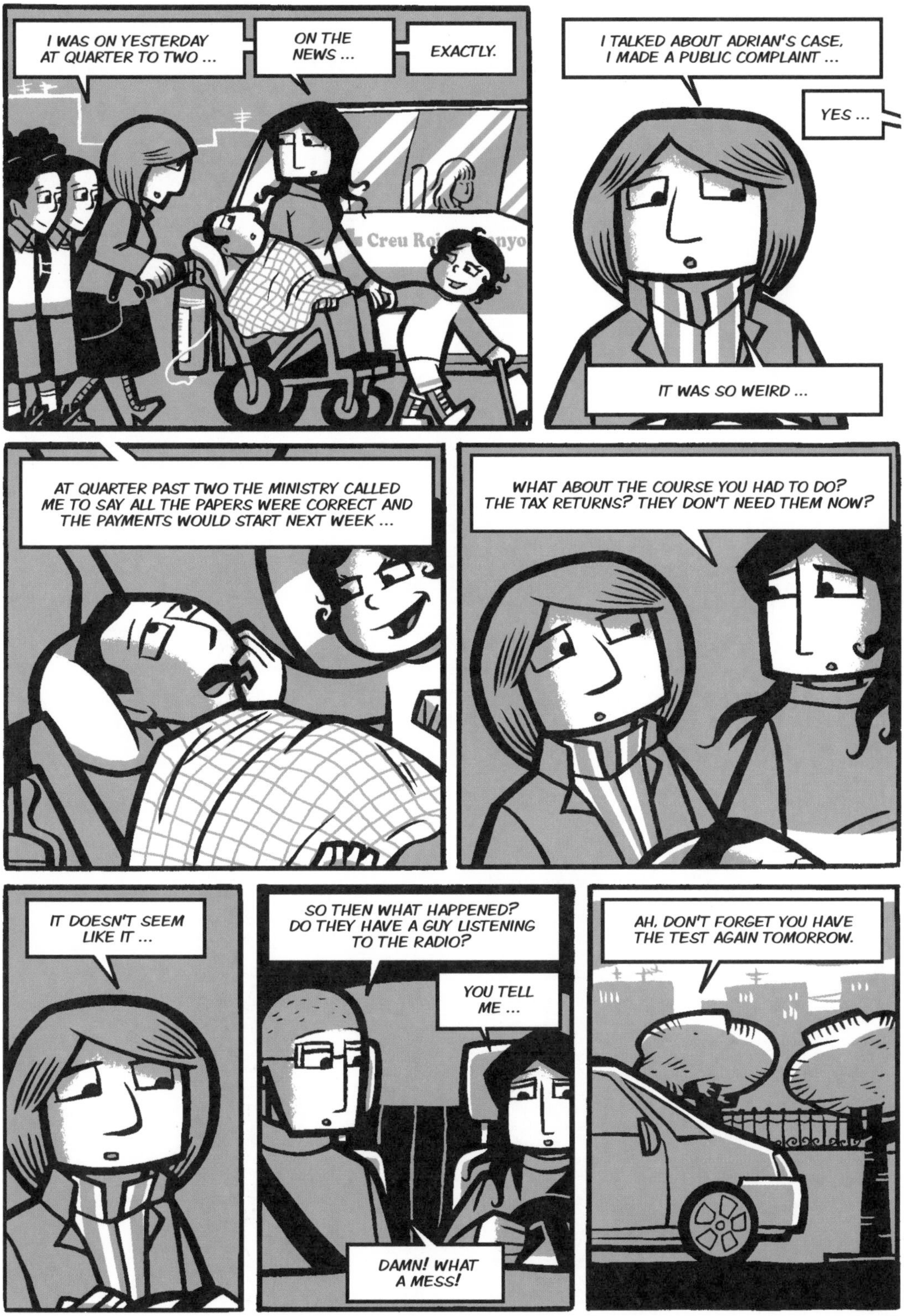
I WAS ON YESTERDAY AT QUARTER TO TWO ...
ON THE NEWS ...
EXACTLY.
I TALKED ABOUT ADRIAN'S CASE, I MADE A PUBLIC COMPLAINT ...
YES ...
IT WAS SO WEIRD ...
AT QUARTER PAST TWO THE MINISTRY CALLED ME TO SAY ALL THE PAPERS WERE CORRECT AND THE PAYMENTS WOULD START NEXT WEEK ...
WHAT ABOUT THE COURSE YOU HAD TO DO? THE TAX RETURNS? THEY DON'T NEED THEM NOW?
IT DOESN'T SEEM LIKE IT ...
SO THEN WHAT HAPPENED? DO THEY HAVE A GUY LISTENING TO THE RADIO?
YOU TELL ME ...
DAMN! WHAT A MESS!
AH, DON'T FORGET YOU HAVE THE TEST AGAIN TOMORROW.

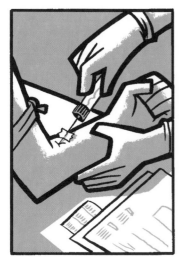

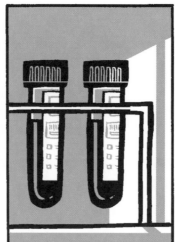

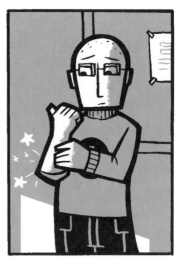

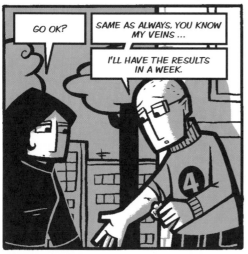

GO OK?

SAME AS ALWAYS, YOU KNOW MY VEINS ...

I'LL HAVE THE RESULTS IN A WEEK.

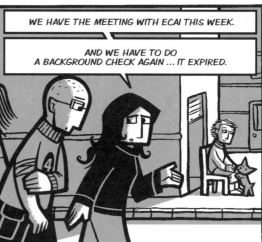

WE HAVE THE MEETING WITH ECAI THIS WEEK.

AND WE HAVE TO DO A BACKGROUND CHECK AGAIN ... IT EXPIRED.

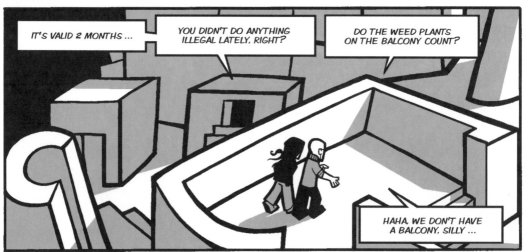

IT'S VALID 2 MONTHS ...

YOU DIDN'T DO ANYTHING ILLEGAL LATELY, RIGHT?

DO THE WEED PLANTS ON THE BALCONY COUNT?

HAHA, WE DON'T HAVE A BALCONY, SILLY ...

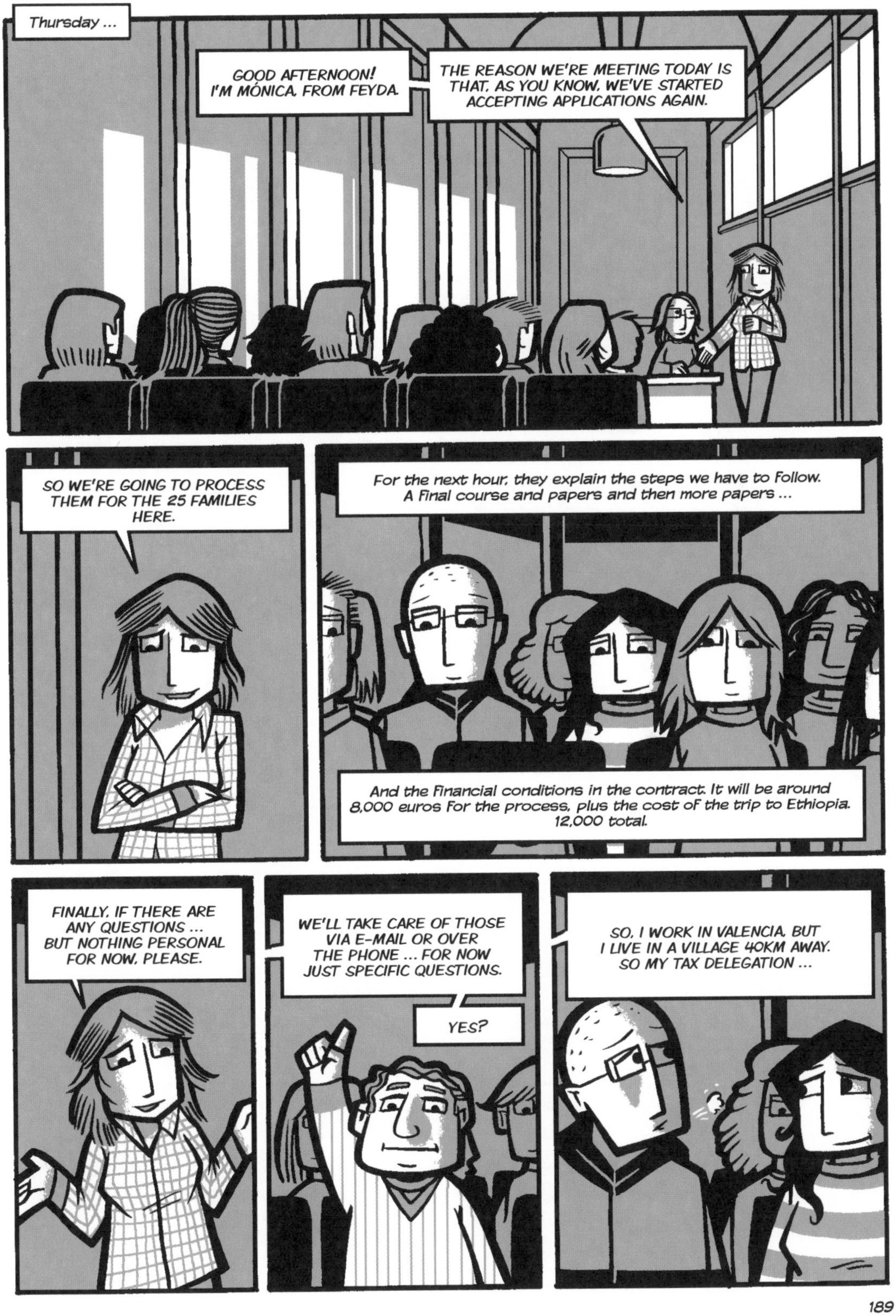
Thursday ...
GOOD AFTERNOON! I'M MÓNICA, FROM FEYDA.
THE REASON WE'RE MEETING TODAY IS THAT, AS YOU KNOW, WE'VE STARTED ACCEPTING APPLICATIONS AGAIN.
SO WE'RE GOING TO PROCESS THEM FOR THE 25 FAMILIES HERE.
For the next hour, they explain the steps we have to follow. A final course and papers and then more papers ...
And the financial conditions in the contract. It will be around 8,000 euros for the process, plus the cost of the trip to Ethiopia. 12,000 total.
FINALLY, IF THERE ARE ANY QUESTIONS ... BUT NOTHING PERSONAL FOR NOW, PLEASE.
WE'LL TAKE CARE OF THOSE VIA E-MAIL OR OVER THE PHONE ... FOR NOW JUST SPECIFIC QUESTIONS.
YES?
SO, I WORK IN VALENCIA, BUT I LIVE IN A VILLAGE 40KM AWAY. SO MY TAX DELEGATION ...

WOW, GOOD THING THEY COULDN'T TAKE PERSONAL QUESTIONS ...
HAHA YEAH ... AT LEAST OUR APPLICATION IS MOVING ...
Medical certification, part 2.
I THINK DR. CASAL WILL BE IN TODAY ...
A bit later ...
CRISTINA, ALL CLEAR ... I'LL DO YOUR CERTIFICATE NOW.
AND MIGUEL ÁNGEL ... HMM ... STRANGE!
WHAT? WHAT IS IT?!
WELL ... THE HIV TEST.

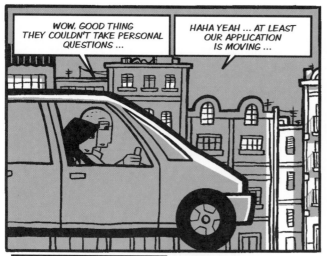

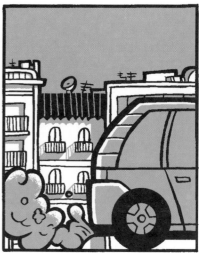

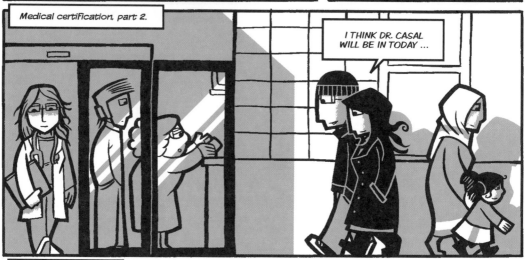

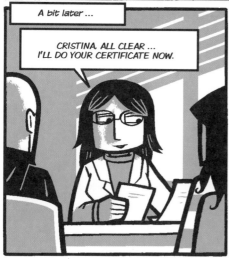

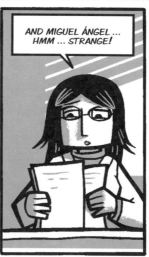

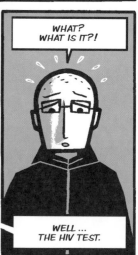

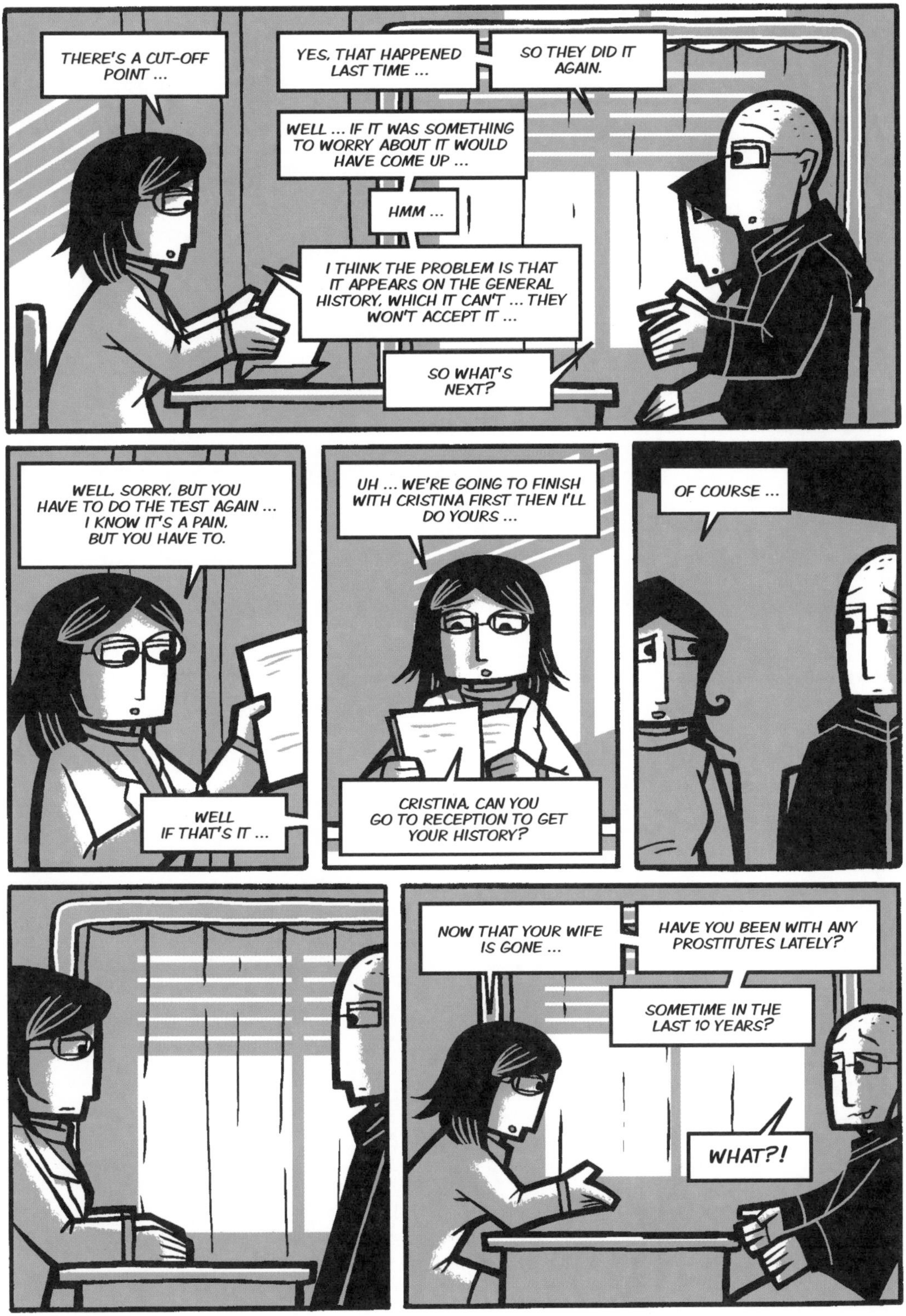
THERE'S A CUT-OFF POINT ...
YES, THAT HAPPENED LAST TIME ...
SO THEY DID IT AGAIN.
WELL ... IF IT WAS SOMETHING TO WORRY ABOUT IT WOULD HAVE COME UP ...
HMM ...
I THINK THE PROBLEM IS THAT IT APPEARS ON THE GENERAL HISTORY, WHICH IT CAN'T ... THEY WON'T ACCEPT IT ...
SO WHAT'S NEXT?
WELL, SORRY, BUT YOU HAVE TO DO THE TEST AGAIN ... I KNOW IT'S A PAIN, BUT YOU HAVE TO.
WELL IF THAT'S IT ...
UH ... WE'RE GOING TO FINISH WITH CRISTINA FIRST THEN I'LL DO YOURS ...
CRISTINA, CAN YOU GO TO RECEPTION TO GET YOUR HISTORY?
OF COURSE ...
NOW THAT YOUR WIFE IS GONE ...
HAVE YOU BEEN WITH ANY PROSTITUTES LATELY?
SOMETIME IN THE LAST 10 YEARS?
WHAT?!

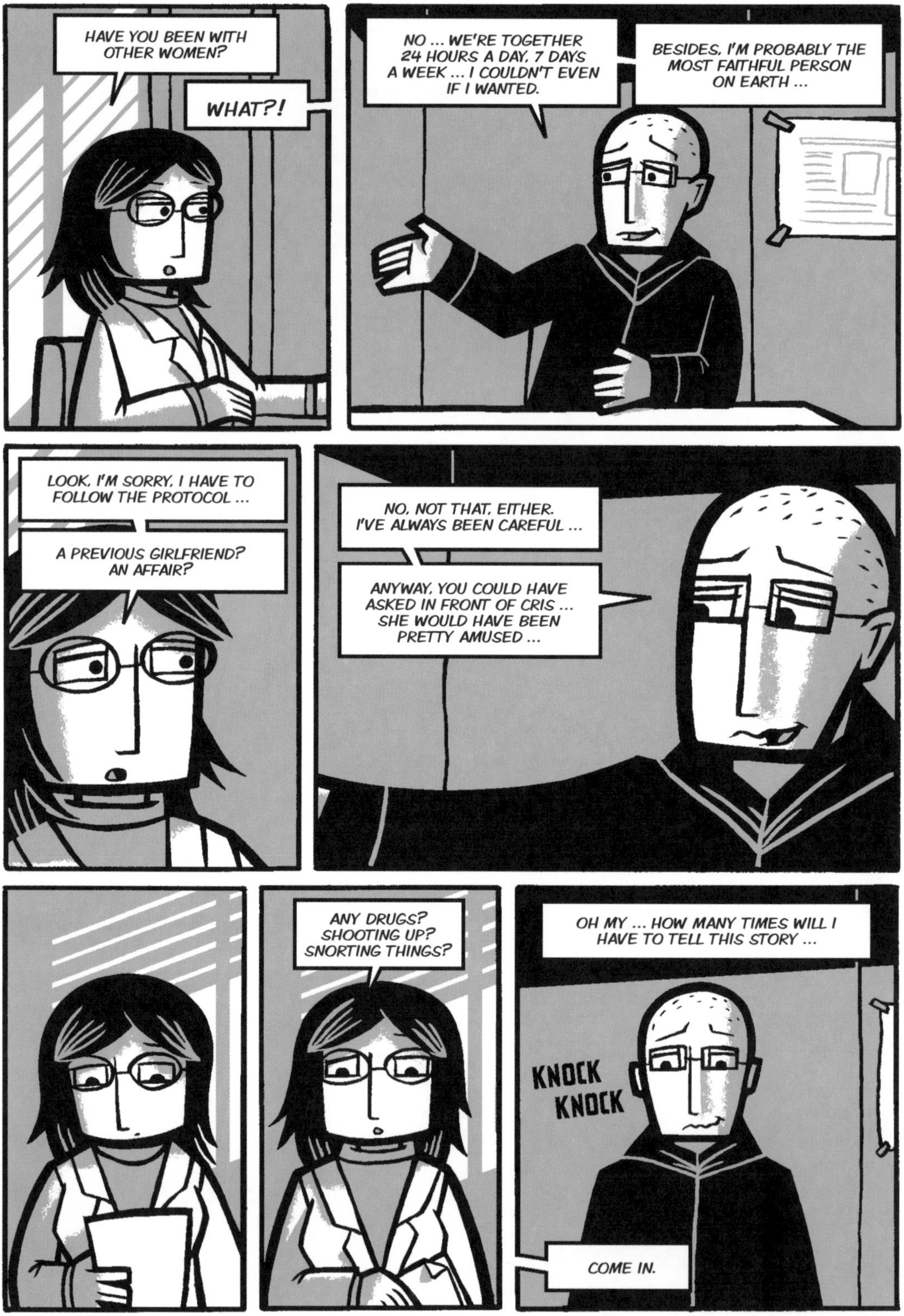
HAVE YOU BEEN WITH OTHER WOMEN?
WHAT?!
NO ... WE'RE TOGETHER 24 HOURS A DAY, 7 DAYS A WEEK ... I COULDN'T EVEN IF I WANTED.
BESIDES, I'M PROBABLY THE MOST FAITHFUL PERSON ON EARTH ...
LOOK, I'M SORRY, I HAVE TO FOLLOW THE PROTOCOL ...
A PREVIOUS GIRLFRIEND? AN AFFAIR?
NO, NOT THAT, EITHER. I'VE ALWAYS BEEN CAREFUL ...
ANYWAY, YOU COULD HAVE ASKED IN FRONT OF CRIS ... SHE WOULD HAVE BEEN PRETTY AMUSED ...
ANY DRUGS? SHOOTING UP? SNORTING THINGS?
OH MY ... HOW MANY TIMES WILL I HAVE TO TELL THIS STORY ...
KNOCK KNOCK
COME IN.

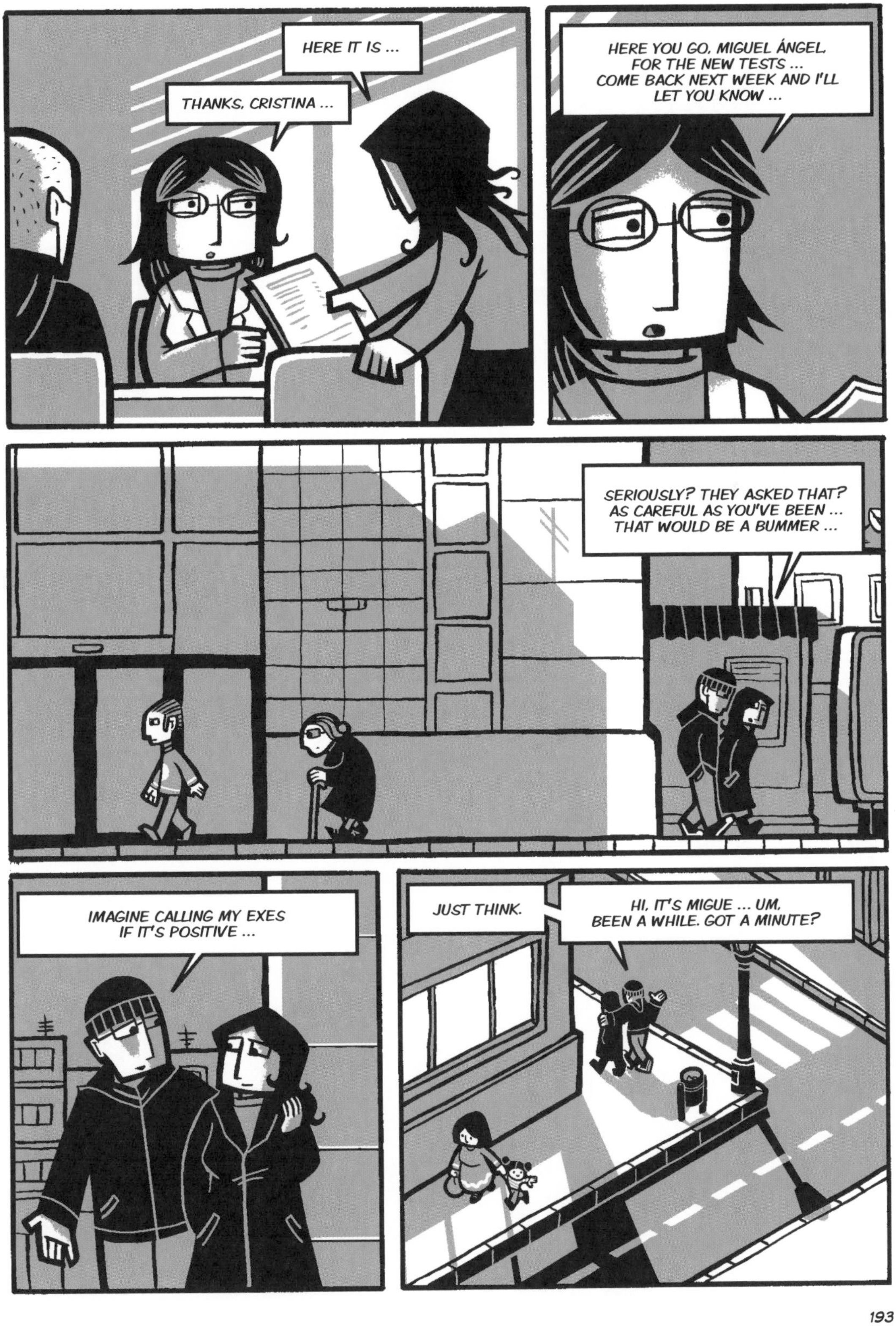
HERE IT IS ...
THANKS, CRISTINA ...
HERE YOU GO, MIGUEL ÁNGEL, FOR THE NEW TESTS ... COME BACK NEXT WEEK AND I'LL LET YOU KNOW ...
SERIOUSLY? THEY ASKED THAT? AS CAREFUL AS YOU'VE BEEN ... THAT WOULD BE A BUMMER ...
IMAGINE CALLING MY EXES IF IT'S POSITIVE ...
JUST THINK.
HI, IT'S MIGUE ... UM, BEEN A WHILE. GOT A MINUTE?

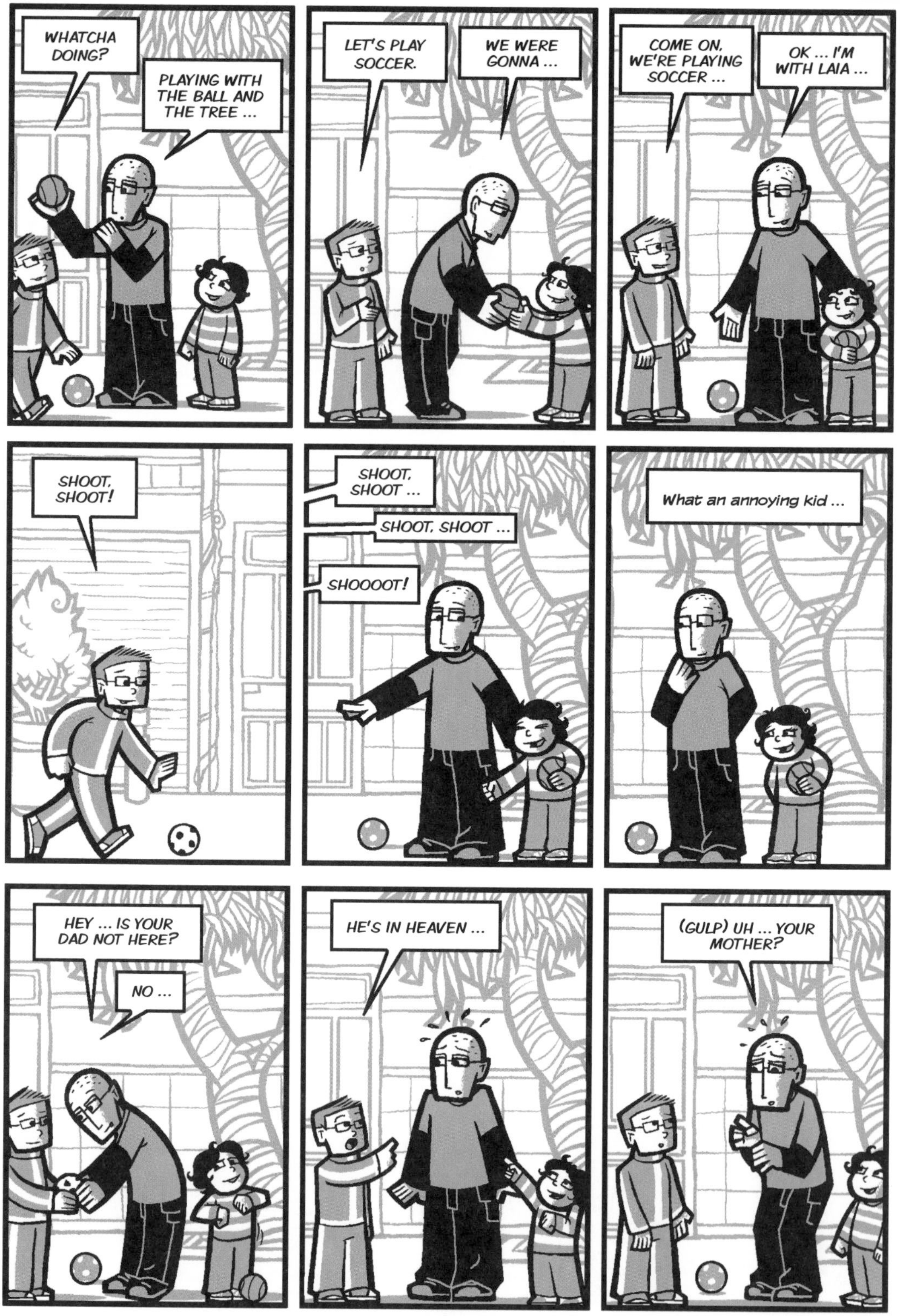
WHATCHA DOING?
PLAYING WITH THE BALL AND THE TREE ...
LET'S PLAY SOCCER.
WE WERE GONNA ...
COME ON, WE'RE PLAYING SOCCER ...
OK ... I'M WITH LAIA ...
SHOOT, SHOOT!
SHOOT, SHOOT ...
SHOOT, SHOOT ...
SHOOOOT!
What an annoying kid ...
HEY ... IS YOUR DAD NOT HERE?
NO ...
HE'S IN HEAVEN ...
(GULP) UH ... YOUR MOTHER?

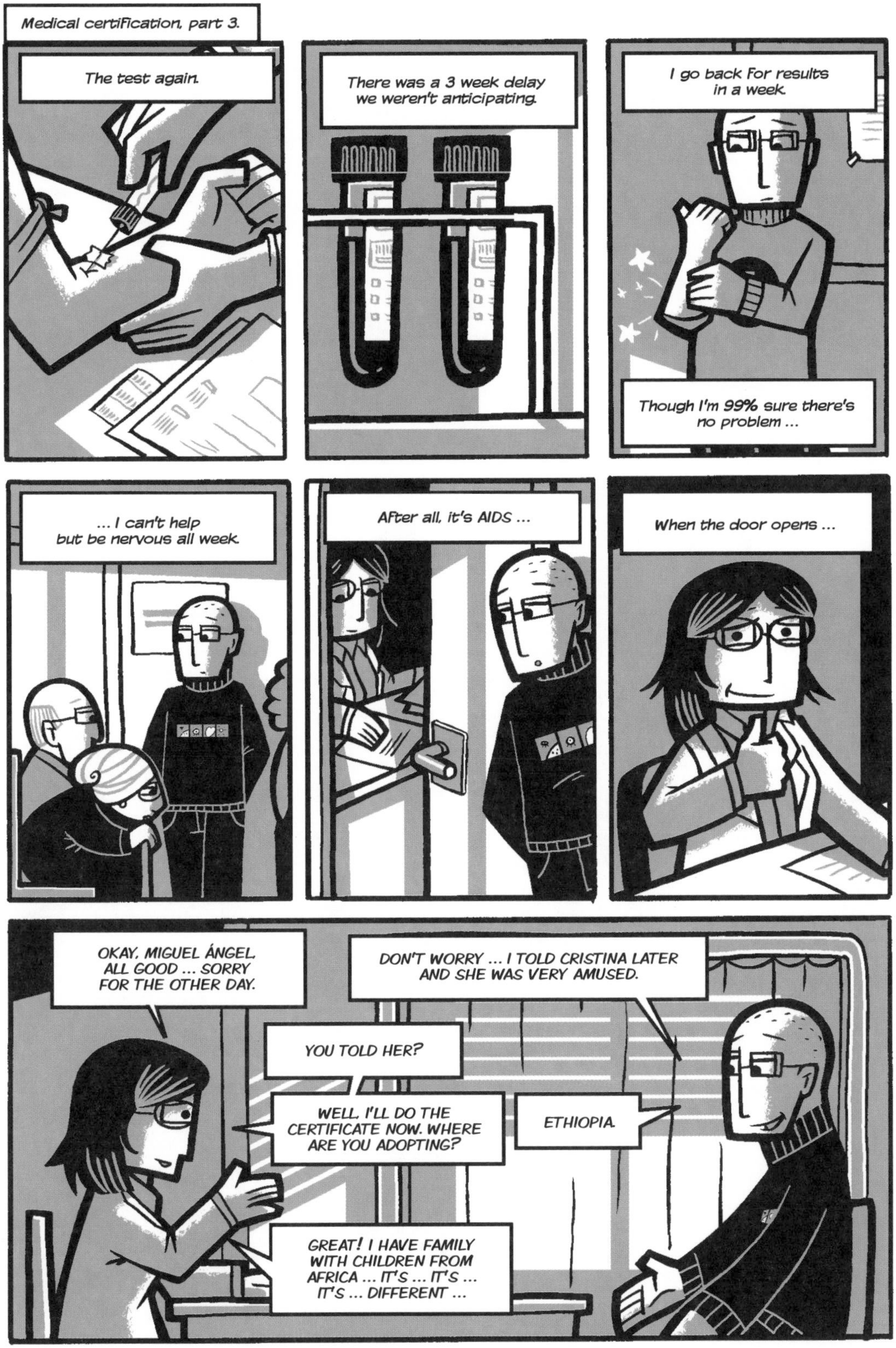
Medical certification, part 3.
The test again.
There was a 3 week delay we weren't anticipating.
I go back for results in a week.
Though I'm 99% sure there's no problem ...
... I can't help but be nervous all week.
After all, it's AIDS ...
When the door opens ...
OKAY, MIGUEL ÁNGEL, ALL GOOD ... SORRY FOR THE OTHER DAY.
DON'T WORRY ... I TOLD CRISTINA LATER AND SHE WAS VERY AMUSED.
YOU TOLD HER?
WELL, I'LL DO THE CERTIFICATE NOW. WHERE ARE YOU ADOPTING?
ETHIOPIA.
GREAT! I HAVE FAMILY WITH CHILDREN FROM AFRICA ... IT'S ... IT'S ... IT'S ... DIFFERENT ...

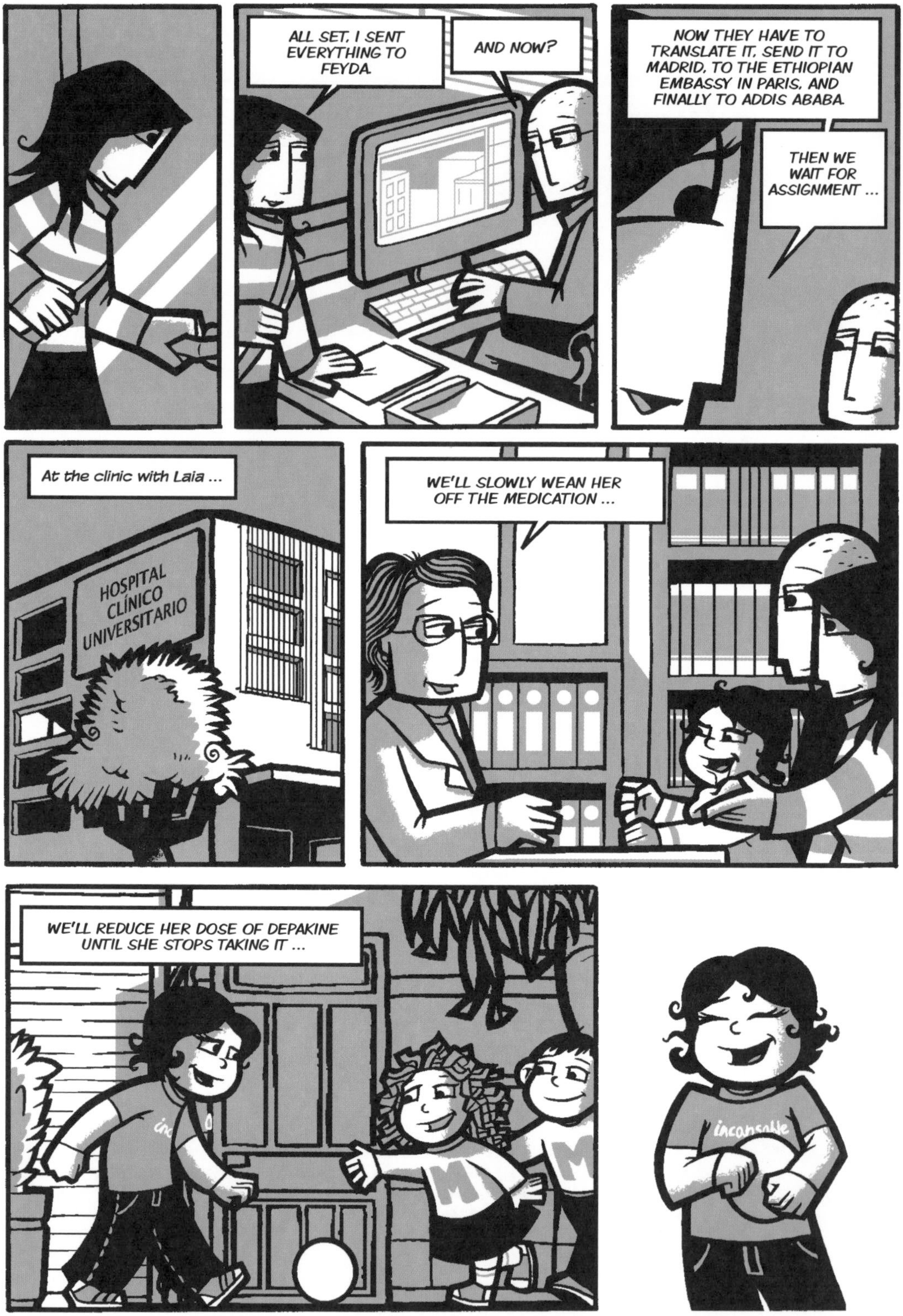
ALL SET, I SENT EVERYTHING TO FEYDA.
AND NOW?
NOW THEY HAVE TO TRANSLATE IT, SEND IT TO MADRID, TO THE ETHIOPIAN EMBASSY IN PARIS, AND FINALLY TO ADDIS ABABA.
THEN WE WAIT FOR ASSIGNMENT ...
At the clinic with Laia ...
HOSPITAL CLÍNICO UNIVERSITARIO
WE'LL SLOWLY WEAN HER OFF THE MEDICATION ...
WE'LL REDUCE HER DOSE OF DEPAKINE UNTIL SHE STOPS TAKING IT ...
incansable

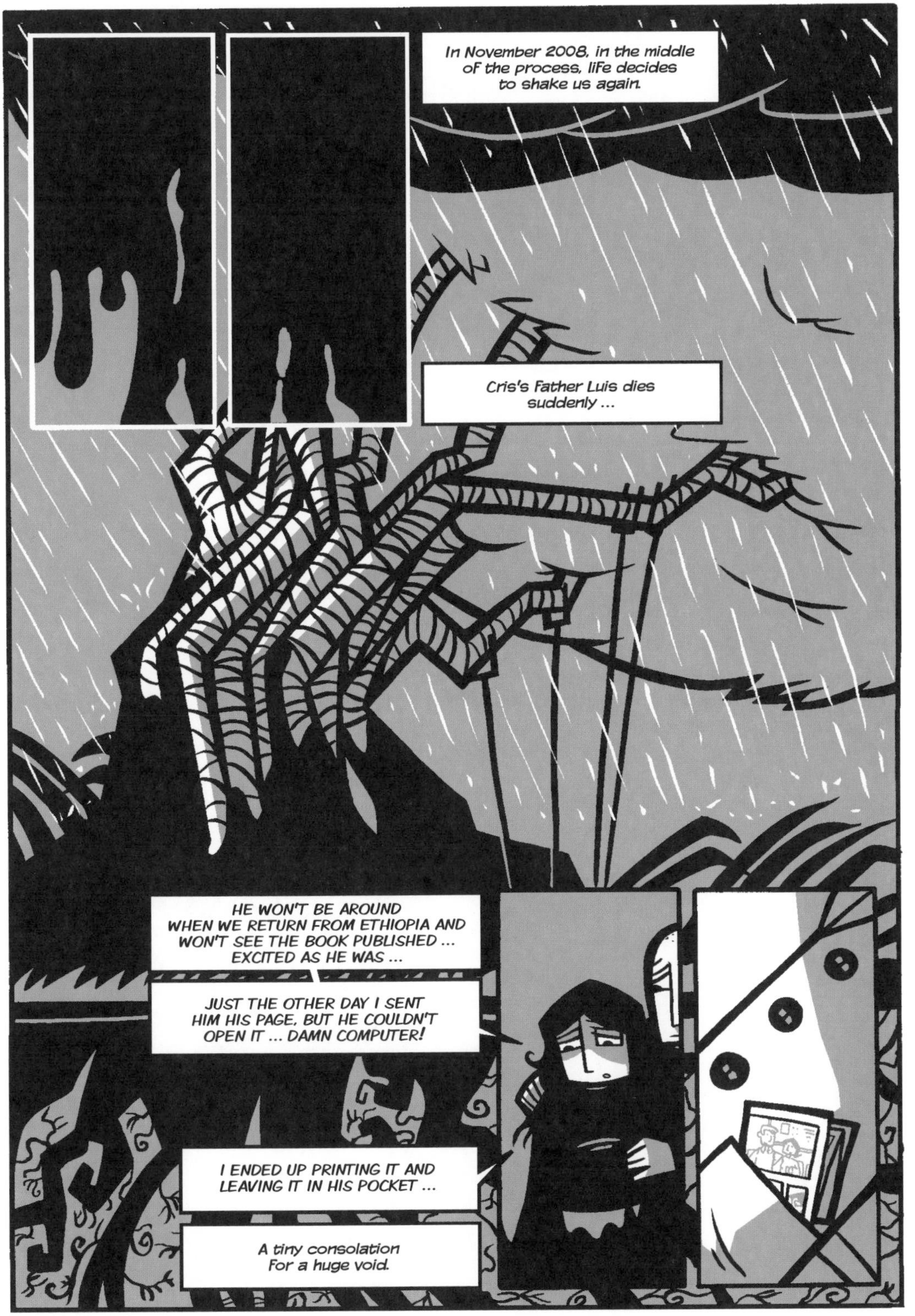
In November 2008, in the middle of the process, life decides to shake us again.
Cris's Father Luis dies suddenly ...
HE WON'T BE AROUND WHEN WE RETURN FROM ETHIOPIA AND WON'T SEE THE BOOK PUBLISHED ... EXCITED AS HE WAS ...
JUST THE OTHER DAY I SENT HIM HIS PAGE, BUT HE COULDN'T OPEN IT ... DAMN COMPUTER!
I ENDED UP PRINTING IT AND LEAVING IT IN HIS POCKET ...
A tiny consolation For a huge void.

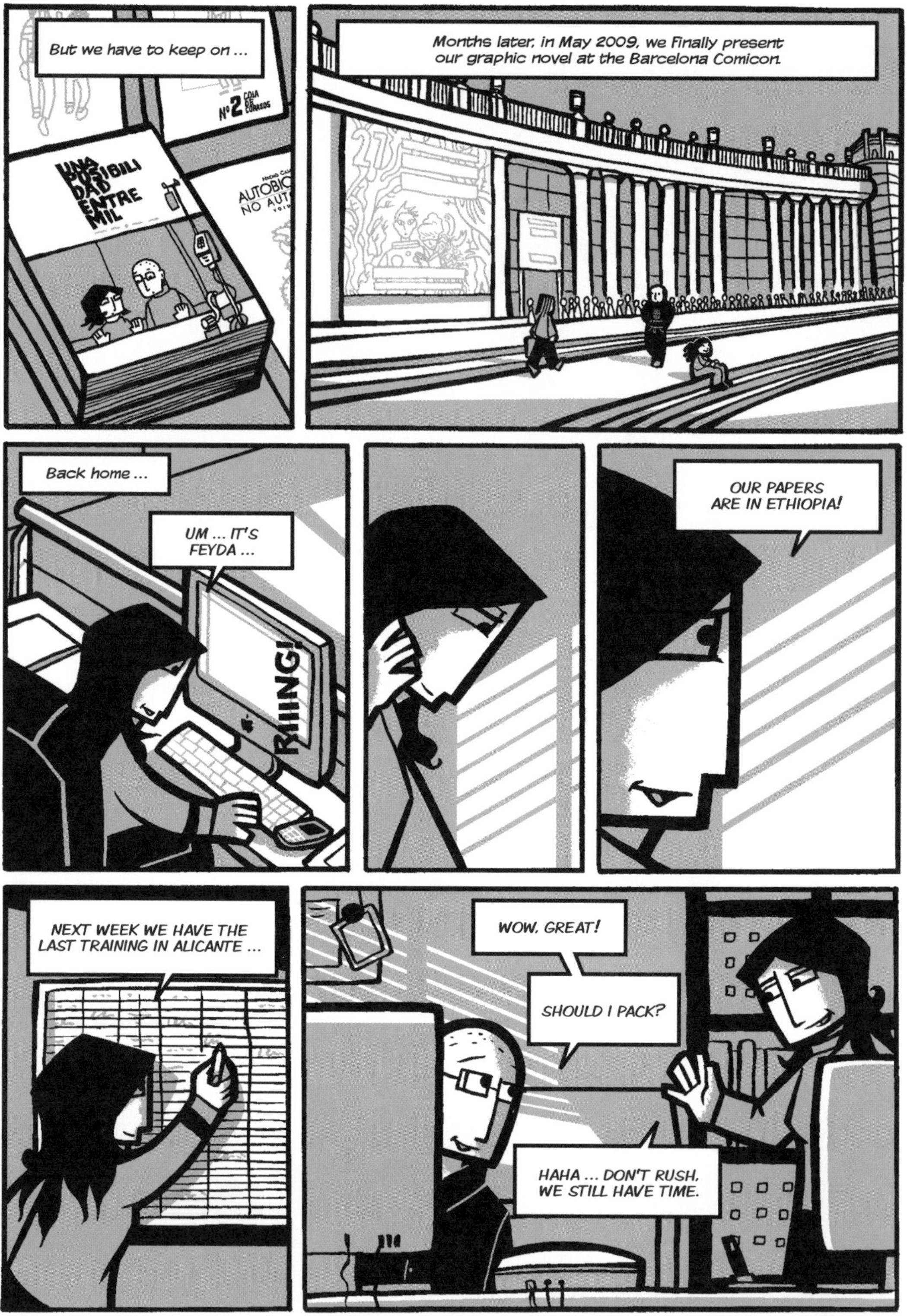
But we have to keep on ...
UNA POSIBILI DAD ENTRE MIL
Months later, in May 2009, we finally present our graphic novel at the Barcelona Comicon.
Back home ...
UM ... IT'S FEYDA ...
RIIIING!
OUR PAPERS ARE IN ETHIOPIA!
NEXT WEEK WE HAVE THE LAST TRAINING IN ALICANTE ...
WOW, GREAT!
SHOULD I PACK?
HAHA ... DON'T RUSH, WE STILL HAVE TIME.

Chapter 5
THE SUITCASE

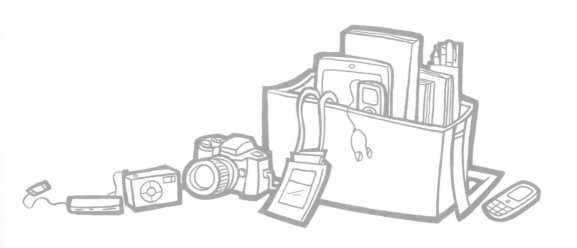

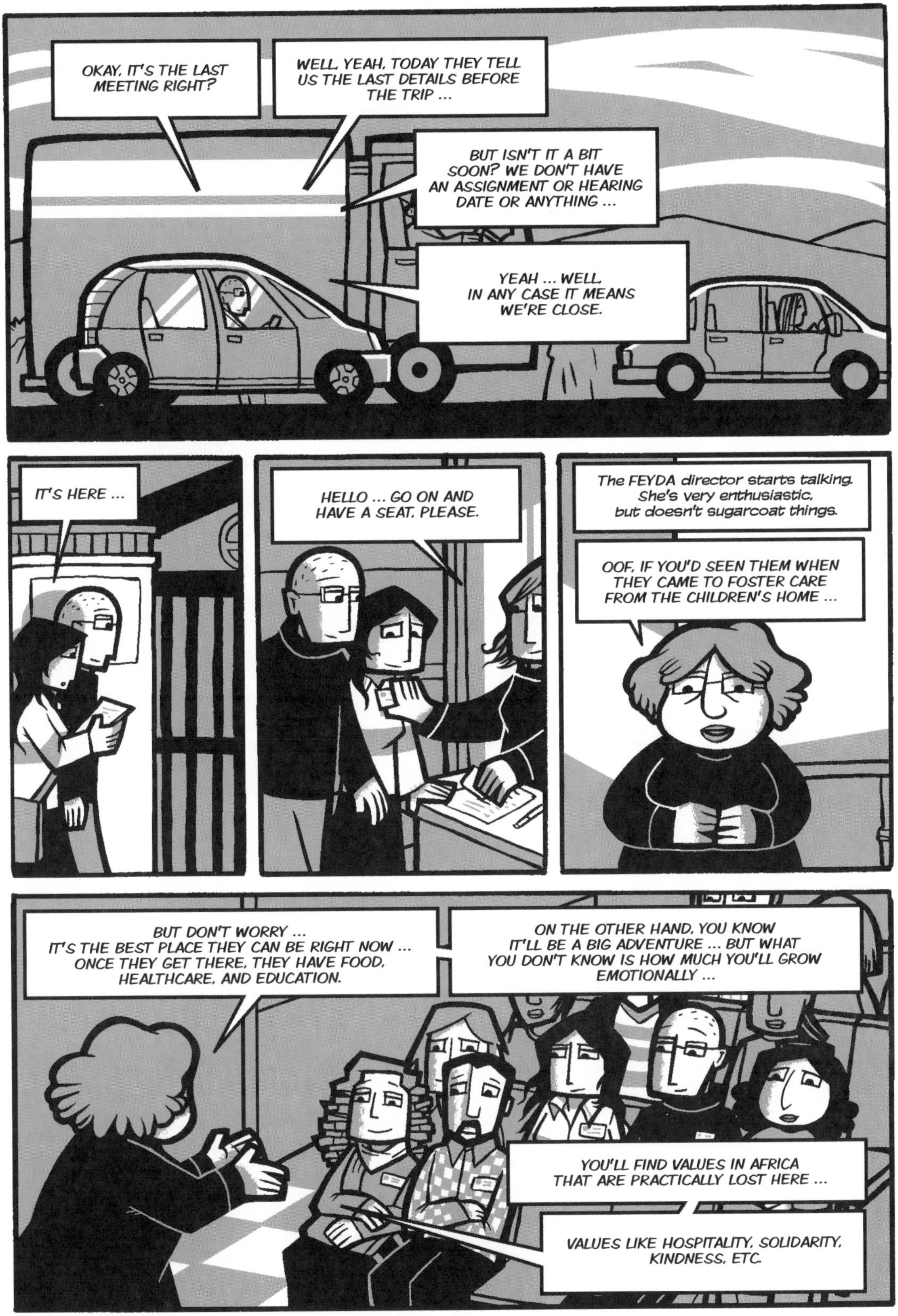
OKAY, IT'S THE LAST MEETING RIGHT?
WELL, YEAH, TODAY THEY TELL US THE LAST DETAILS BEFORE THE TRIP ...
BUT ISN'T IT A BIT SOON? WE DON'T HAVE AN ASSIGNMENT OR HEARING DATE OR ANYTHING ...
YEAH ... WELL, IN ANY CASE IT MEANS WE'RE CLOSE.
IT'S HERE ...
HELLO ... GO ON AND HAVE A SEAT, PLEASE.
The FEYDA director starts talking. She's very enthusiastic, but doesn't sugarcoat things.
OOF, IF YOU'D SEEN THEM WHEN THEY CAME TO FOSTER CARE FROM THE CHILDREN'S HOME ...
BUT DON'T WORRY ... IT'S THE BEST PLACE THEY CAN BE RIGHT NOW ... ONCE THEY GET THERE, THEY HAVE FOOD, HEALTHCARE, AND EDUCATION.
ON THE OTHER HAND, YOU KNOW IT'LL BE A BIG ADVENTURE ... BUT WHAT YOU DON'T KNOW IS HOW MUCH YOU'LL GROW EMOTIONALLY ...
YOU'LL FIND VALUES IN AFRICA THAT ARE PRACTICALLY LOST HERE ...
VALUES LIKE HOSPITALITY, SOLIDARITY, KINDNESS, ETC.

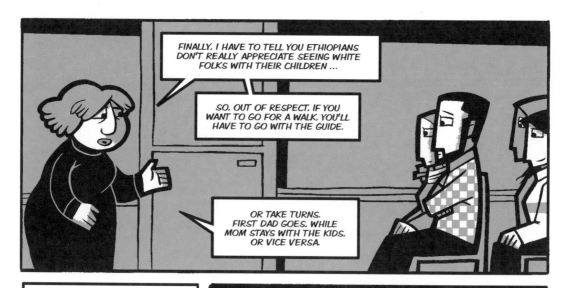

FINALLY, I HAVE TO TELL YOU ETHIOPIANS DON'T REALLY APPRECIATE SEEING WHITE FOLKS WITH THEIR CHILDREN ...

SO, OUT OF RESPECT, IF YOU WANT TO GO FOR A WALK, YOU'LL HAVE TO GO WITH THE GUIDE.

OR TAKE TURNS. FIRST DAD GOES, WHILE MOM STAYS WITH THE KIDS, OR VICE VERSA.

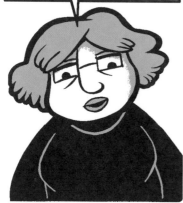

WE, AS ECAI, ARE CONTROLLED BY THE SPANISH AND ETHIOPIAN GOVERNMENTS ...

THEY REQUIRE US TO SEND MONEY TO BUILD HOSPITALS, SCHOOLS, RETIREMENT HOMES ...

ACCORDING TO OUR STATUTES, ALL OUR SURPLUS HAS TO GO TO INTERNATIONAL AID.

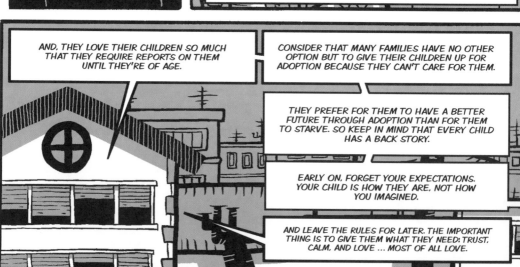

AND, THEY LOVE THEIR CHILDREN SO MUCH THAT THEY REQUIRE REPORTS ON THEM UNTIL THEY'RE OF AGE.

CONSIDER THAT MANY FAMILIES HAVE NO OTHER OPTION BUT TO GIVE THEIR CHILDREN UP FOR ADOPTION BECAUSE THEY CAN'T CARE FOR THEM.

THEY PREFER FOR THEM TO HAVE A BETTER FUTURE THROUGH ADOPTION THAN FOR THEM TO STARVE. SO KEEP IN MIND THAT EVERY CHILD HAS A BACK STORY.

EARLY ON, FORGET YOUR EXPECTATIONS. YOUR CHILD IS HOW THEY ARE, NOT HOW YOU IMAGINED.

AND LEAVE THE RULES FOR LATER. THE IMPORTANT THING IS TO GIVE THEM WHAT THEY NEED: TRUST, CALM, AND LOVE ... MOST OF ALL LOVE.

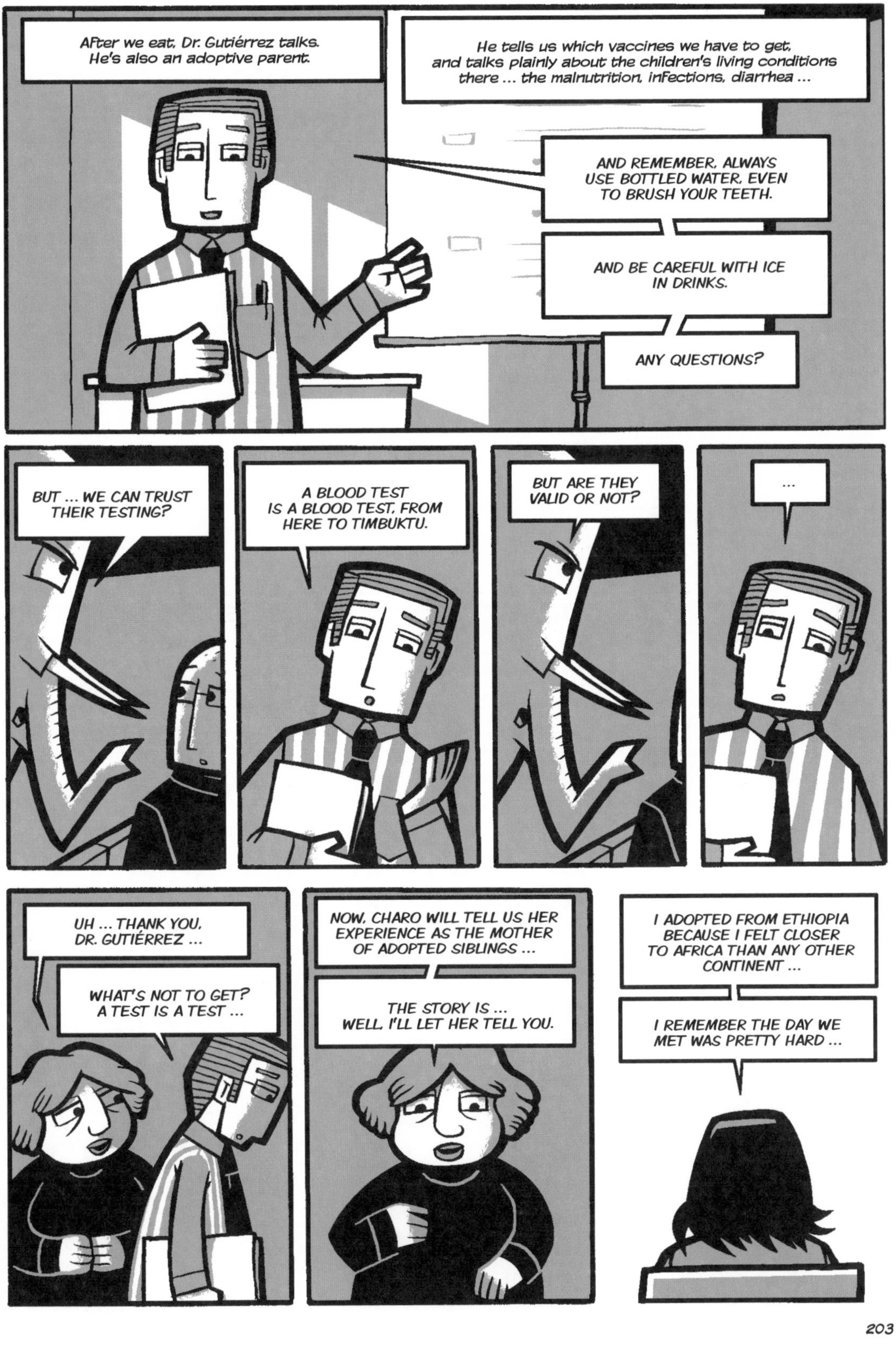
After we eat, Dr. Gutiérrez talks. He's also an adoptive parent.
He tells us which vaccines we have to get, and talks plainly about the children's living conditions there ... the malnutrition, infections, diarrhea ...
AND REMEMBER, ALWAYS USE BOTTLED WATER, EVEN TO BRUSH YOUR TEETH.
AND BE CAREFUL WITH ICE IN DRINKS.
ANY QUESTIONS?
BUT ... WE CAN TRUST THEIR TESTING?
A BLOOD TEST IS A BLOOD TEST, FROM HERE TO TIMBUKTU.
BUT ARE THEY VALID OR NOT?
...
UH ... THANK YOU, DR. GUTIÉRREZ ...
WHAT'S NOT TO GET? A TEST IS A TEST ...
NOW, CHARO WILL TELL US HER EXPERIENCE AS THE MOTHER OF ADOPTED SIBLINGS ...
THE STORY IS ... WELL, I'LL LET HER TELL YOU.
I ADOPTED FROM ETHIOPIA BECAUSE I FELT CLOSER TO AFRICA THAN ANY OTHER CONTINENT ...
I REMEMBER THE DAY WE MET WAS PRETTY HARD ...

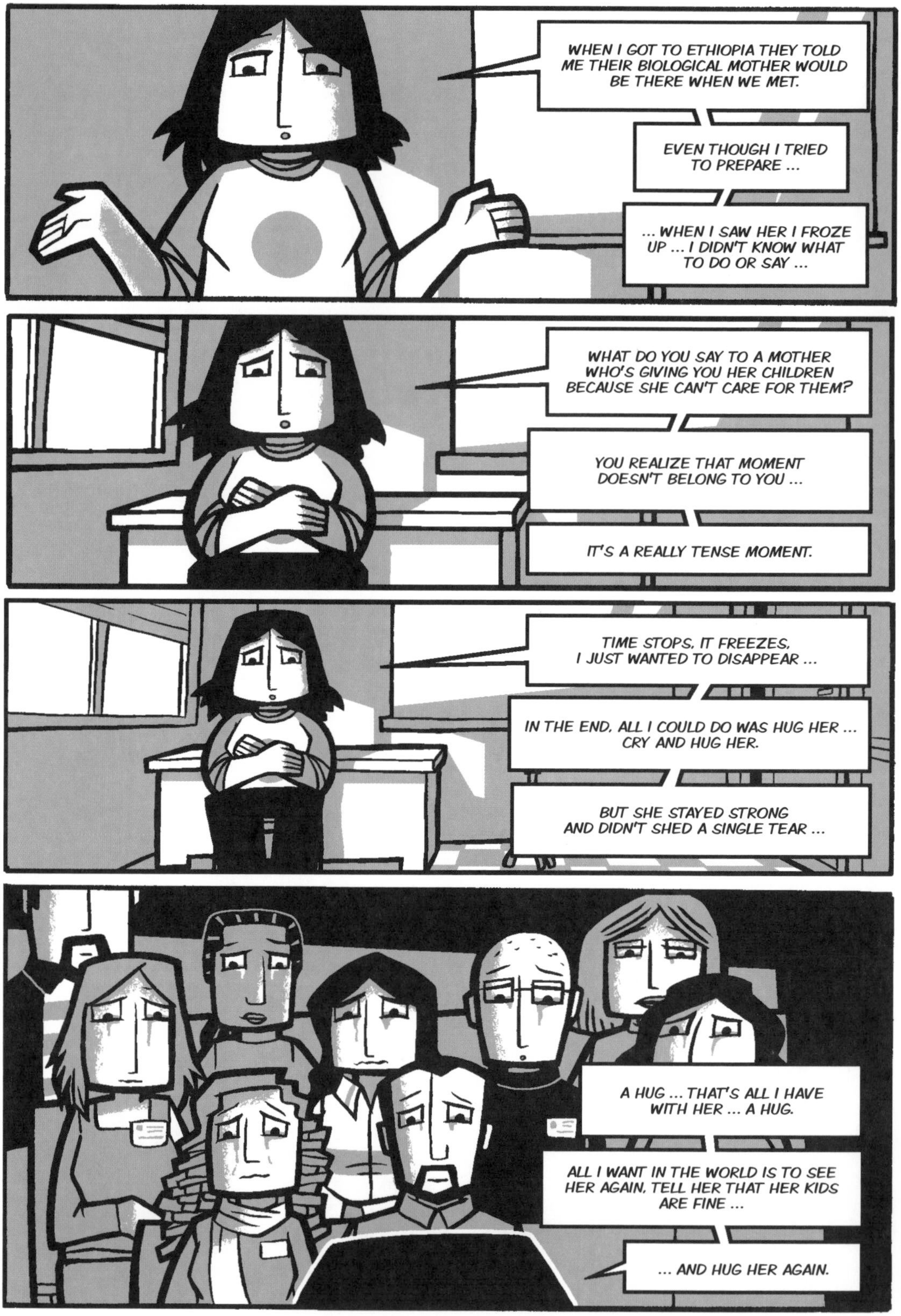
WHEN I GOT TO ETHIOPIA THEY TOLD ME THEIR BIOLOGICAL MOTHER WOULD BE THERE WHEN WE MET.
EVEN THOUGH I TRIED TO PREPARE ...
... WHEN I SAW HER I FROZE UP ... I DIDN'T KNOW WHAT TO DO OR SAY ...
WHAT DO YOU SAY TO A MOTHER WHO'S GIVING YOU HER CHILDREN BECAUSE SHE CAN'T CARE FOR THEM?
YOU REALIZE THAT MOMENT DOESN'T BELONG TO YOU ...
IT'S A REALLY TENSE MOMENT.
TIME STOPS, IT FREEZES, I JUST WANTED TO DISAPPEAR ...
IN THE END, ALL I COULD DO WAS HUG HER ... CRY AND HUG HER.
BUT SHE STAYED STRONG AND DIDN'T SHED A SINGLE TEAR ...
A HUG ... THAT'S ALL I HAVE WITH HER ... A HUG.
ALL I WANT IN THE WORLD IS TO SEE HER AGAIN, TELL HER THAT HER KIDS ARE FINE ...
... AND HUG HER AGAIN.

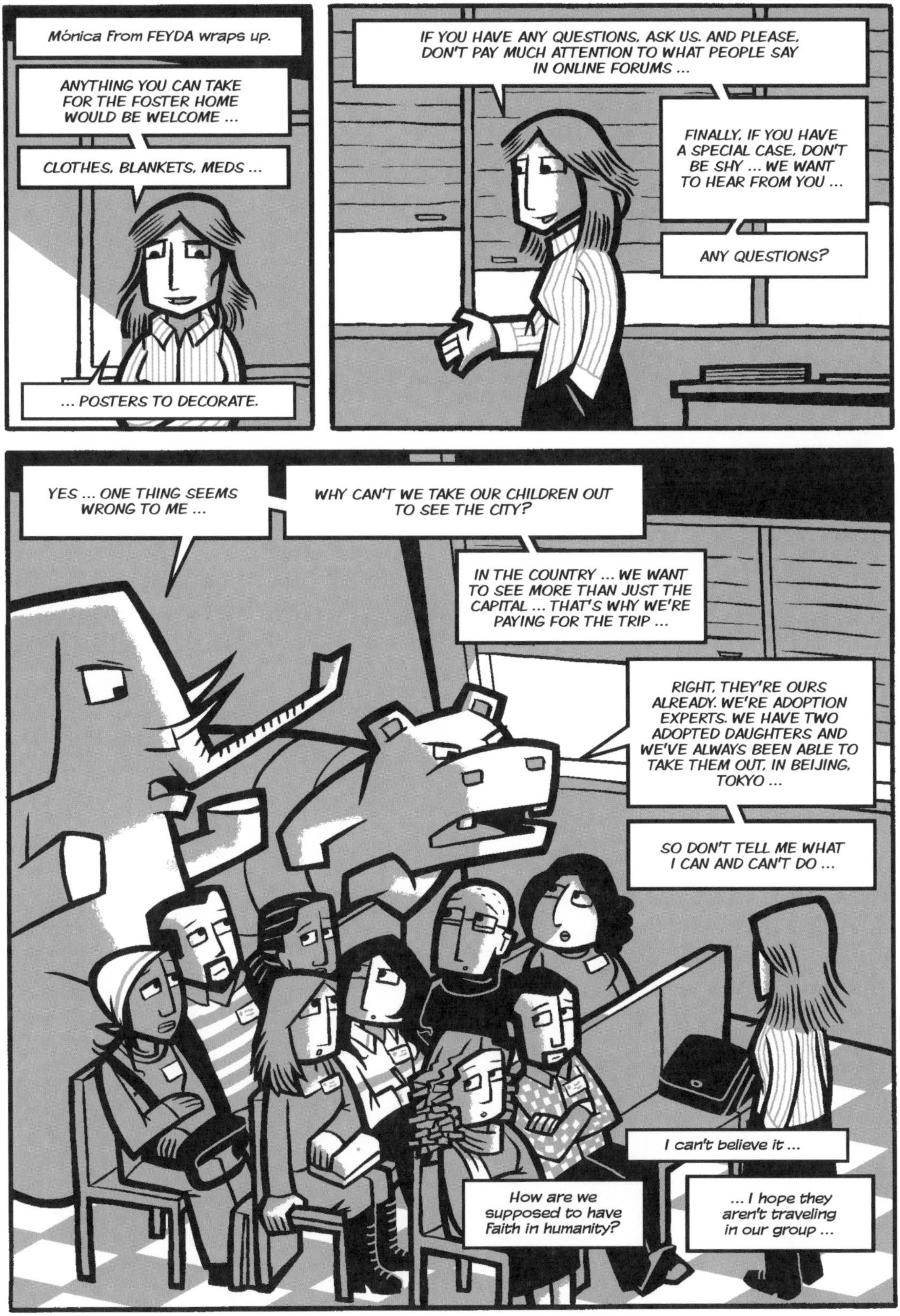
Mónica from FEYDA wraps up.
ANYTHING YOU CAN TAKE FOR THE FOSTER HOME WOULD BE WELCOME ...
CLOTHES, BLANKETS, MEDS ...
... POSTERS TO DECORATE.
IF YOU HAVE ANY QUESTIONS, ASK US. AND PLEASE, DON'T PAY MUCH ATTENTION TO WHAT PEOPLE SAY IN ONLINE FORUMS ...
FINALLY, IF YOU HAVE A SPECIAL CASE, DON'T BE SHY ... WE WANT TO HEAR FROM YOU ...
ANY QUESTIONS?
YES ... ONE THING SEEMS WRONG TO ME ...
WHY CAN'T WE TAKE OUR CHILDREN OUT TO SEE THE CITY?
IN THE COUNTRY ... WE WANT TO SEE MORE THAN JUST THE CAPITAL ... THAT'S WHY WE'RE PAYING FOR THE TRIP ...
RIGHT, THEY'RE OURS ALREADY. WE'RE ADOPTION EXPERTS. WE HAVE TWO ADOPTED DAUGHTERS AND WE'VE ALWAYS BEEN ABLE TO TAKE THEM OUT, IN BEIJING, TOKYO ...
SO DON'T TELL ME WHAT I CAN AND CAN'T DO ...
I can't believe it ...
How are we supposed to have faith in humanity?
... I hope they aren't traveling in our group ...

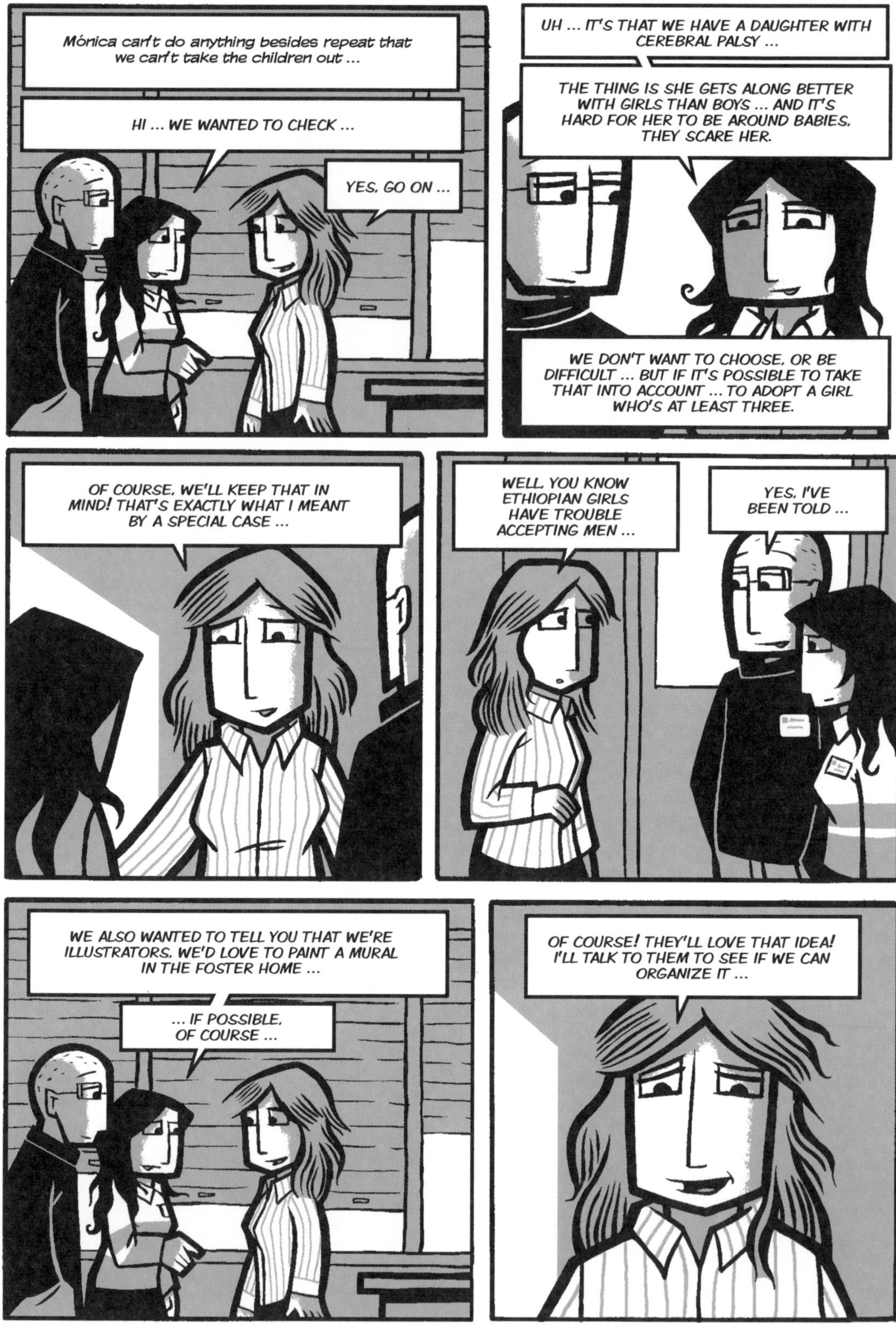
Mónica can't do anything besides repeat that we can't take the children out ...
HI ... WE WANTED TO CHECK ...
YES, GO ON ...
UH ... IT'S THAT WE HAVE A DAUGHTER WITH CEREBRAL PALSY ...
THE THING IS SHE GETS ALONG BETTER WITH GIRLS THAN BOYS ... AND IT'S HARD FOR HER TO BE AROUND BABIES, THEY SCARE HER.
WE DON'T WANT TO CHOOSE, OR BE DIFFICULT ... BUT IF IT'S POSSIBLE TO TAKE THAT INTO ACCOUNT ... TO ADOPT A GIRL WHO'S AT LEAST THREE.
OF COURSE, WE'LL KEEP THAT IN MIND! THAT'S EXACTLY WHAT I MEANT BY A SPECIAL CASE ...
WELL, YOU KNOW ETHIOPIAN GIRLS HAVE TROUBLE ACCEPTING MEN ...
YES, I'VE BEEN TOLD ...
WE ALSO WANTED TO TELL YOU THAT WE'RE ILLUSTRATORS, WE'D LOVE TO PAINT A MURAL IN THE FOSTER HOME ...
... IF POSSIBLE, OF COURSE ...
OF COURSE! THEY'LL LOVE THAT IDEA! I'LL TALK TO THEM TO SEE IF WE CAN ORGANIZE IT ...

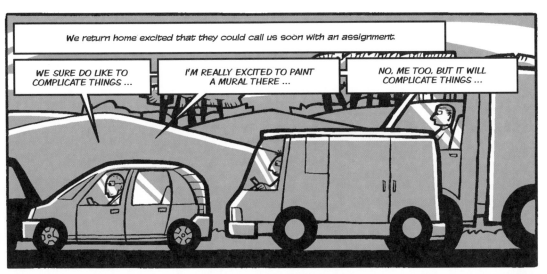

We return home excited that they could call us soon with an assignment.

WE SURE DO LIKE TO COMPLICATE THINGS ...

I'M REALLY EXCITED TO PAINT A MURAL THERE ...

NO, ME TOO, BUT IT WILL COMPLICATE THINGS ...

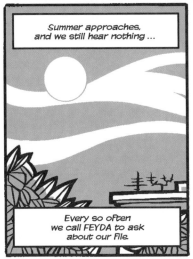

Summer approaches, and we still hear nothing ...

Every so often we call FEYDA to ask about our File.

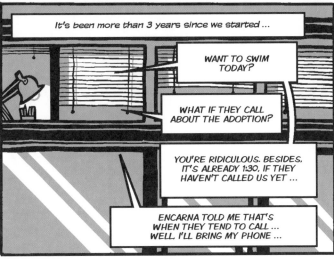

It's been more than 3 years since we started ...

WANT TO SWIM TODAY?

WHAT IF THEY CALL ABOUT THE ADOPTION?

YOU'RE RIDICULOUS. BESIDES, IT'S ALREADY 1:30, IF THEY HAVEN'T CALLED US YET ...

ENCARNA TOLD ME THAT'S WHEN THEY TEND TO CALL ... WELL I'LL BRING MY PHONE ...

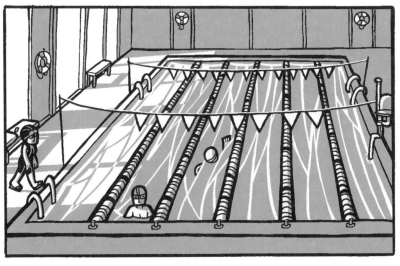

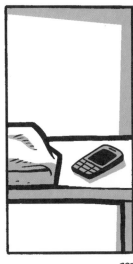

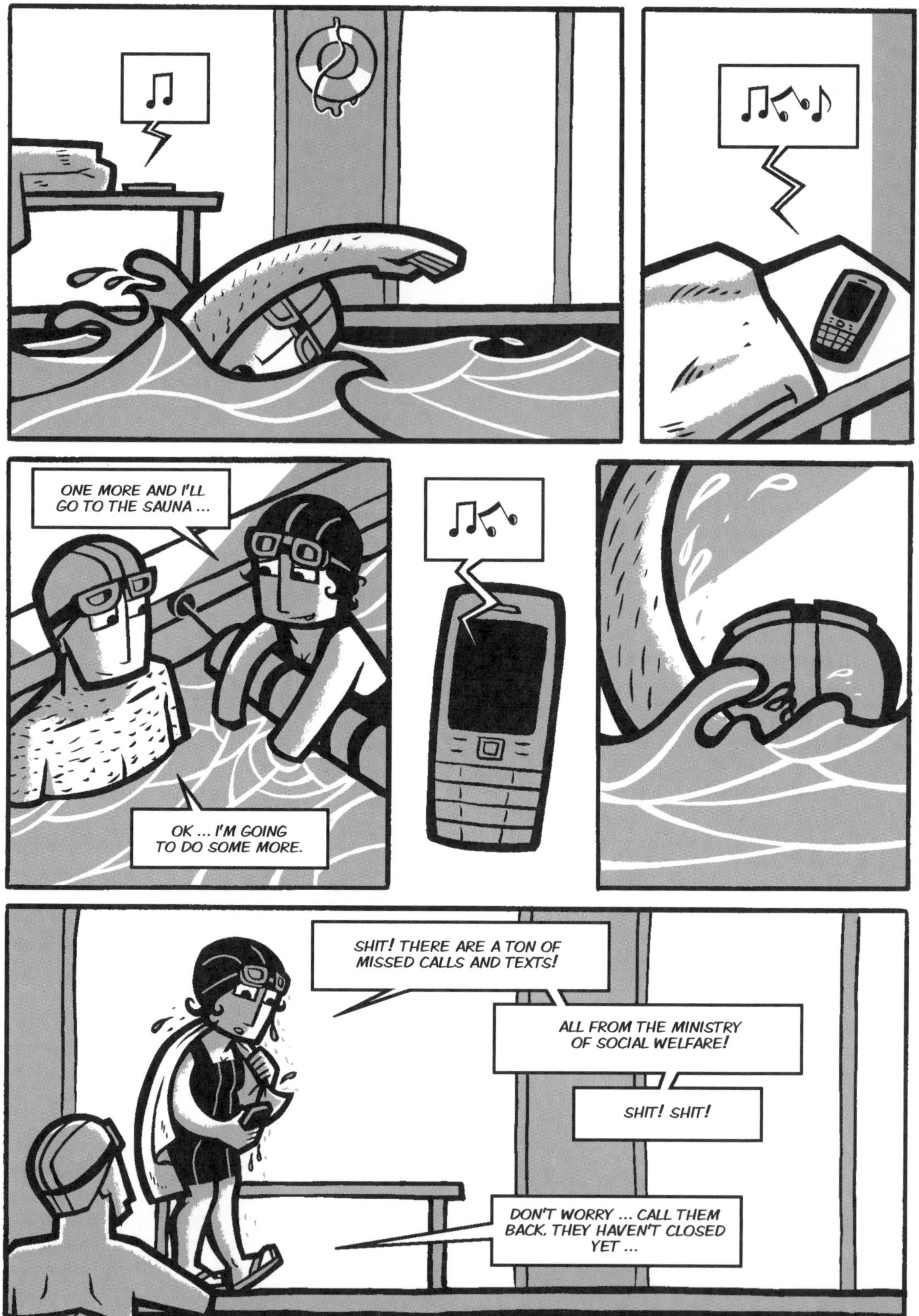
ONE MORE AND I'LL GO TO THE SAUNA ...
OK ... I'M GOING TO DO SOME MORE.
SHIT! THERE ARE A TON OF MISSED CALLS AND TEXTS!
ALL FROM THE MINISTRY OF SOCIAL WELFARE!
SHIT! SHIT!
DON'T WORRY ... CALL THEM BACK. THEY HAVEN'T CLOSED YET ...

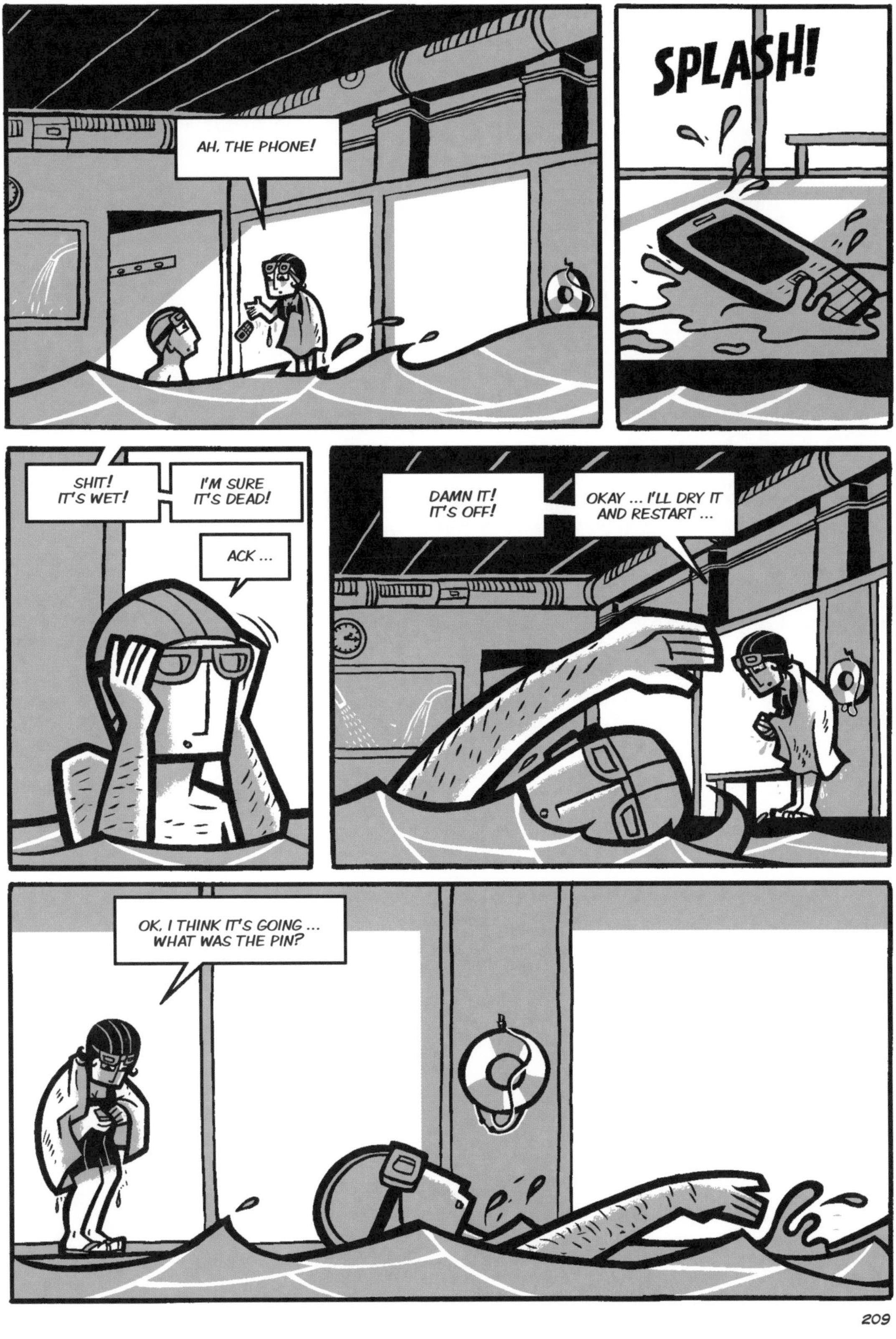
AH, THE PHONE!
SPLASH!
SHIT! IT'S WET!
I'M SURE IT'S DEAD!
ACK ...
DAMN IT! IT'S OFF!
OKAY ... I'LL DRY IT AND RESTART ...
OK, I THINK IT'S GOING ... WHAT WAS THE PIN?

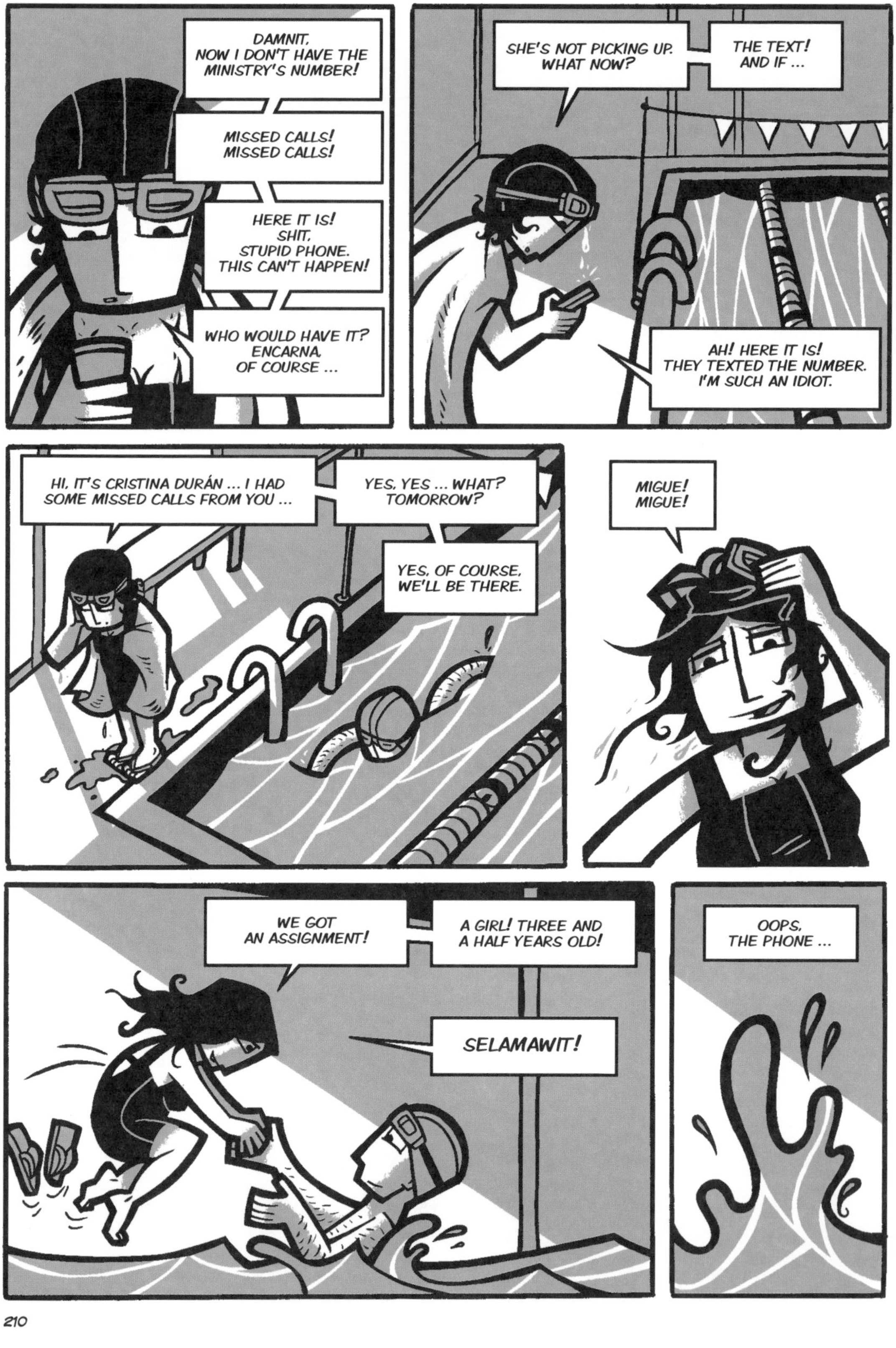
DAMNIT, NOW I DON'T HAVE THE MINISTRY'S NUMBER!
MISSED CALLS! MISSED CALLS!
HERE IT IS! SHIT, STUPID PHONE. THIS CAN'T HAPPEN!
WHO WOULD HAVE IT? ENCARNA, OF COURSE ...
SHE'S NOT PICKING UP. WHAT NOW?
THE TEXT! AND IF ...
AH! HERE IT IS! THEY TEXTED THE NUMBER. I'M SUCH AN IDIOT.
HI, IT'S CRISTINA DURÁN ... I HAD SOME MISSED CALLS FROM YOU ...
YES, YES ... WHAT? TOMORROW?
YES, OF COURSE, WE'LL BE THERE.
MIGUE! MIGUE!
WE GOT AN ASSIGNMENT!
A GIRL! THREE AND A HALF YEARS OLD!
SELAMAWIT!
OOPS, THE PHONE ...

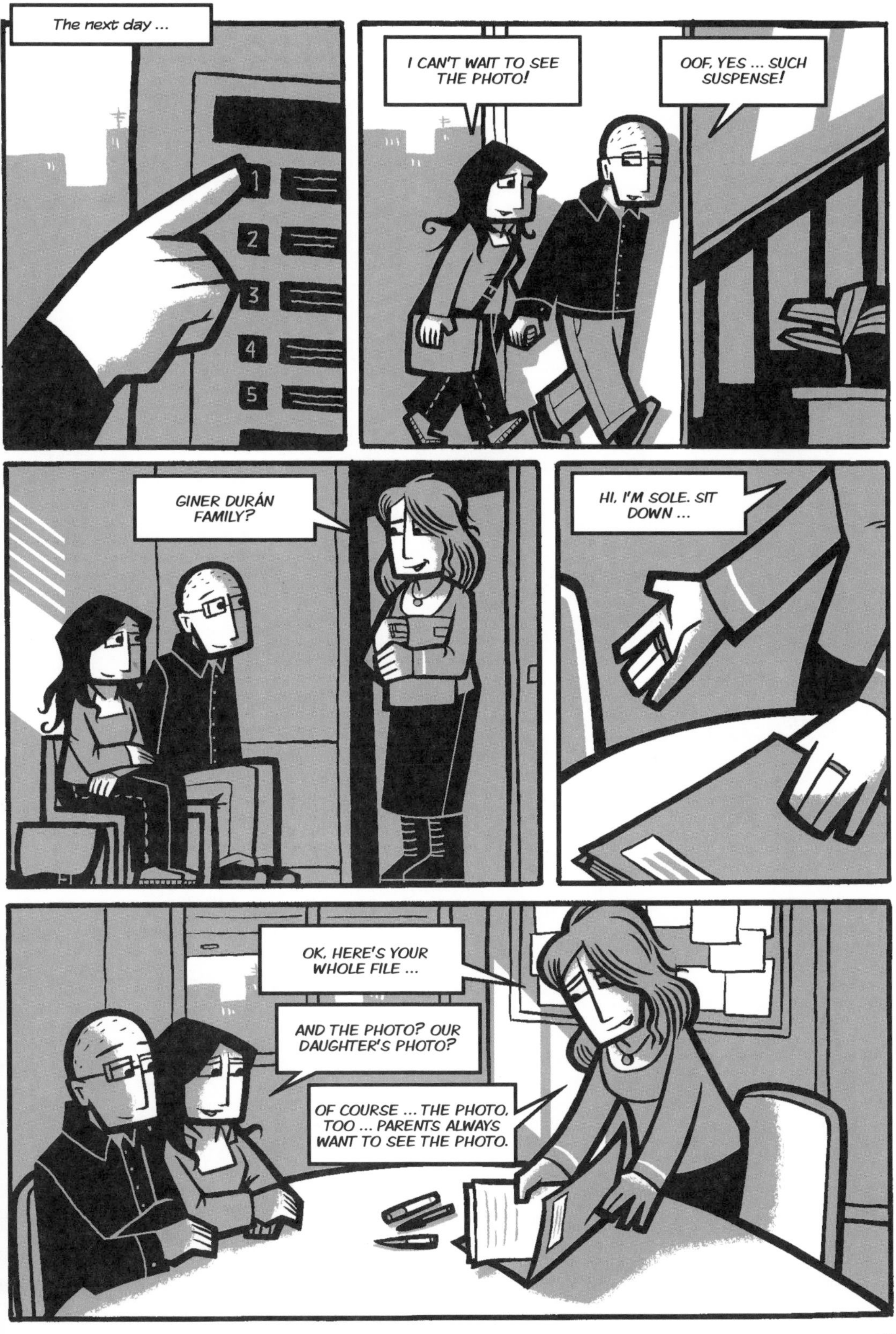
The next day ...
I CAN'T WAIT TO SEE THE PHOTO!
OOF, YES ... SUCH SUSPENSE!
GINER DURÁN FAMILY?
HI, I'M SOLE. SIT DOWN ...
OK, HERE'S YOUR WHOLE FILE ...
AND THE PHOTO? OUR DAUGHTER'S PHOTO?
OF COURSE ... THE PHOTO, TOO ... PARENTS ALWAYS WANT TO SEE THE PHOTO.

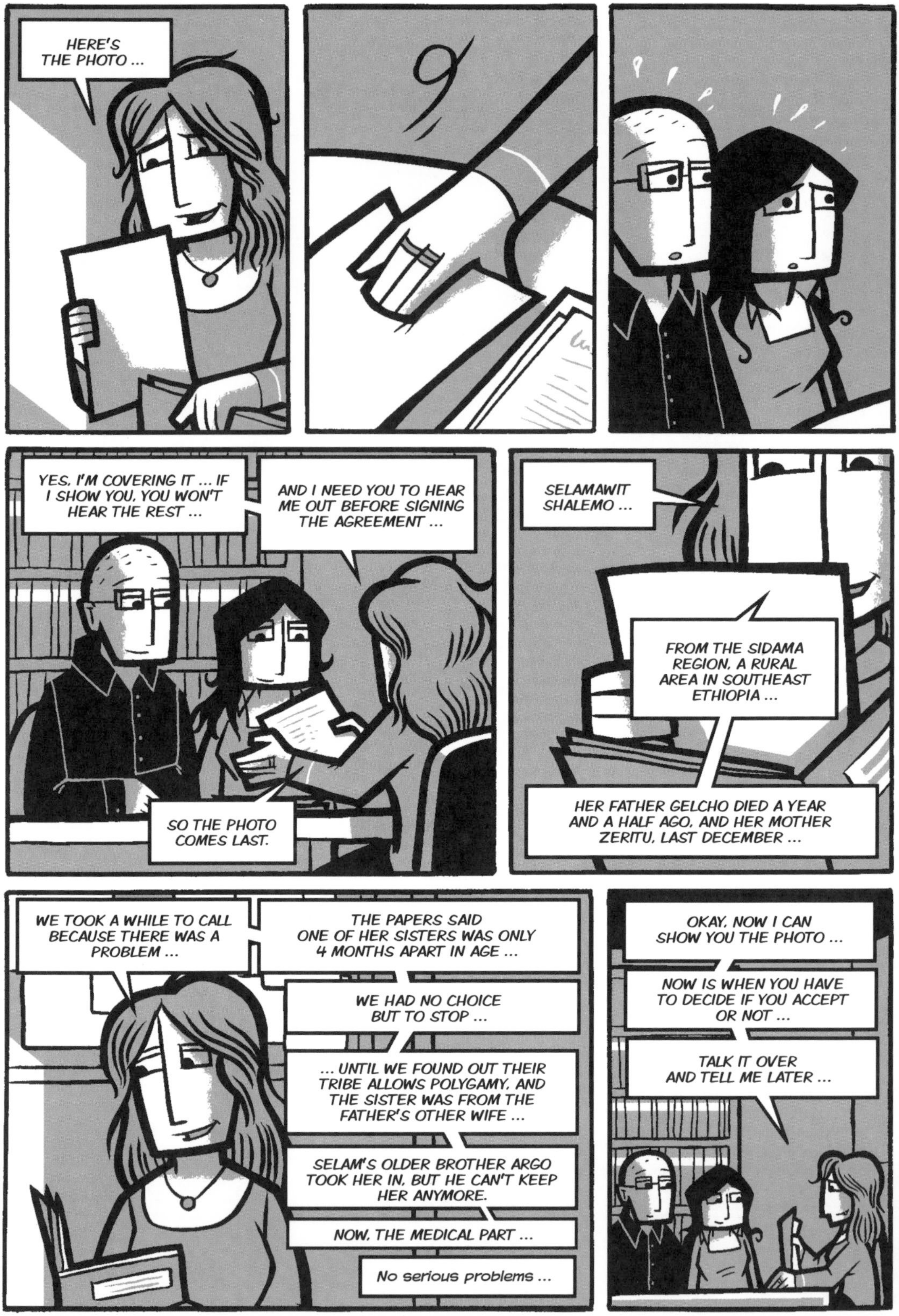
HERE'S THE PHOTO ...
YES, I'M COVERING IT ... IF I SHOW YOU, YOU WON'T HEAR THE REST ...
AND I NEED YOU TO HEAR ME OUT BEFORE SIGNING THE AGREEMENT ...
SO THE PHOTO COMES LAST.
SELAMAWIT SHALEMO ...
FROM THE SIDAMA REGION, A RURAL AREA IN SOUTHEAST ETHIOPIA ...
HER FATHER GELCHO DIED A YEAR AND A HALF AGO, AND HER MOTHER ZERITU, LAST DECEMBER ...
WE TOOK A WHILE TO CALL BECAUSE THERE WAS A PROBLEM ...
THE PAPERS SAID ONE OF HER SISTERS WAS ONLY 4 MONTHS APART IN AGE ...
WE HAD NO CHOICE BUT TO STOP ...
... UNTIL WE FOUND OUT THEIR TRIBE ALLOWS POLYGAMY, AND THE SISTER WAS FROM THE FATHER'S OTHER WIFE ...
SELAM'S OLDER BROTHER ARGO TOOK HER IN, BUT HE CAN'T KEEP HER ANYMORE.
NOW, THE MEDICAL PART ...
No serious problems ...
OKAY, NOW I CAN SHOW YOU THE PHOTO ...
NOW IS WHEN YOU HAVE TO DECIDE IF YOU ACCEPT OR NOT ...
TALK IT OVER AND TELL ME LATER ...

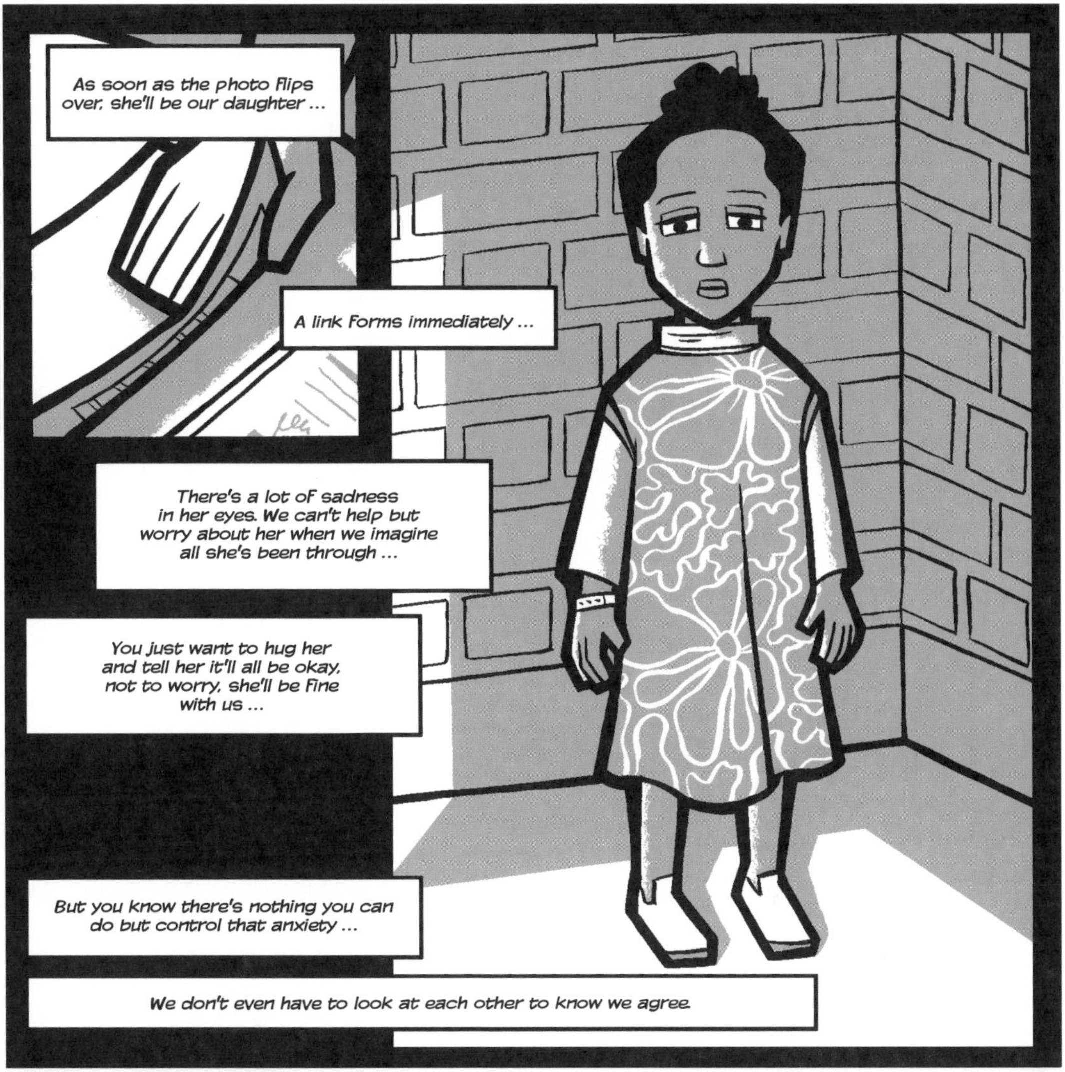
As soon as the photo flips over, she'll be our daughter ...
A link forms immediately ...
There's a lot of sadness in her eyes. We can't help but worry about her when we imagine all she's been through ...
You just want to hug her and tell her it'll all be okay, not to worry, she'll be fine with us ...
But you know there's nothing you can do but control that anxiety ...
We don't even have to look at each other to know we agree.

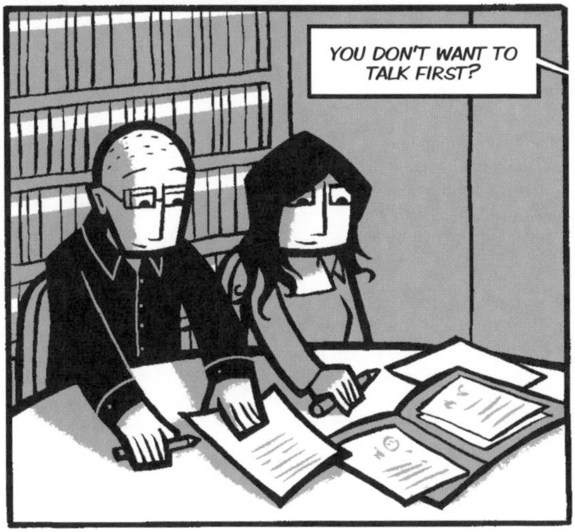
YOU DON'T WANT TO TALK FIRST?

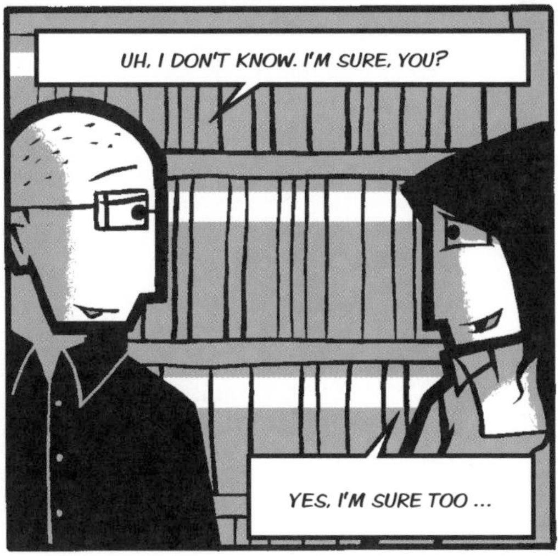
UH, I DON'T KNOW. I'M SURE, YOU?
YES, I'M SURE TOO ...

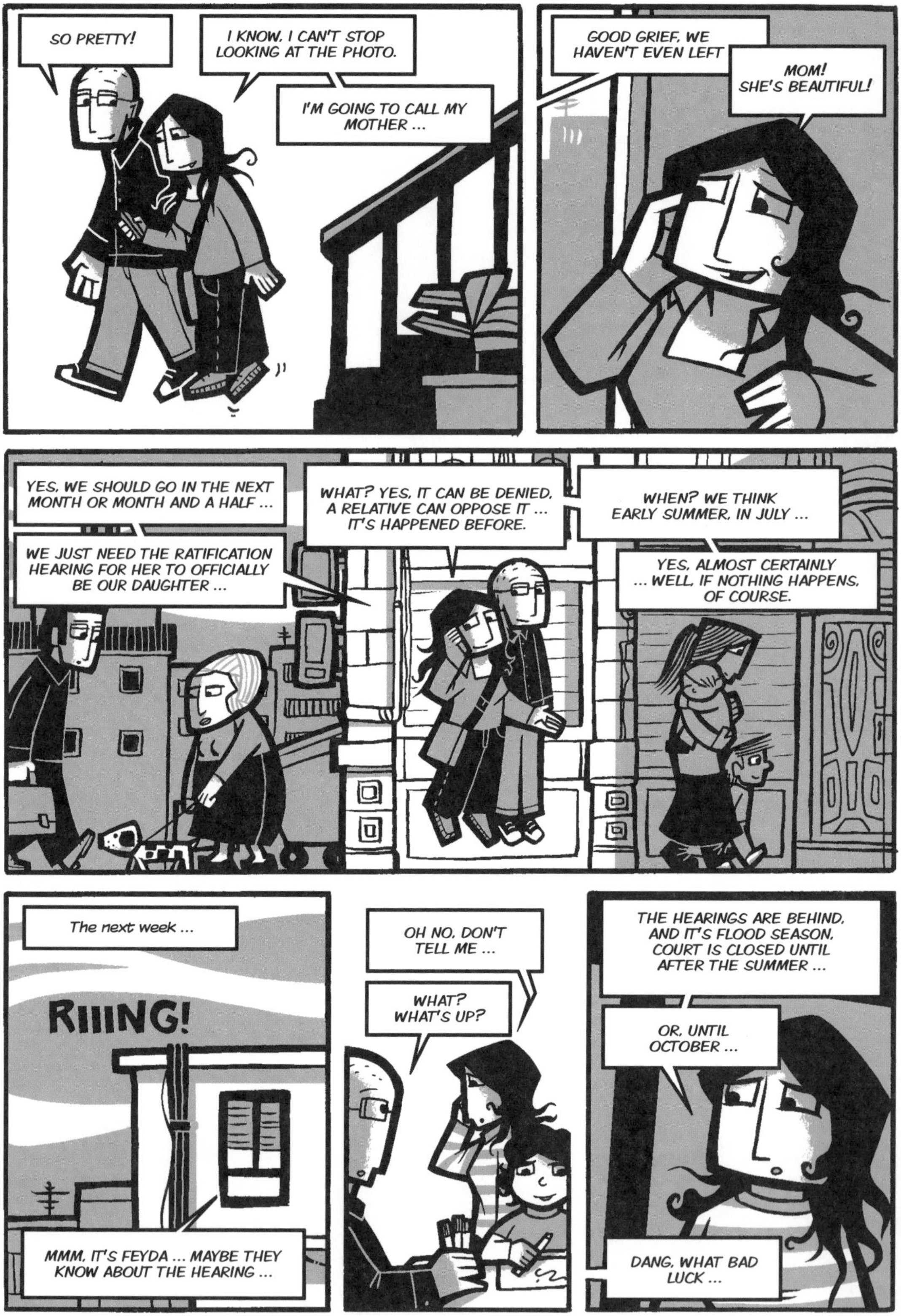
SO PRETTY!
I KNOW, I CAN'T STOP LOOKING AT THE PHOTO.
I'M GOING TO CALL MY MOTHER ...
GOOD GRIEF, WE HAVEN'T EVEN LEFT
MOM! SHE'S BEAUTIFUL!
YES, WE SHOULD GO IN THE NEXT MONTH OR MONTH AND A HALF ...
WE JUST NEED THE RATIFICATION HEARING FOR HER TO OFFICIALLY BE OUR DAUGHTER ...
WHAT? YES, IT CAN BE DENIED, A RELATIVE CAN OPPOSE IT ... IT'S HAPPENED BEFORE.
WHEN? WE THINK EARLY SUMMER, IN JULY ...
YES, ALMOST CERTAINLY ... WELL, IF NOTHING HAPPENS, OF COURSE.
The next week ...
RIIING!
MMM, IT'S FEYDA ... MAYBE THEY KNOW ABOUT THE HEARING ...
OH NO, DON'T TELL ME ...
WHAT? WHAT'S UP?
THE HEARINGS ARE BEHIND, AND IT'S FLOOD SEASON, COURT IS CLOSED UNTIL AFTER THE SUMMER ...
OR, UNTIL OCTOBER ...
DANG, WHAT BAD LUCK ...

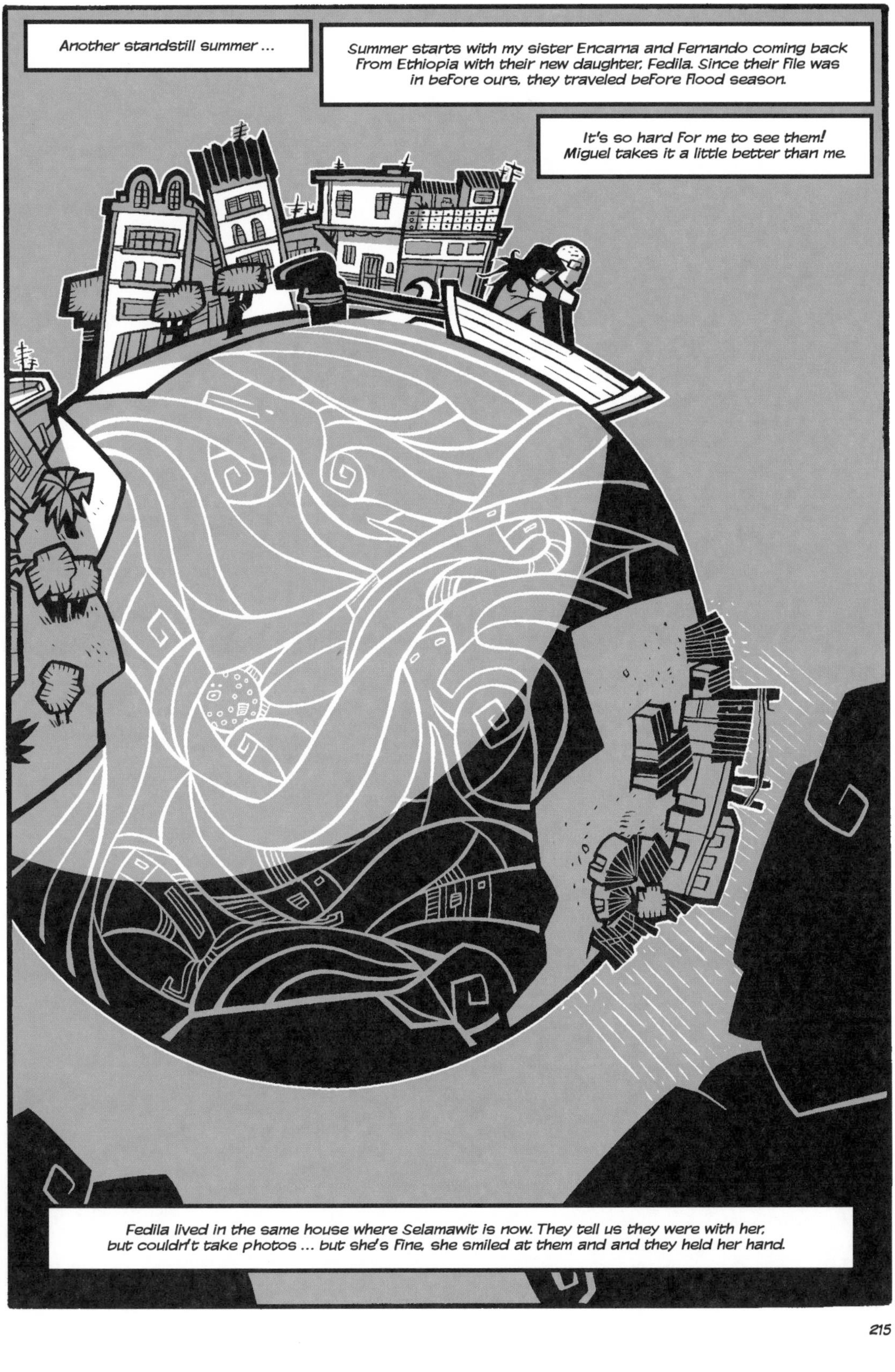
Another standstill summer ...
Summer starts with my sister Encarna and Fernando coming back from Ethiopia with their new daughter, Fedila. Since their file was in before ours, they traveled before flood season.
It's so hard for me to see them! Miguel takes it a little better than me.
Fedila lived in the same house where Selamawit is now. They tell us they were with her, but couldn't take photos ... but she's fine, she smiled at them and and they held her hand.

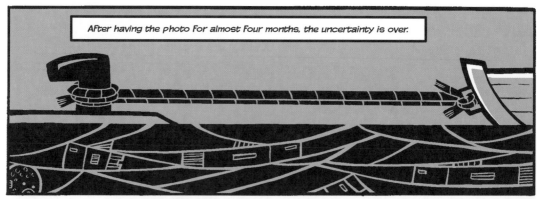

After having the photo for almost four months, the uncertainty is over.

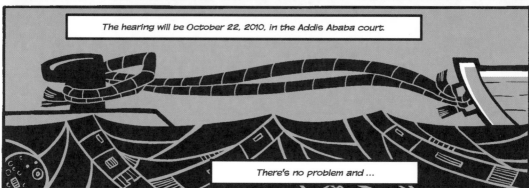

The hearing will be October 22, 2010, in the Addis Ababa court.

There's no problem and ...

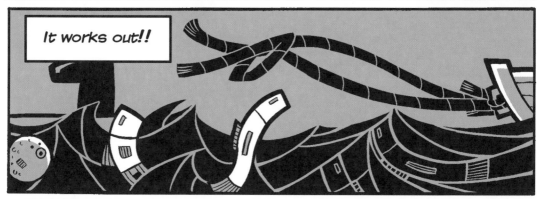

It works out!!

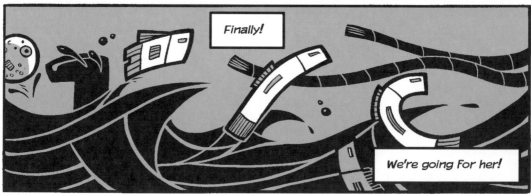

Finally!

We're going for her!

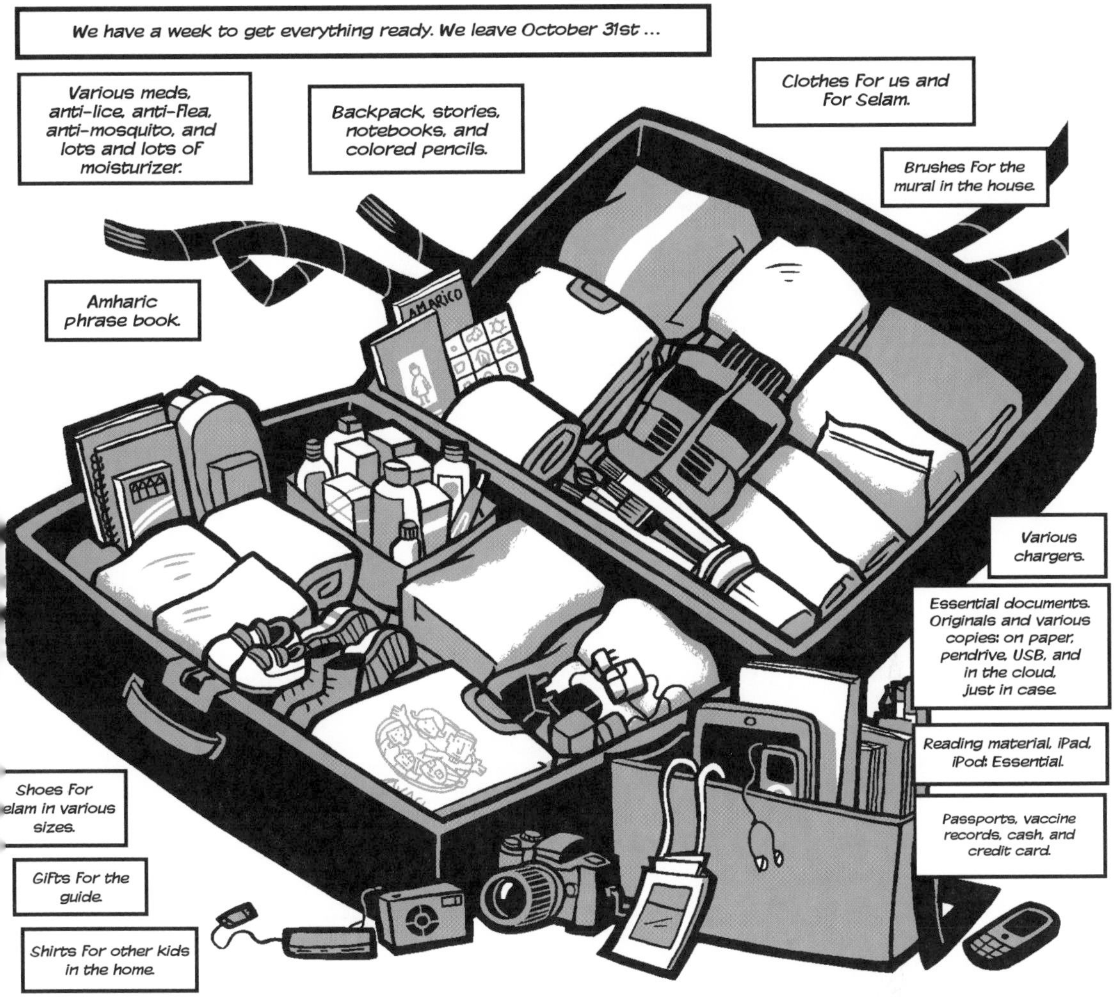
We have a week to get everything ready. We leave October 31st ...
Various meds, anti-lice, anti-flea, anti-mosquito, and lots and lots of moisturizer.
Backpack, stories, notebooks, and colored pencils.
Clothes for us and for Selam.
Brushes for the mural in the house.
Amharic phrase book.
AMARICO
Various chargers.
Essential documents. Originals and various copies: on paper, pendrive, USB, and in the cloud, just in case.
Reading material, iPad, iPod: Essential.
Passports, vaccine records, cash, and credit card.
Shoes for elam in various sizes.
Gifts for the guide.
Shirts for other kids in the home.

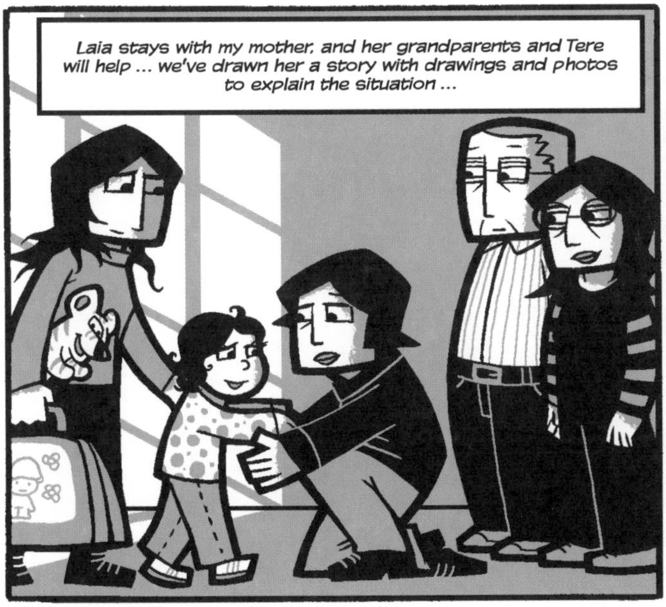
Laia stays with my mother, and her grandparents and Tere will help ... we've drawn her a story with drawings and photos to explain the situation ...

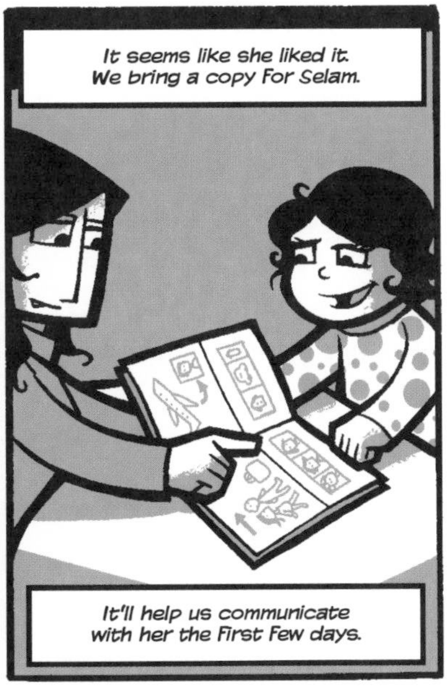
It seems like she liked it. We bring a copy for Selam.
It'll help us communicate with her the first few days.

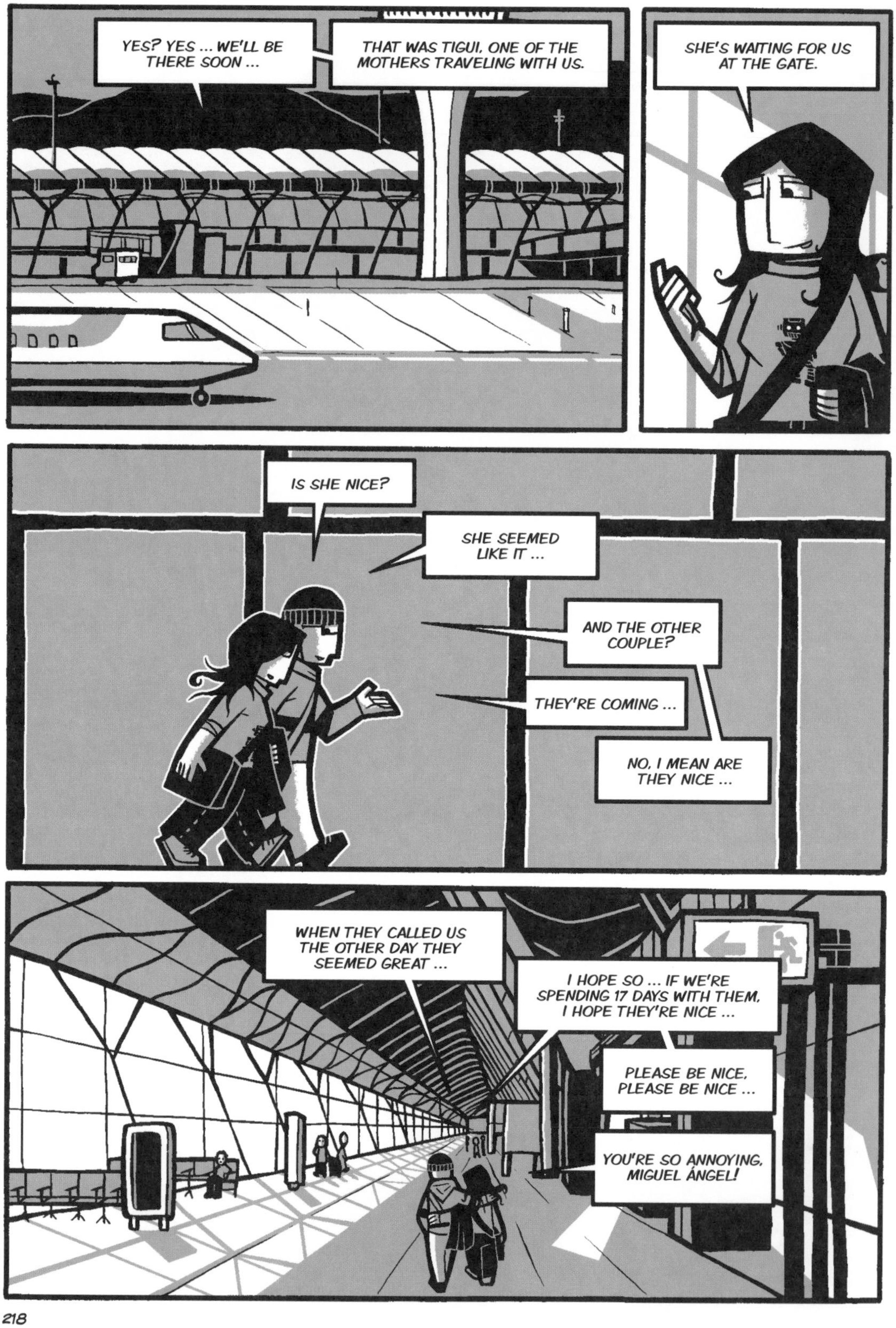
YES? YES ... WE'LL BE THERE SOON ...
THAT WAS TIGUI, ONE OF THE MOTHERS TRAVELING WITH US.
SHE'S WAITING FOR US AT THE GATE.
IS SHE NICE?
SHE SEEMED LIKE IT ...
AND THE OTHER COUPLE?
THEY'RE COMING ...
NO, I MEAN ARE THEY NICE ...
WHEN THEY CALLED US THE OTHER DAY THEY SEEMED GREAT ...
I HOPE SO ... IF WE'RE SPENDING 17 DAYS WITH THEM, I HOPE THEY'RE NICE ...
PLEASE BE NICE, PLEASE BE NICE ...
YOU'RE SO ANNOYING, MIGUEL ÁNGEL!

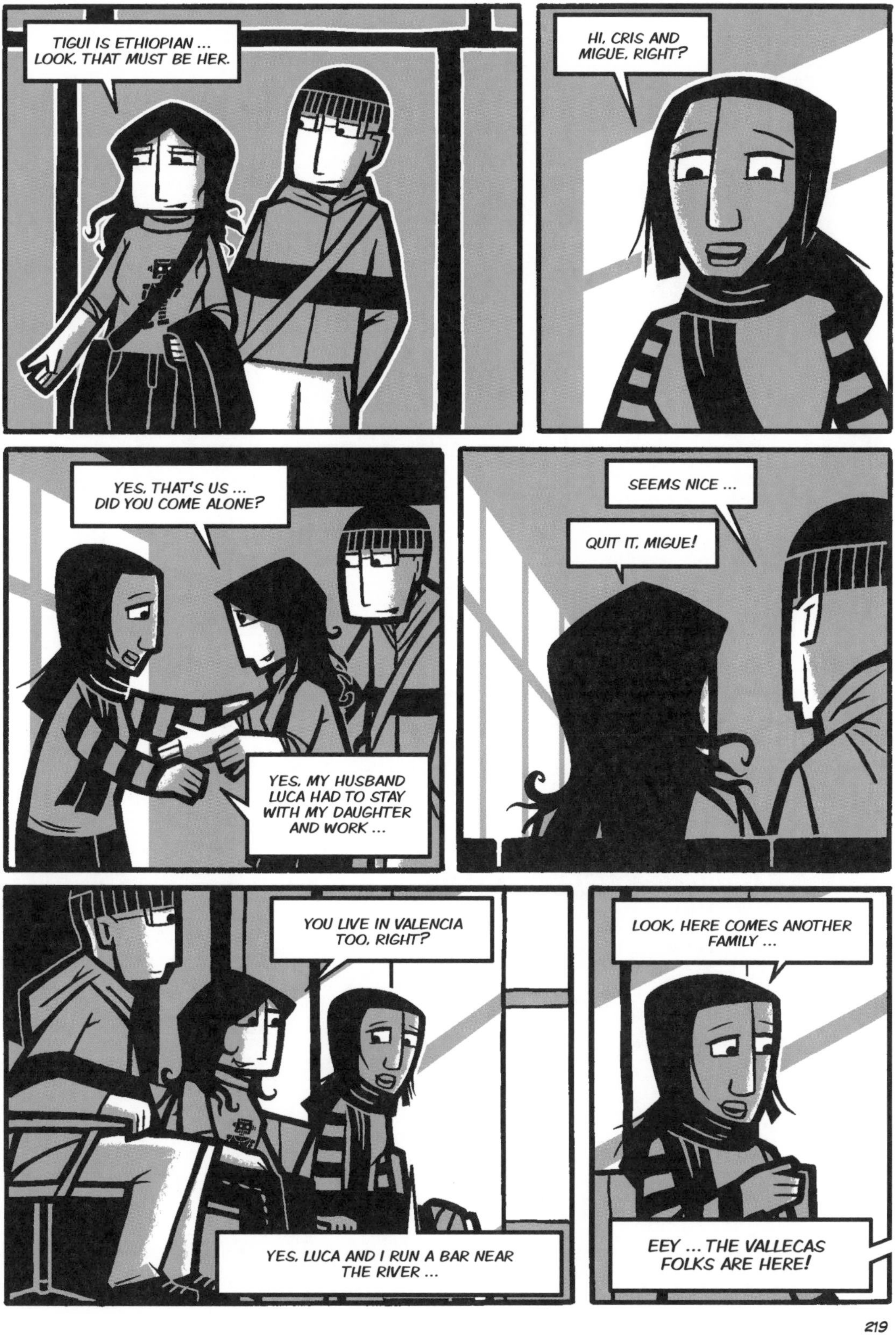
TIGUI IS ETHIOPIAN ... LOOK, THAT MUST BE HER.
HI, CRIS AND MIGUE, RIGHT?
YES, THAT'S US ... DID YOU COME ALONE?
YES, MY HUSBAND LUCA HAD TO STAY WITH MY DAUGHTER AND WORK ...
SEEMS NICE ...
QUIT IT, MIGUE!
YOU LIVE IN VALENCIA TOO, RIGHT?
YES, LUCA AND I RUN A BAR NEAR THE RIVER ...
LOOK, HERE COMES ANOTHER FAMILY ...
EEY ... THE VALLECAS FOLKS ARE HERE!

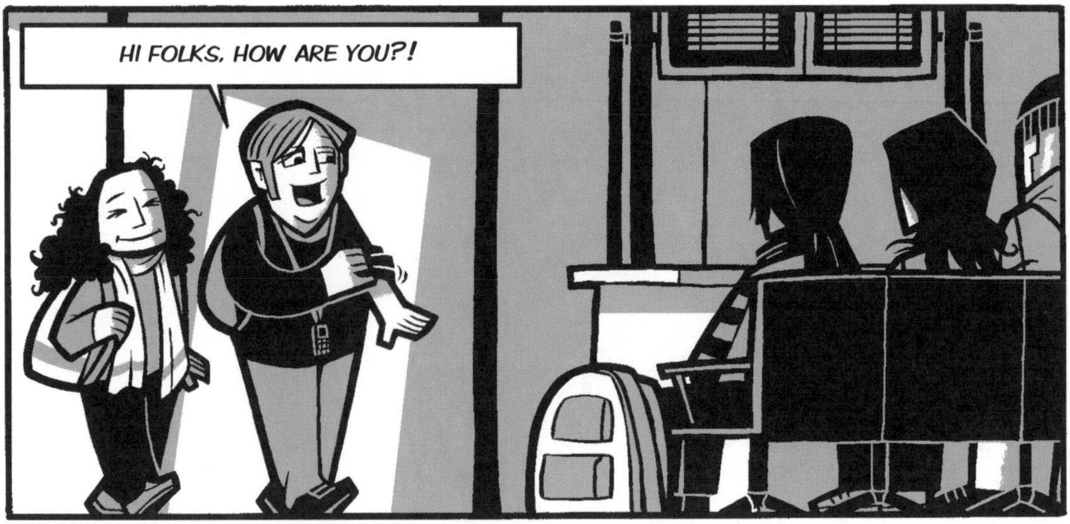
HI FOLKS, HOW ARE YOU?!

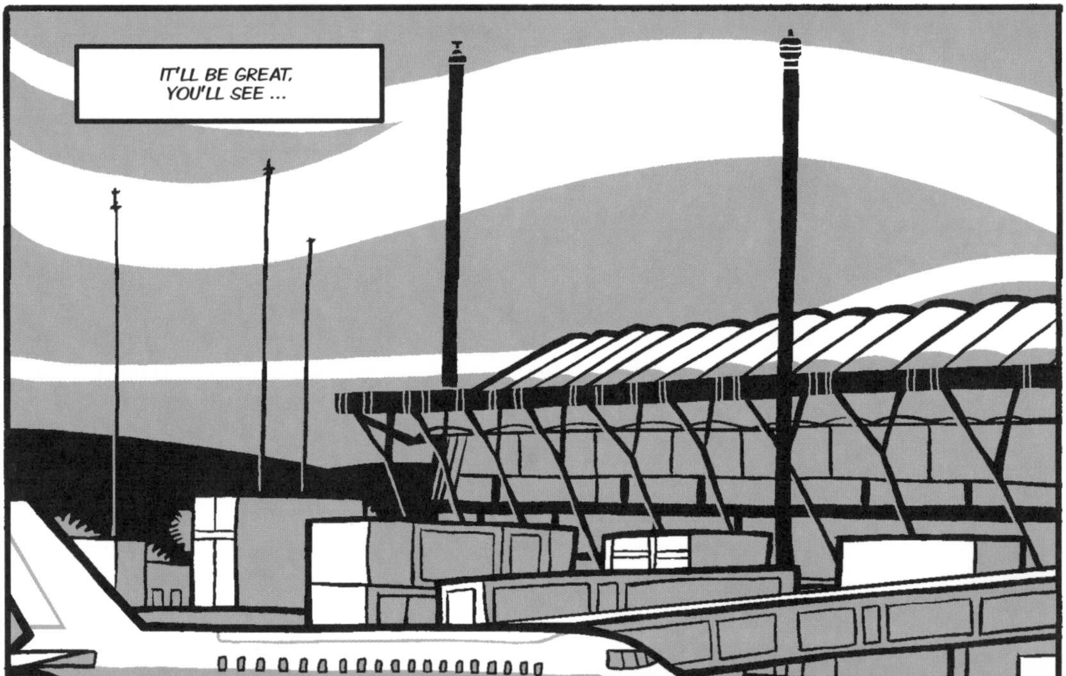
IT'LL BE GREAT, YOU'LL SEE ...

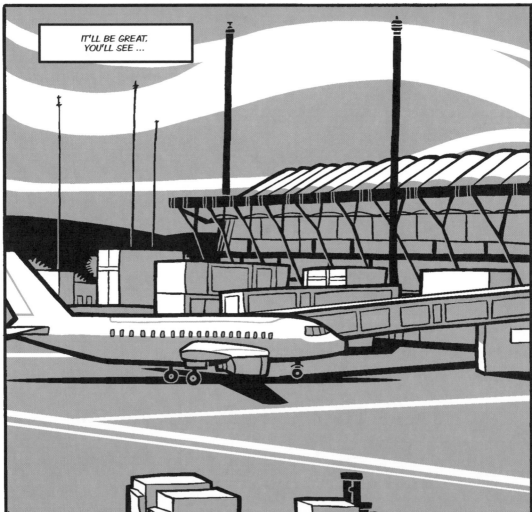

Chapter 6
THE MEET-UP

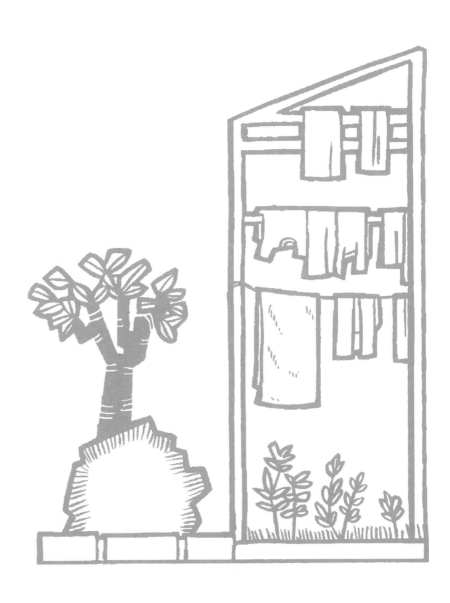

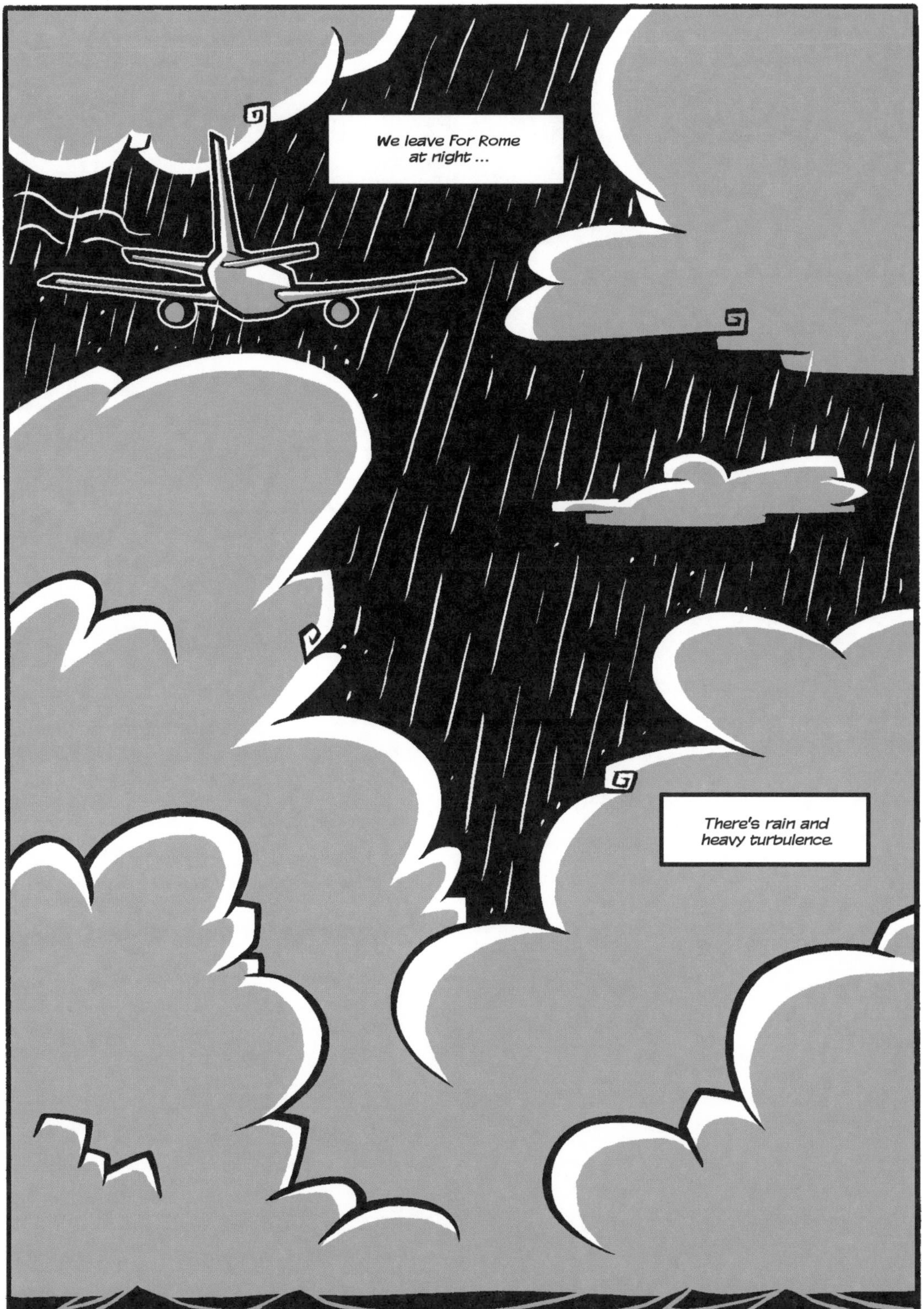
We leave for Rome at night ...
There's rain and heavy turbulence.

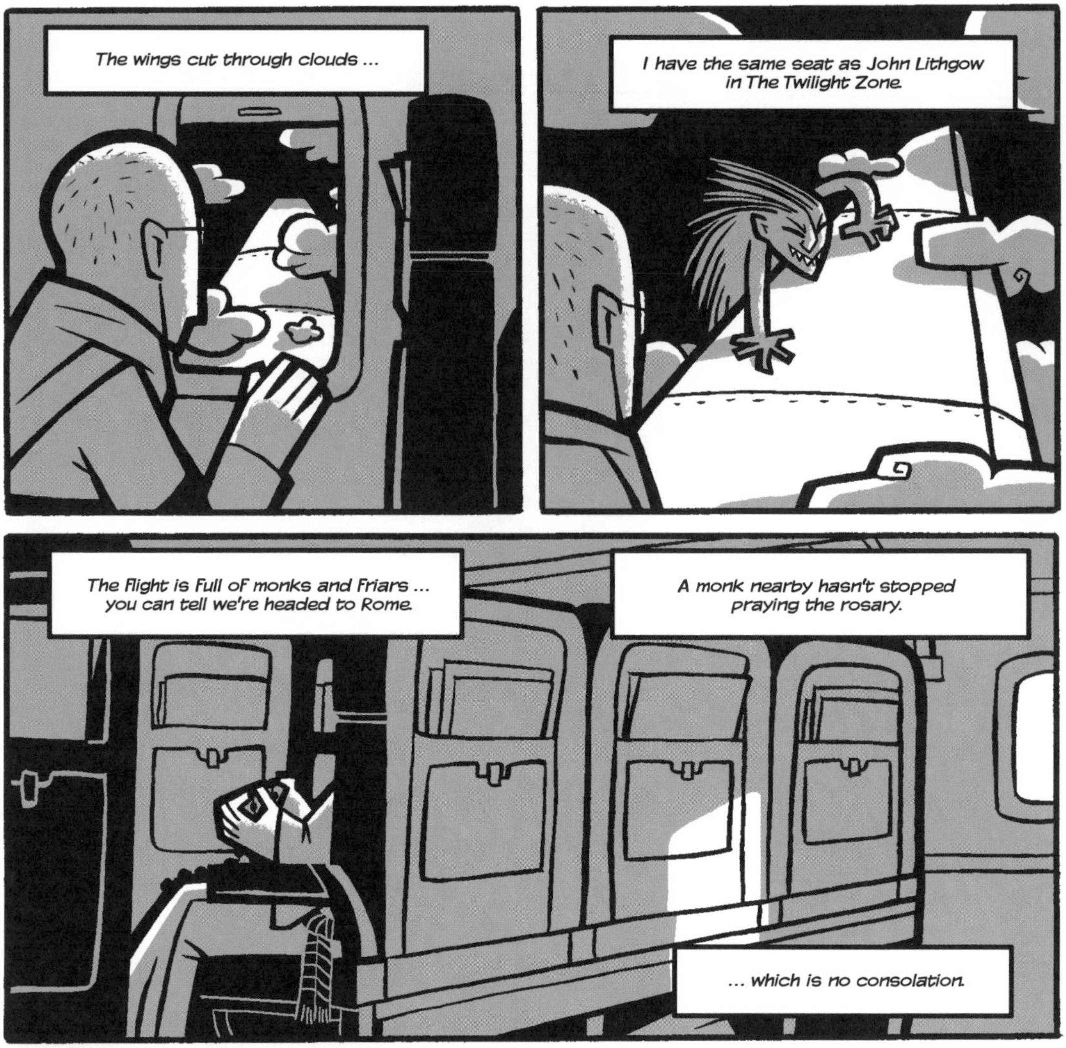
The wings cut through clouds ...
I have the same seat as John Lithgow in The Twilight Zone.
The flight is full of monks and friars ... you can tell we're headed to Rome.
A monk nearby hasn't stopped praying the rosary.
... which is no consolation.
IF something happens, I'll make his boss answer for it ...

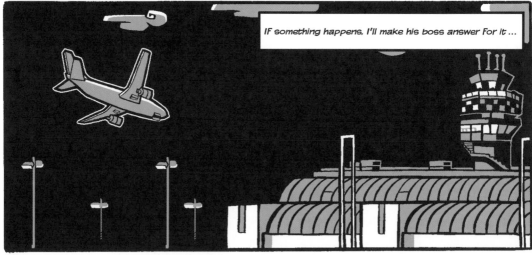

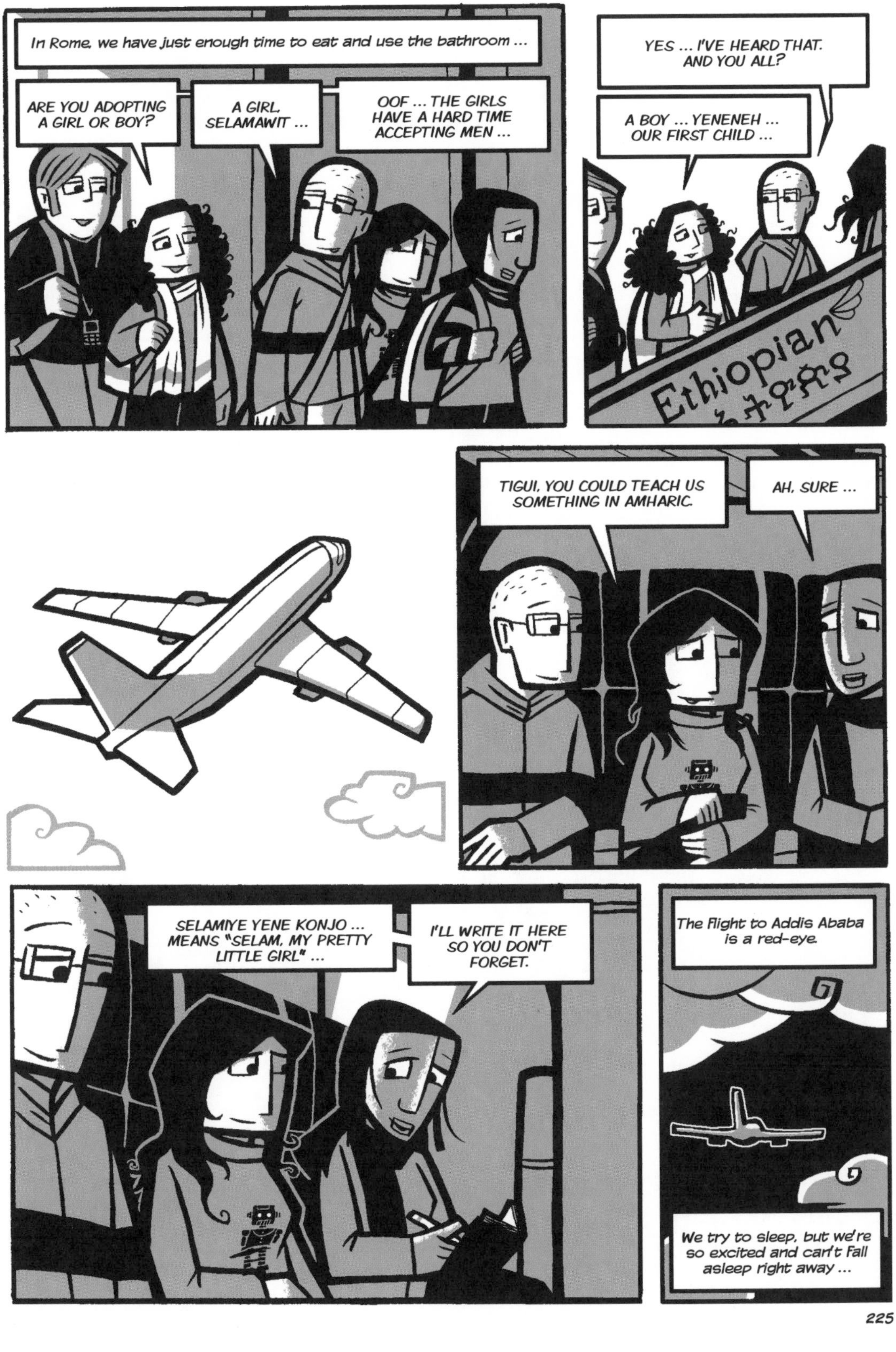
In Rome, we have just enough time to eat and use the bathroom ...
ARE YOU ADOPTING A GIRL OR BOY?
A GIRL, SELAMAWIT ...
OOF ... THE GIRLS HAVE A HARD TIME ACCEPTING MEN ...
YES ... I'VE HEARD THAT. AND YOU ALL?
A BOY ... YENENEH ... OUR FIRST CHILD ...
Ethiopian
TIGUI, YOU COULD TEACH US SOMETHING IN AMHARIC.
AH, SURE ...
SELAMIYE YENE KONJO ... MEANS "SELAM, MY PRETTY LITTLE GIRL" ...
I'LL WRITE IT HERE SO YOU DON'T FORGET.
The flight to Addis Ababa is a red-eye.
We try to sleep, but we're so excited and can't fall asleep right away ...

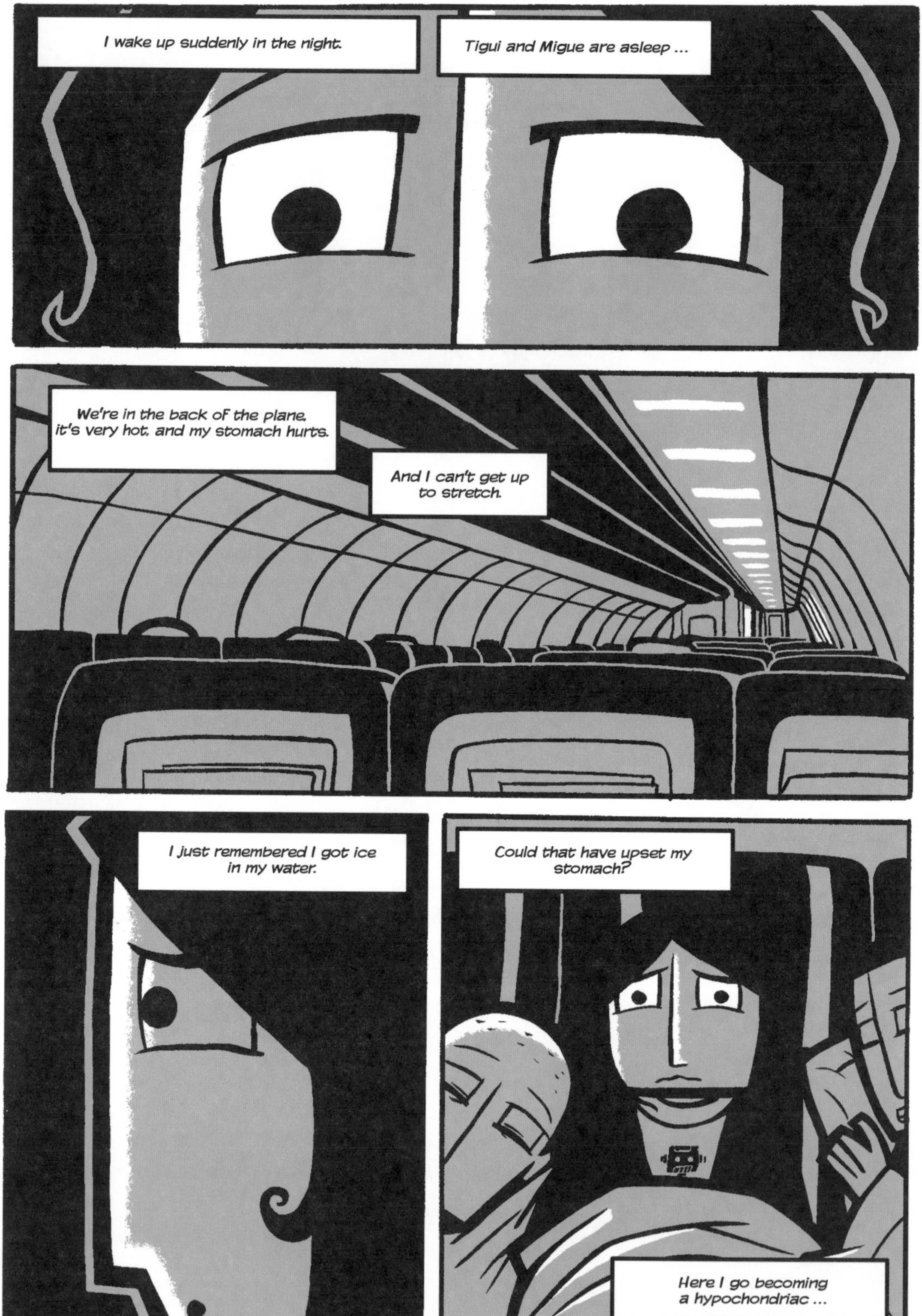
I wake up suddenly in the night.
Tigui and Migue are asleep ...
We're in the back of the plane, it's very hot, and my stomach hurts.
And I can't get up to stretch.
I just remembered I got ice in my water.
Could that have upset my stomach?
Here I go becoming a hypochondriac ...

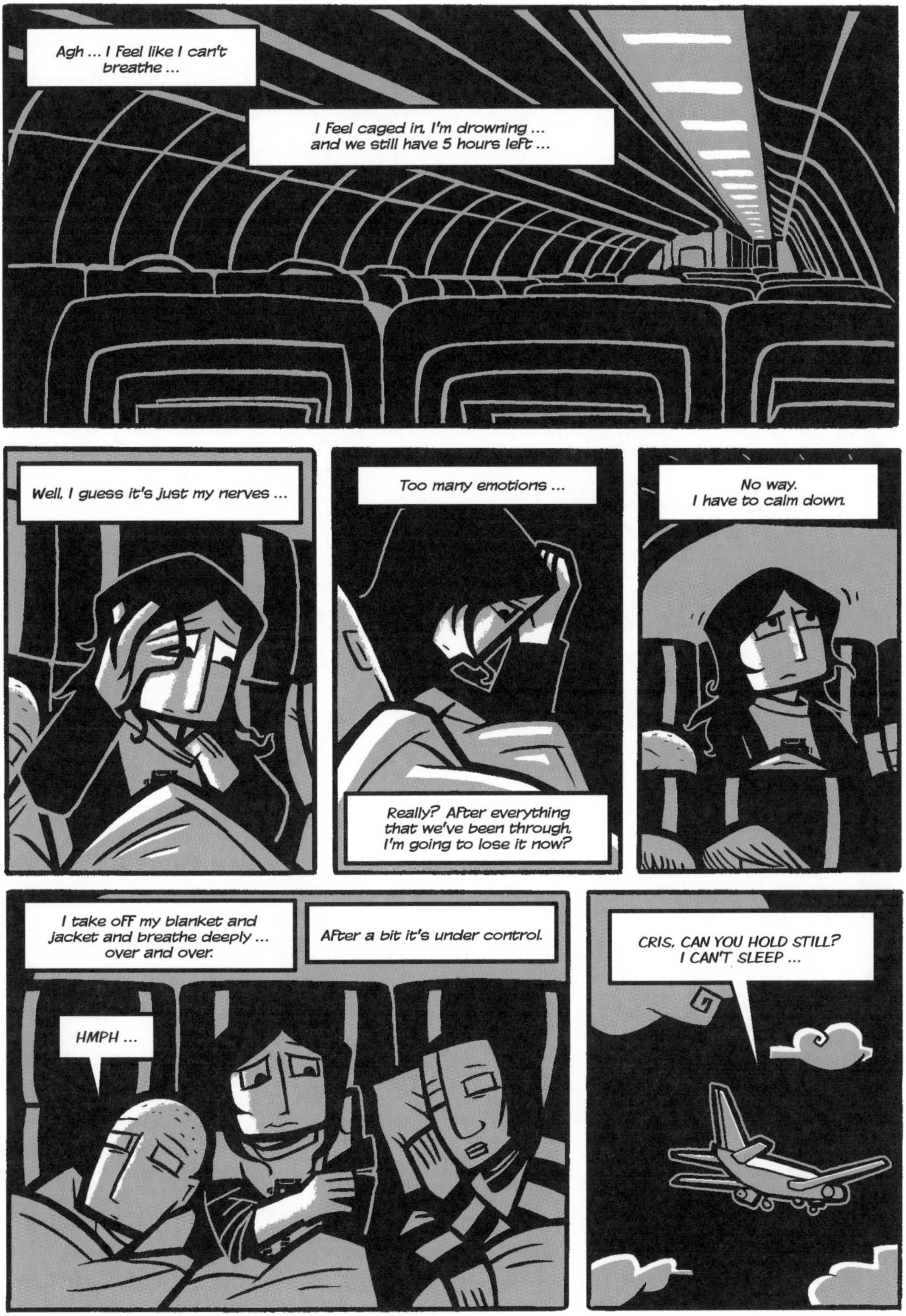
Agh ... I Feel like I can't breathe ...
I Feel caged in, I'm drowning ... and we still have 5 hours left ...
Well, I guess it's just my nerves ...
Too many emotions ...
Really? After everything that we've been through, I'm going to lose it now?
No way. I have to calm down.
I take off my blanket and jacket and breathe deeply ... over and over.
After a bit it's under control.
HMPH ...
CRIS, CAN YOU HOLD STILL? I CAN'T SLEEP ...

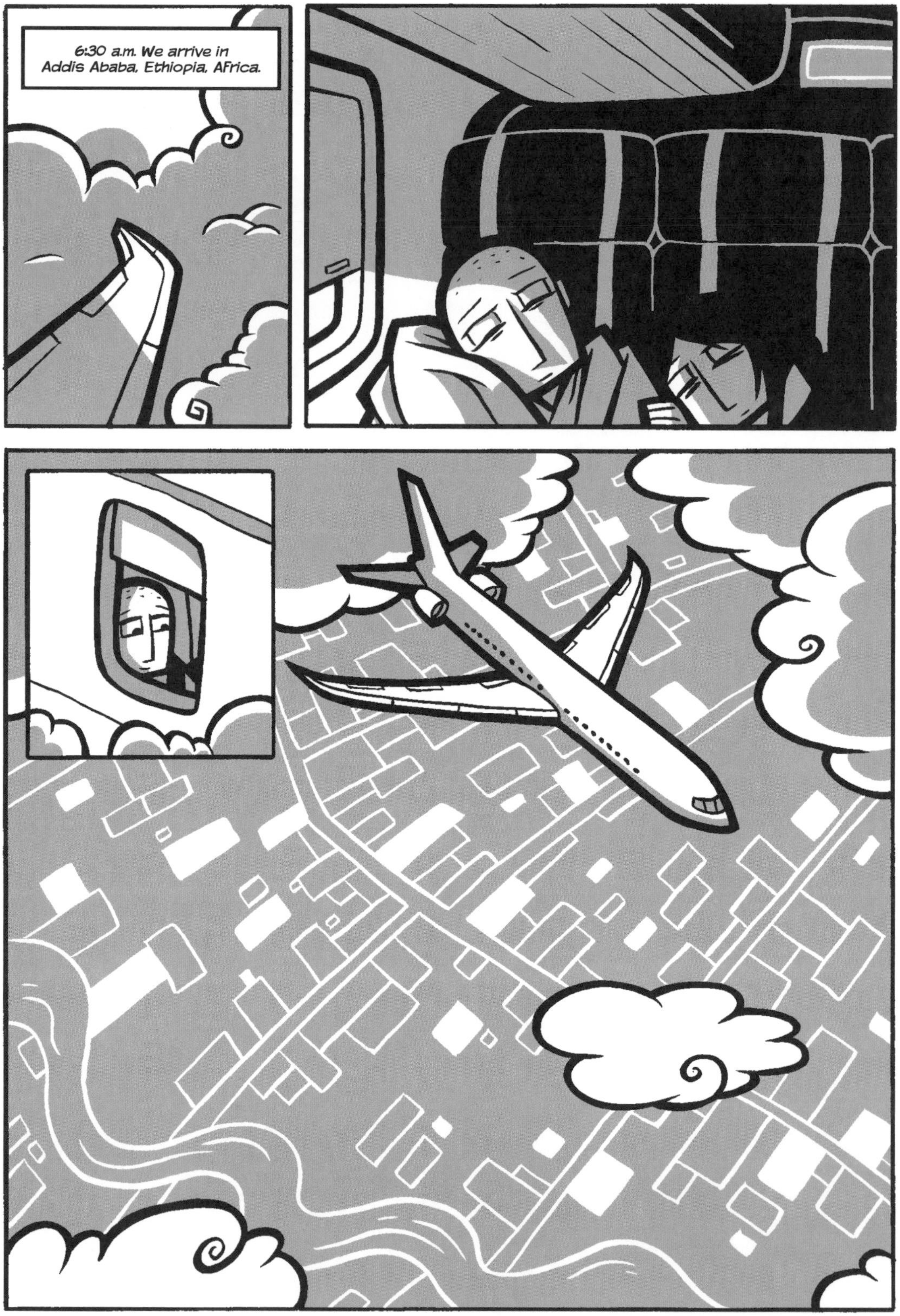
6:30 a.m. We arrive in Addis Ababa, Ethiopia, Africa.

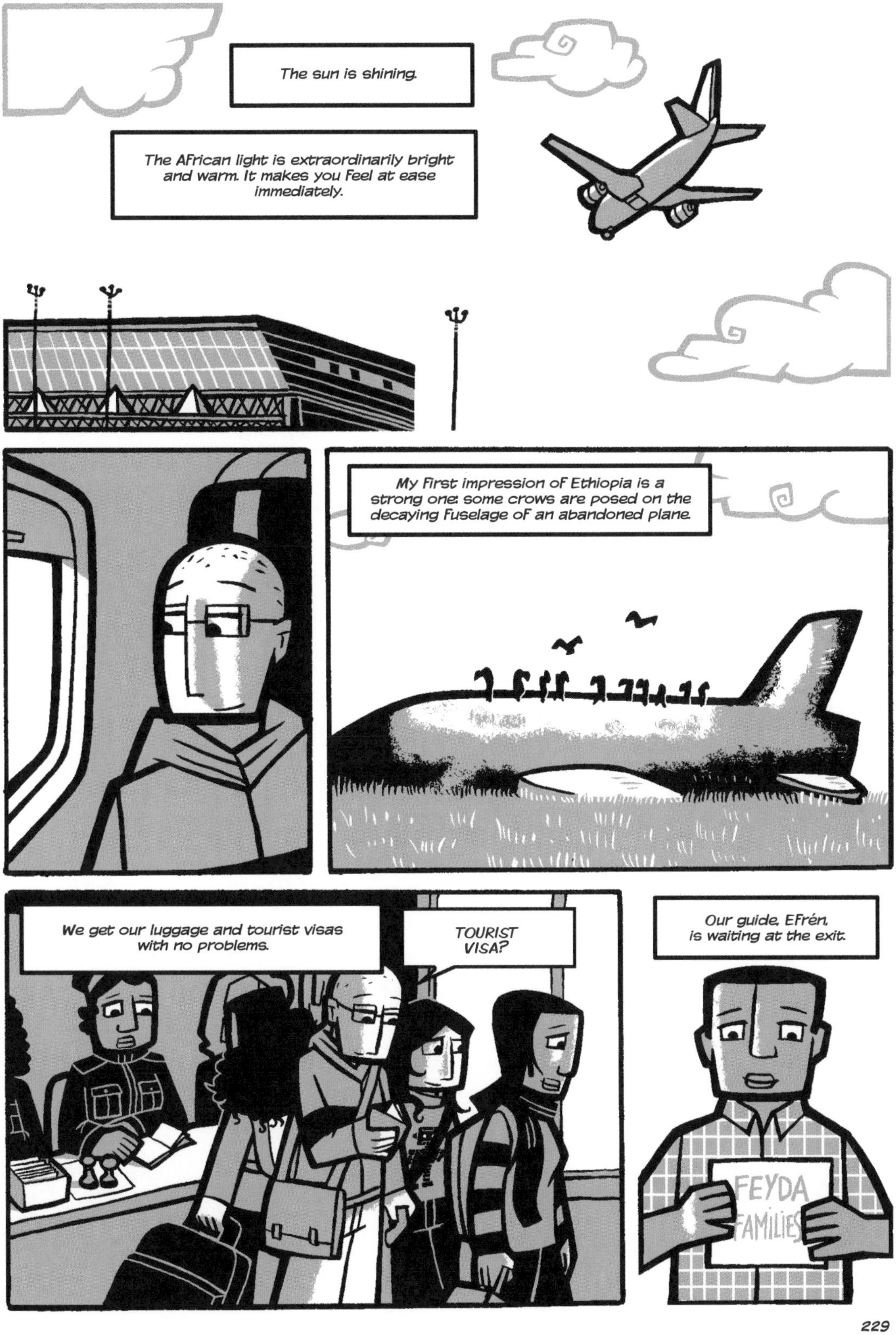
The sun is shining.
The African light is extraordinarily bright and warm. It makes you feel at ease immediately.
My first impression of Ethiopia is a strong one: some crows are posed on the decaying fuselage of an abandoned plane.
We get our luggage and tourist visas with no problems.
TOURIST VISA?
Our guide, Efrén, is waiting at the exit.
FEYDA FAMILIES

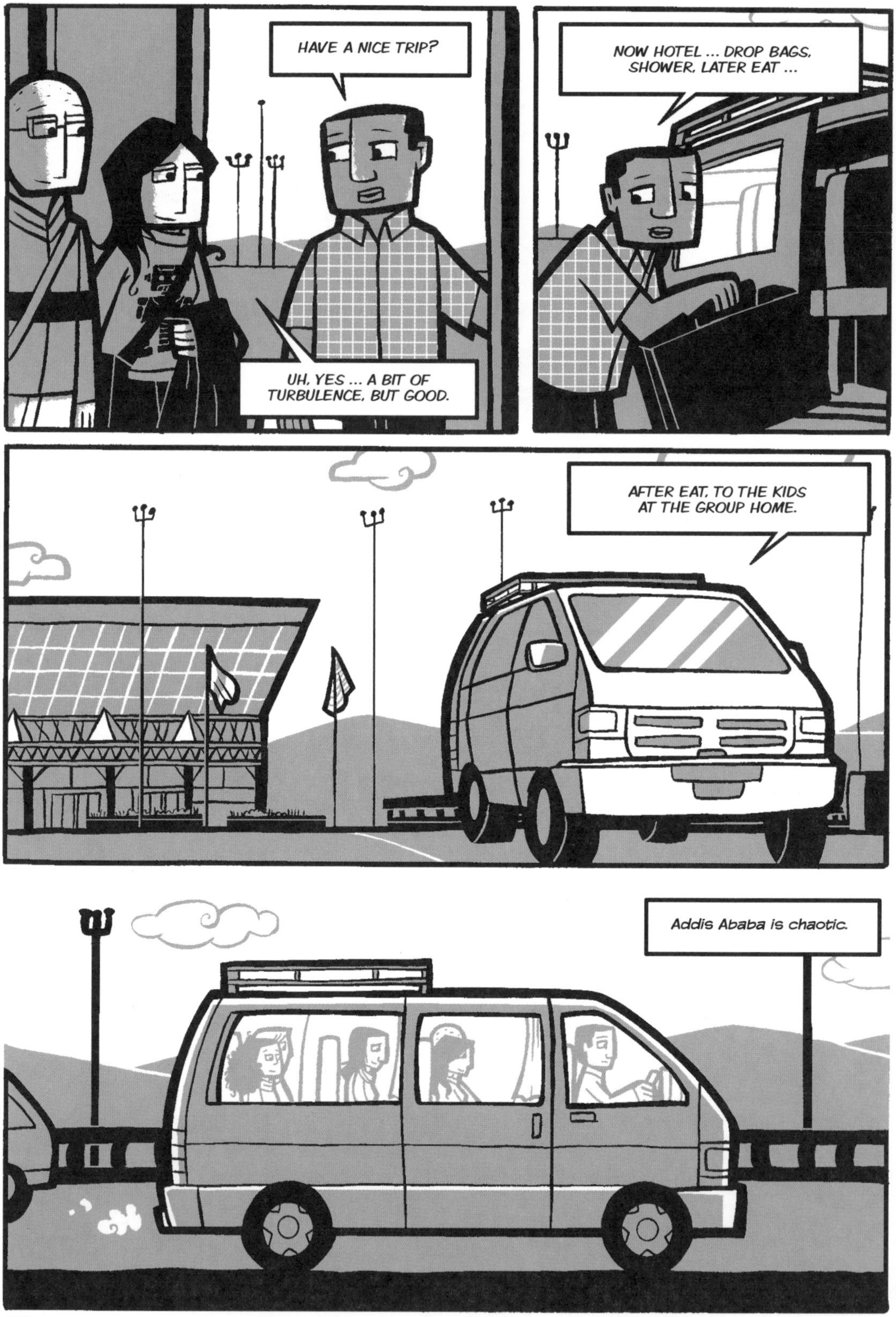
HAVE A NICE TRIP?
UH, YES ... A BIT OF TURBULENCE, BUT GOOD.
NOW HOTEL ... DROP BAGS, SHOWER, LATER EAT ...
AFTER EAT, TO THE KIDS AT THE GROUP HOME.
Addis Ababa is chaotic.

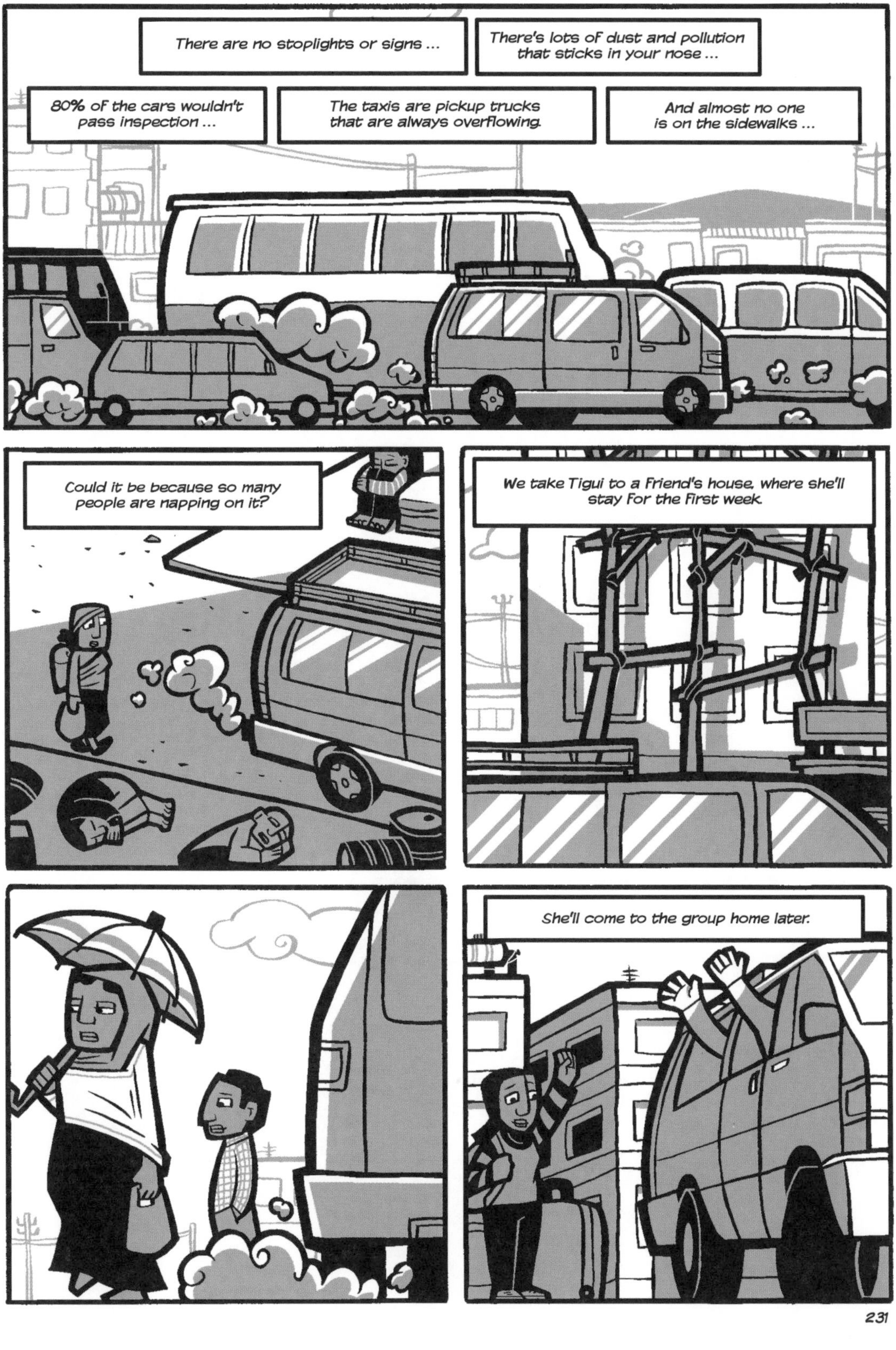
There are no stoplights or signs ...
There's lots of dust and pollution that sticks in your nose ...
80% of the cars wouldn't pass inspection ...
The taxis are pickup trucks that are always overflowing.
And almost no one is on the sidewalks ...
Could it be because so many people are napping on it?
We take Tigui to a friend's house, where she'll stay for the first week.
She'll come to the group home later.

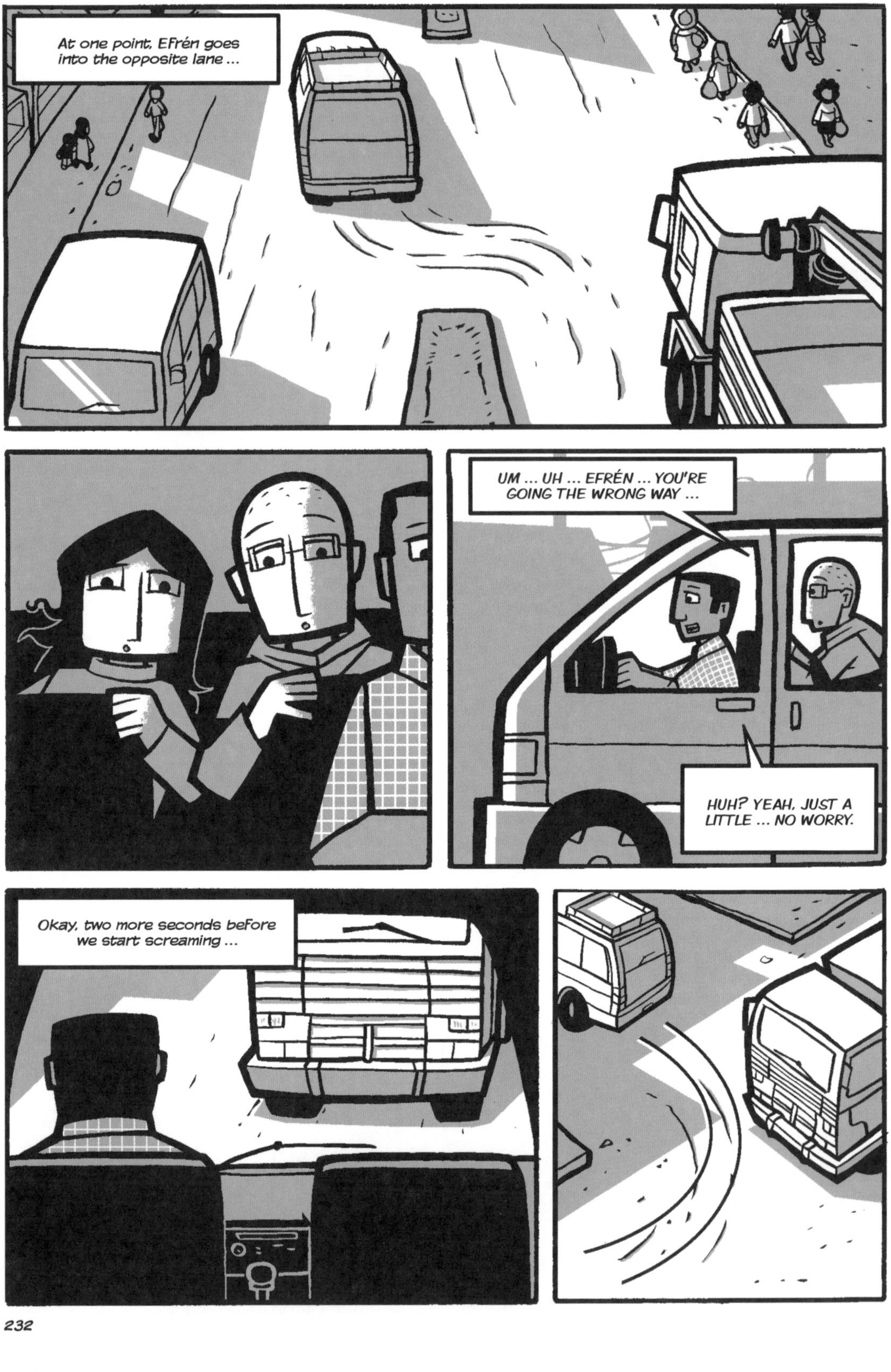
At one point, Efrén goes into the opposite lane ...
UM ... UH ... EFRÉN ... YOU'RE GOING THE WRONG WAY ...
HUH? YEAH, JUST A LITTLE ... NO WORRY.
Okay, two more seconds before we start screaming ...

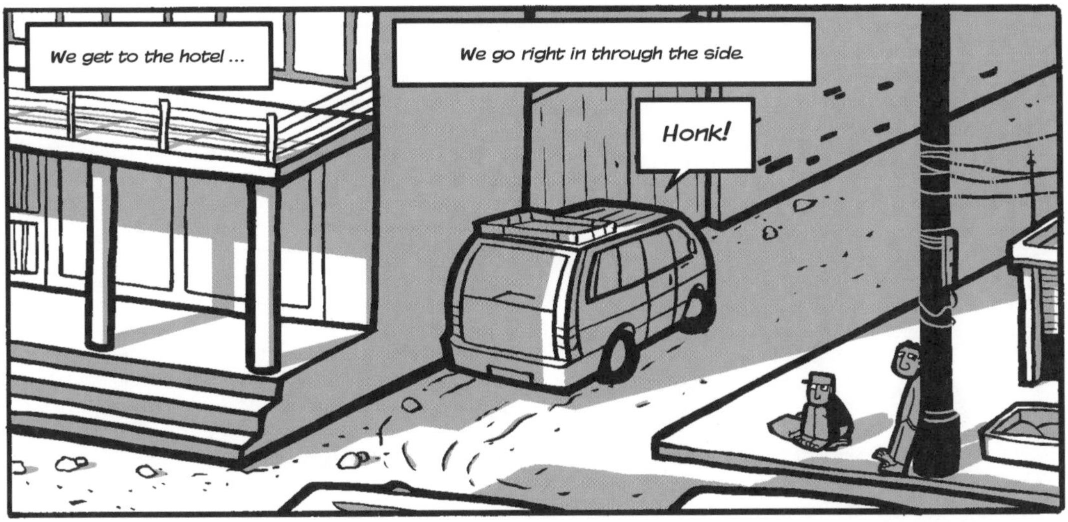
We get to the hotel ...
We go right in through the side.
Honk!

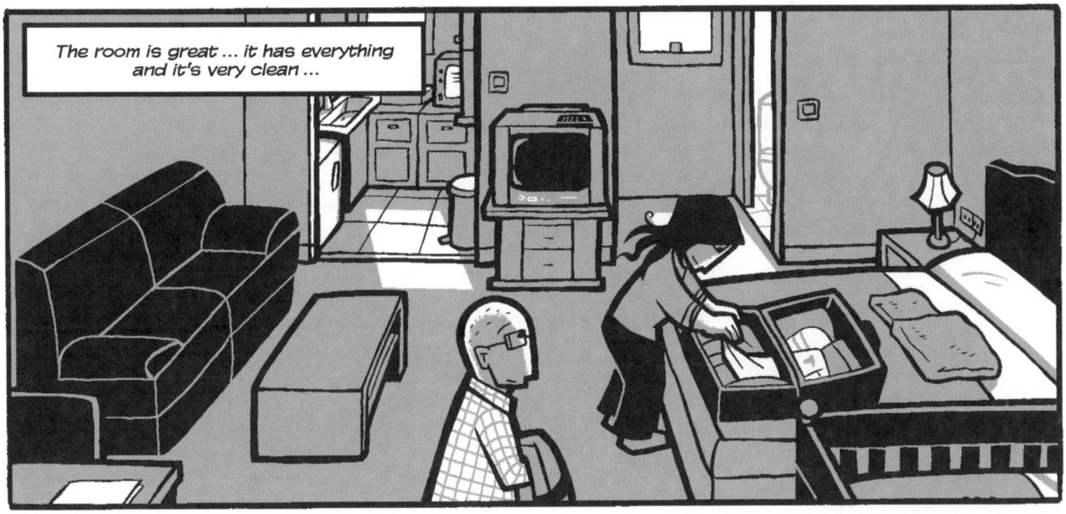
The room is great ... it has everything and it's very clean ...

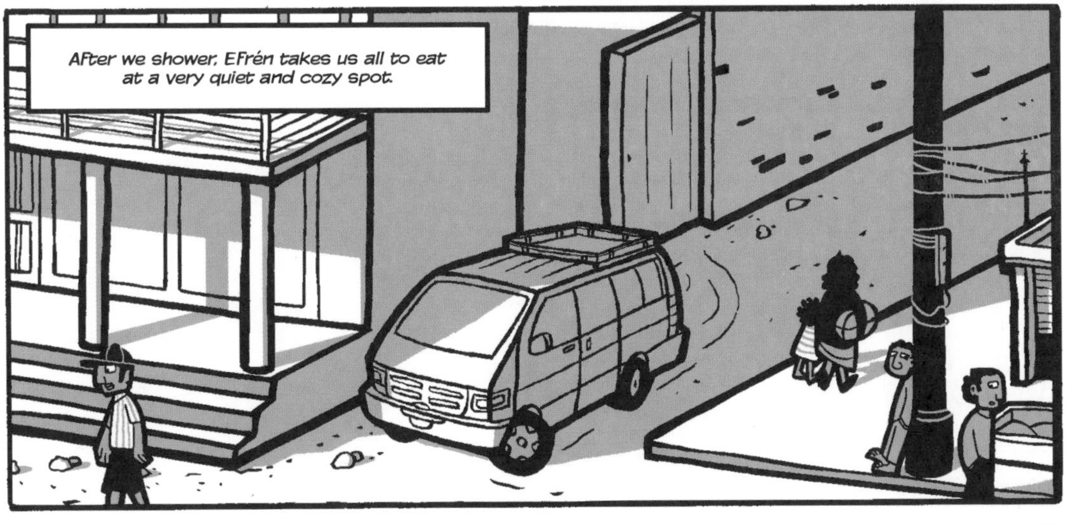
After we shower, Efrén takes us all to eat at a very quiet and cozy spot.

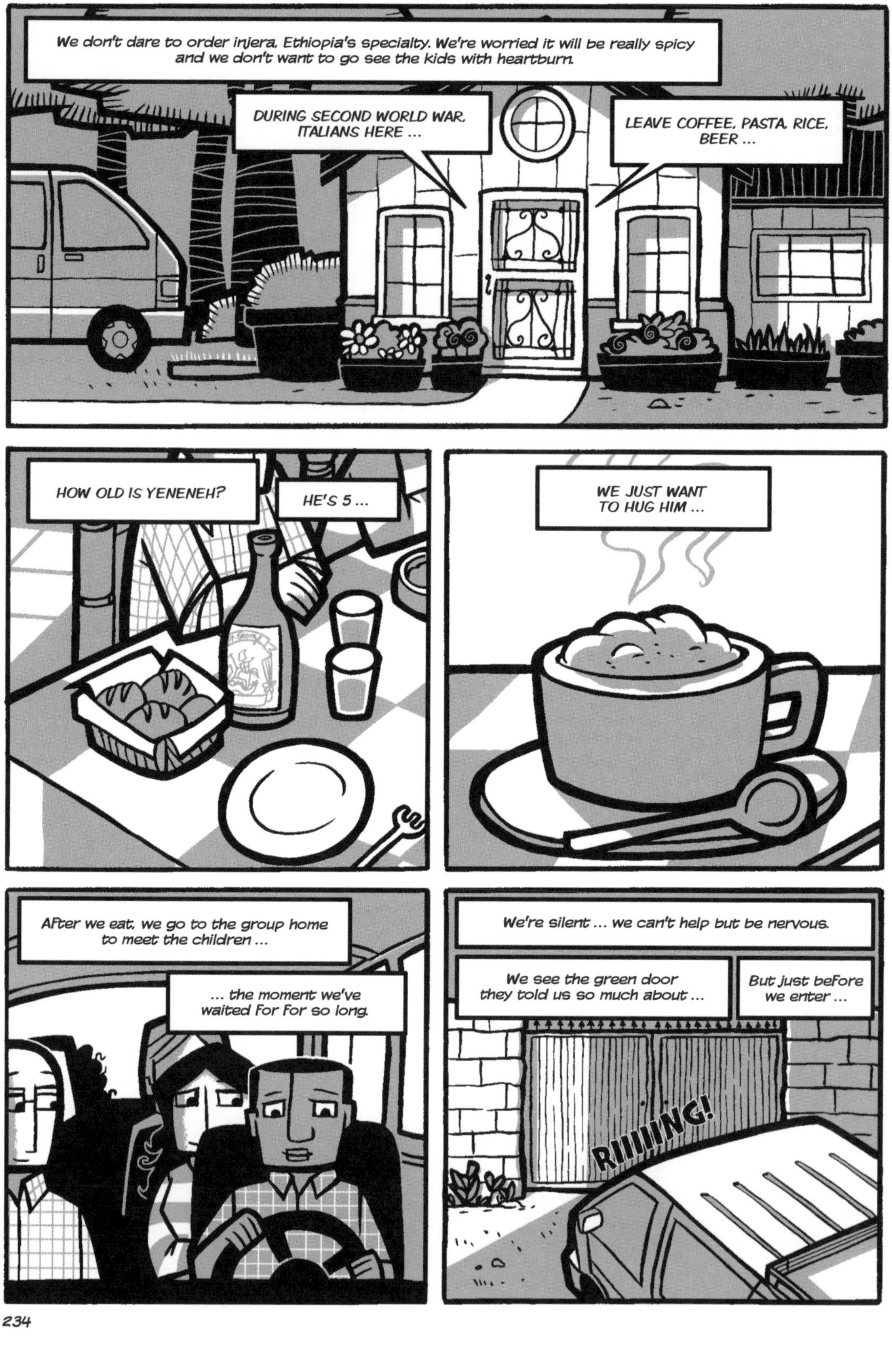
We don't dare to order injera, Ethiopia's specialty. We're worried it will be really spicy and we don't want to go see the kids with heartburn.
DURING SECOND WORLD WAR, ITALIANS HERE ...
LEAVE COFFEE, PASTA, RICE, BEER ...
HOW OLD IS YENENEH?
HE'S 5 ...
WE JUST WANT TO HUG HIM ...
After we eat, we go to the group home to meet the children ...
... the moment we've waited for for so long.
We're silent ... we can't help but be nervous.
We see the green door they told us so much about ...
But just before we enter ...
RIIIIING!

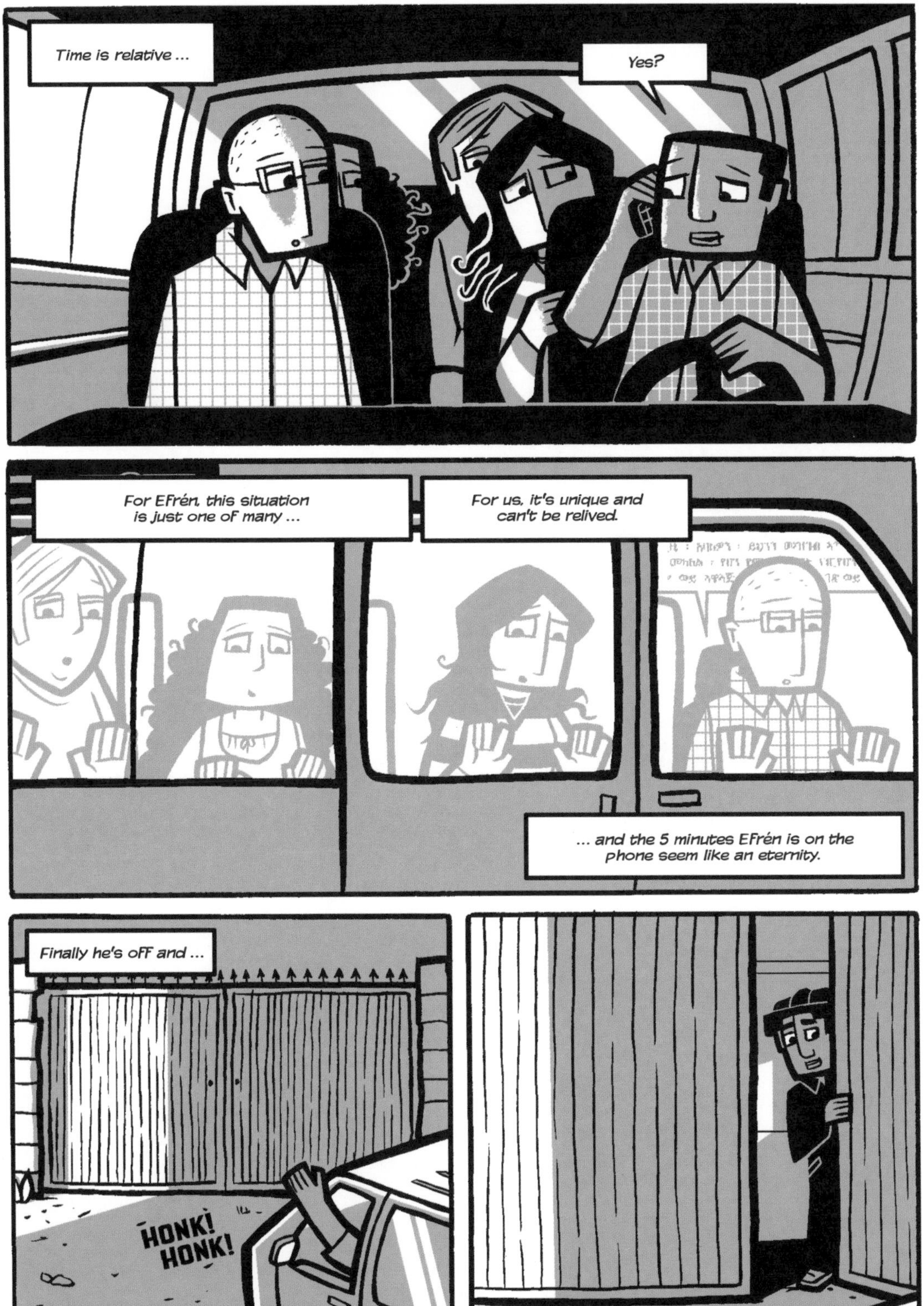
Time is relative ...
Yes?
For Efrén, this situation is just one of many ...
For us, it's unique and can't be relived.
... and the 5 minutes Efrén is on the phone seem like an eternity.
Finally he's off and ...
HONK! HONK!

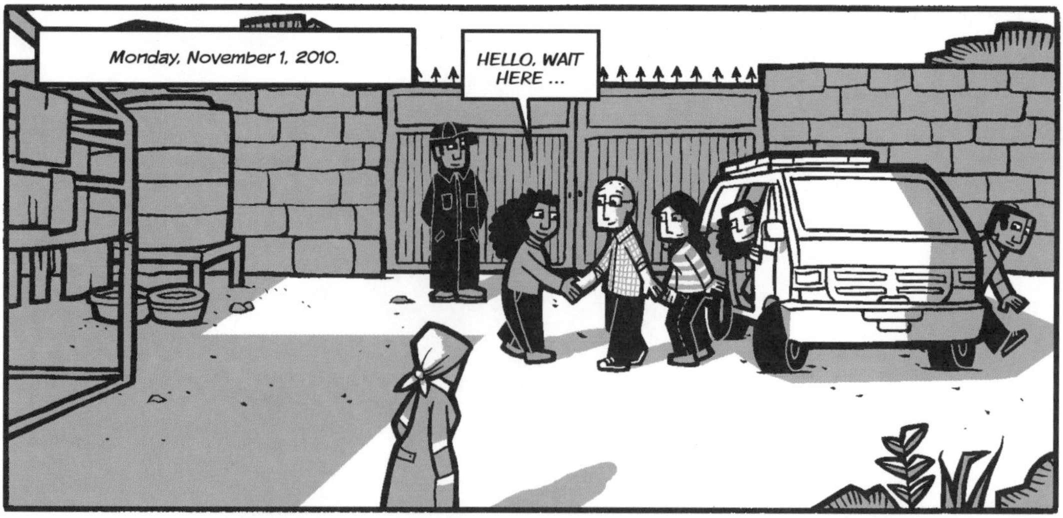
Monday, November 1, 2010.
HELLO, WAIT HERE ...

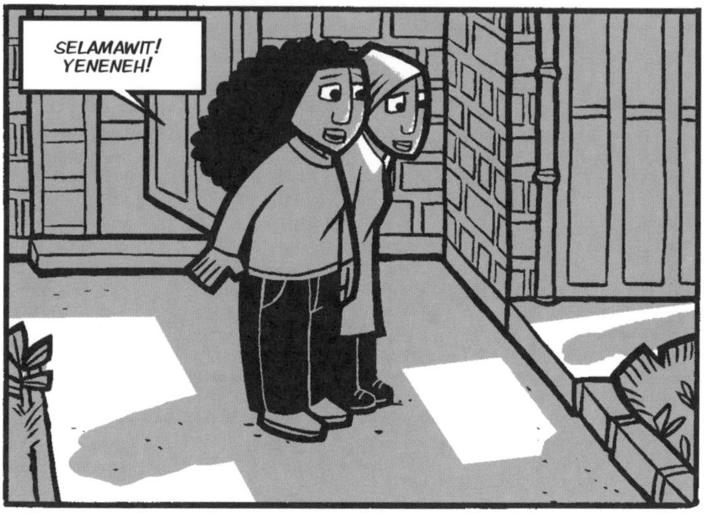
SELAMAWIT! YENENEH!

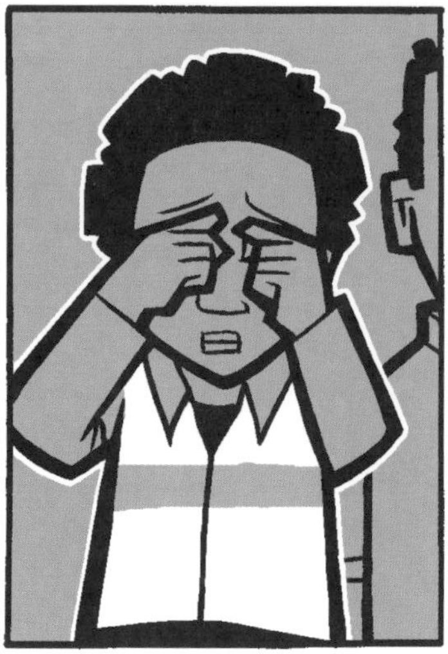

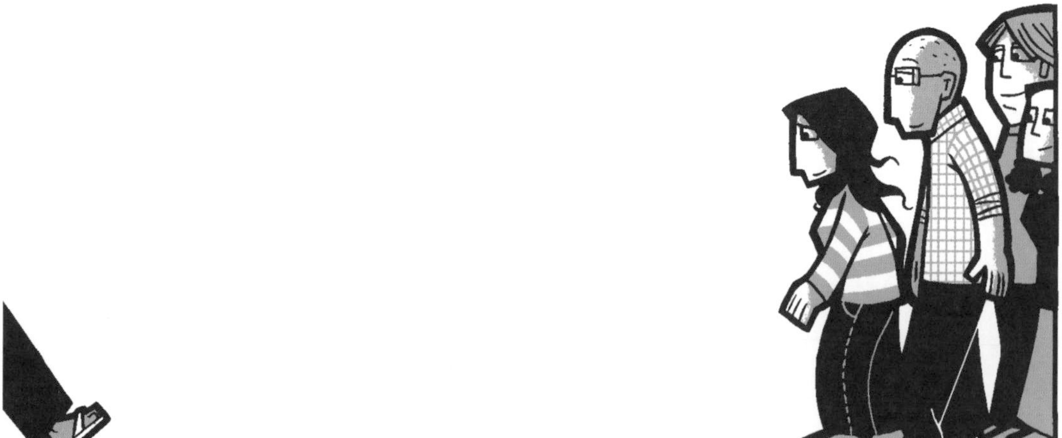

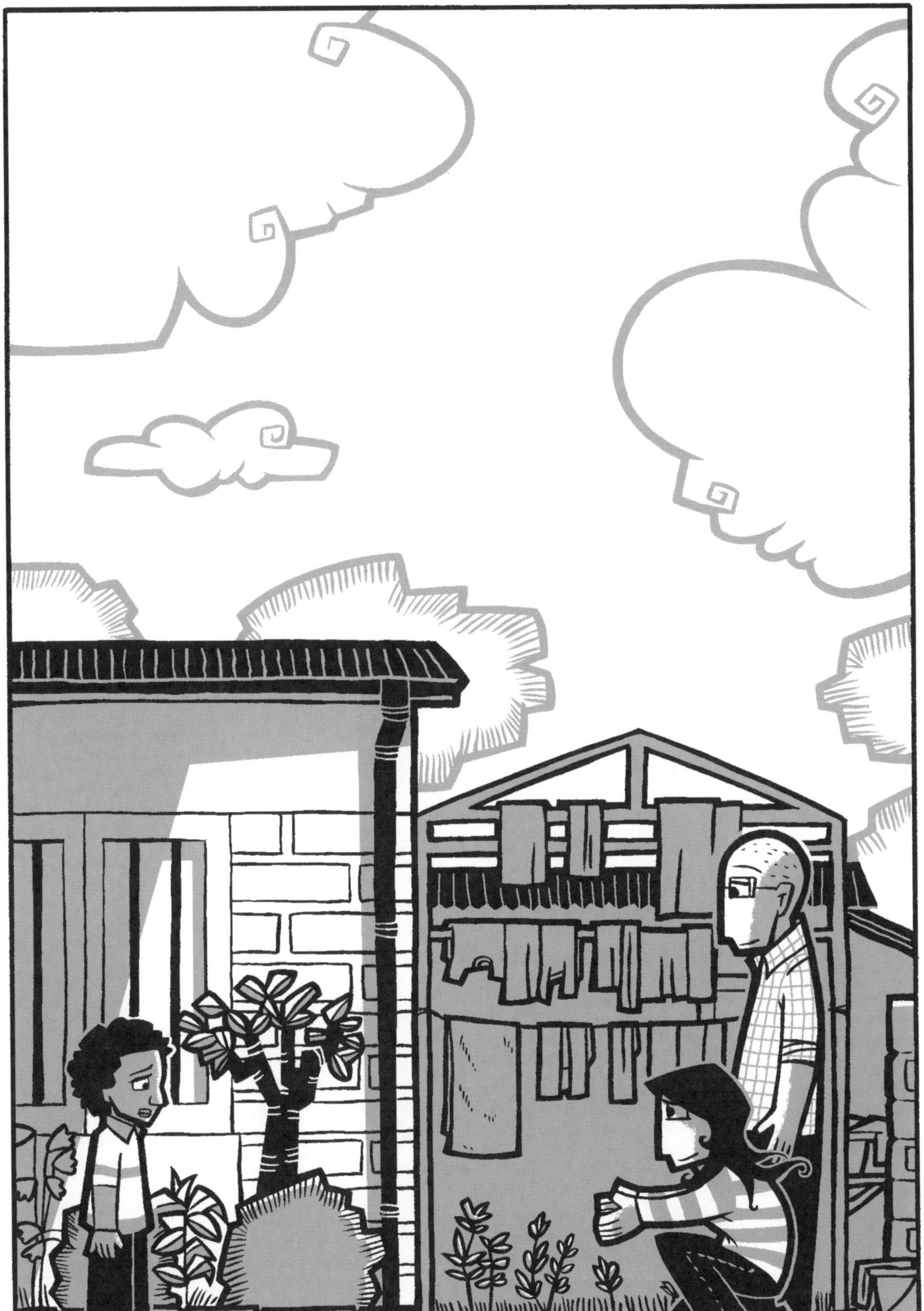

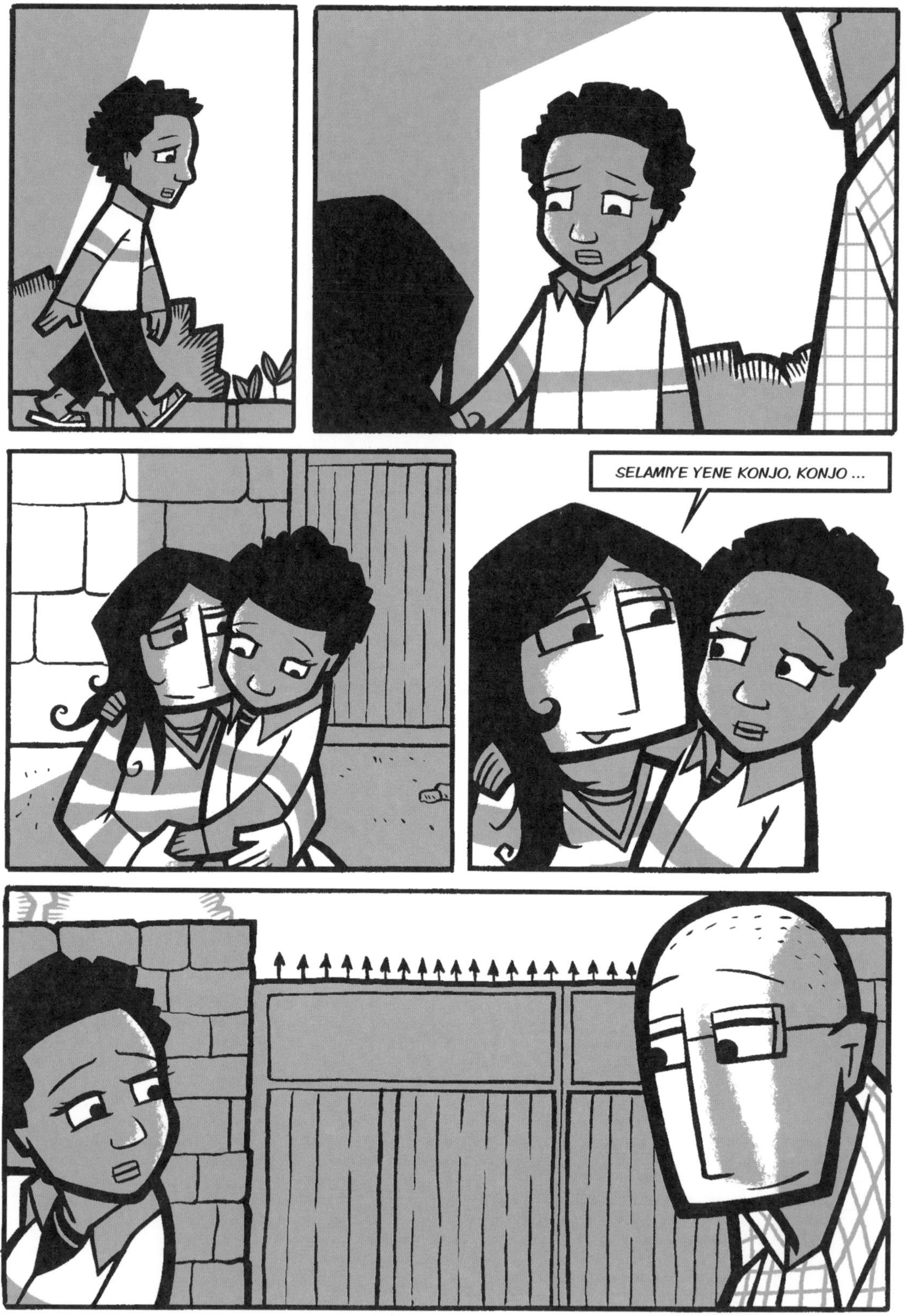
SELAMIYE YENE KONJO, KONJO ...

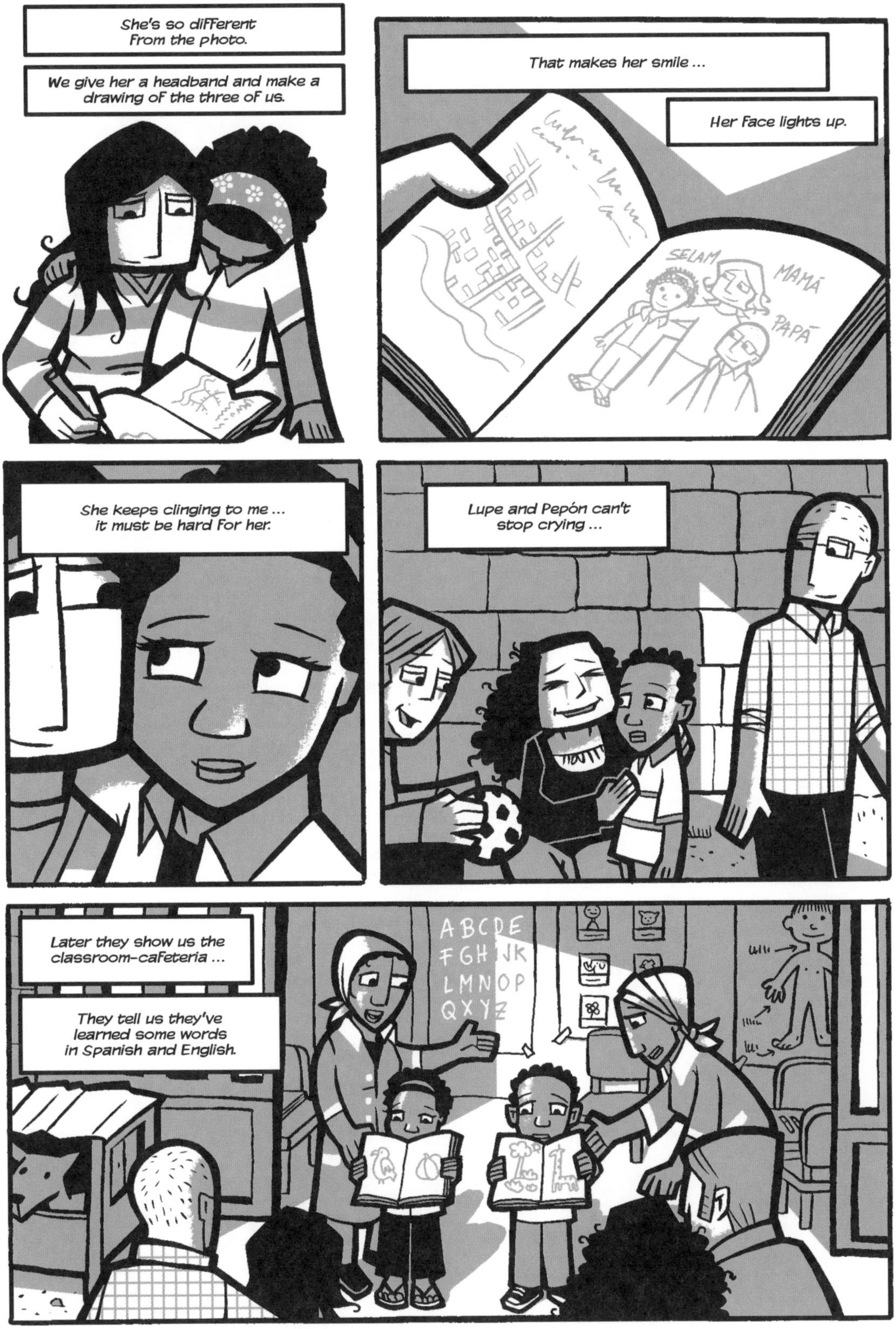
She's so different from the photo.
We give her a headband and make a drawing of the three of us.
That makes her smile ...
Her face lights up.
SELAM
MAMÁ
PAPÁ
She keeps clinging to me ... it must be hard for her.
Lupe and Pepón can't stop crying ...
Later they show us the classroom-cafeteria ...
They tell us they've learned some words in Spanish and English.

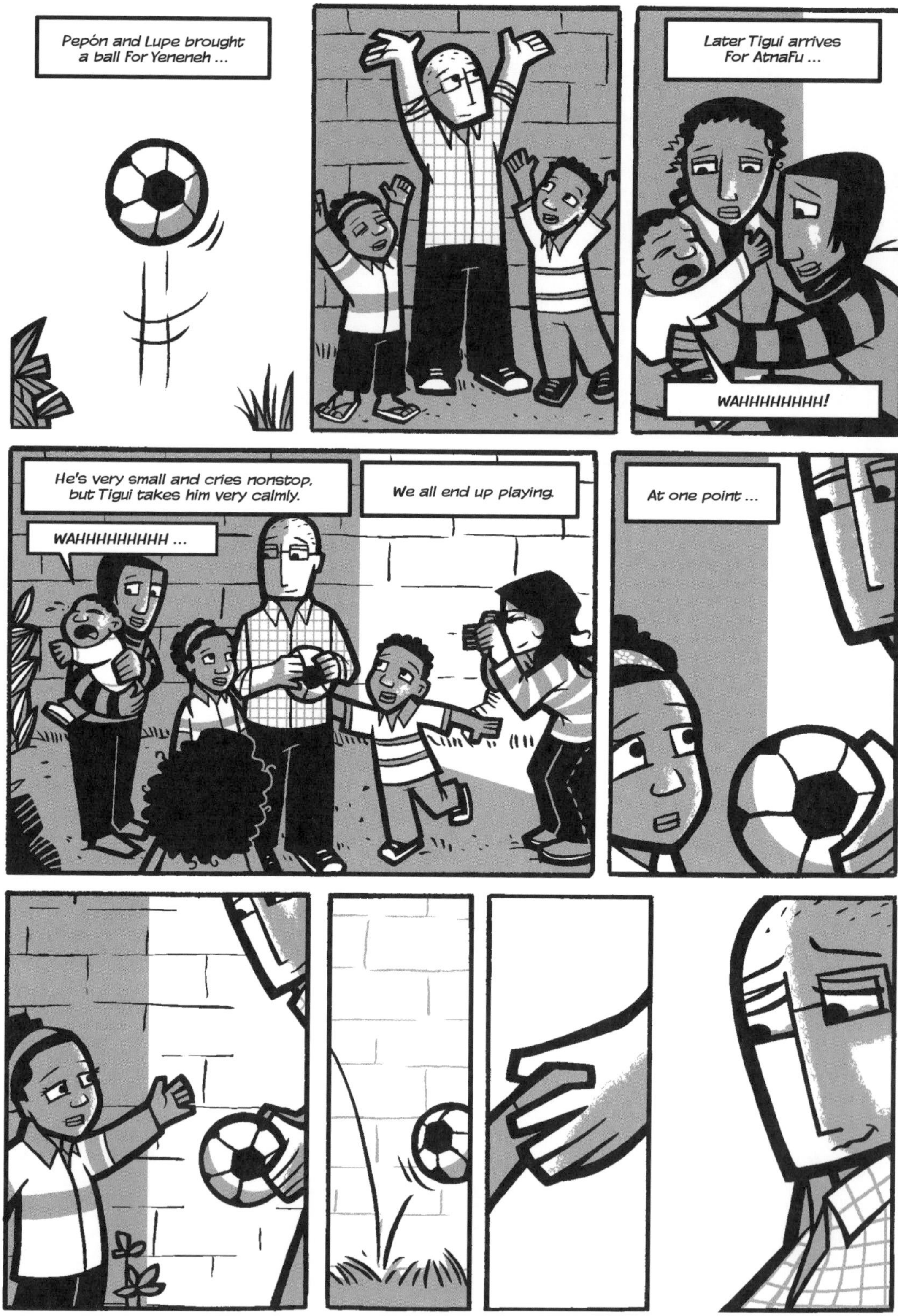
Pepón and Lupe brought a ball for Yeneneh ...
Later Tigui arrives for Atnafu ...
WAHHHHHHHH!
He's very small and cries nonstop, but Tigui takes him very calmly.
WAHHHHHHHHH ...
We all end up playing.
At one point ...

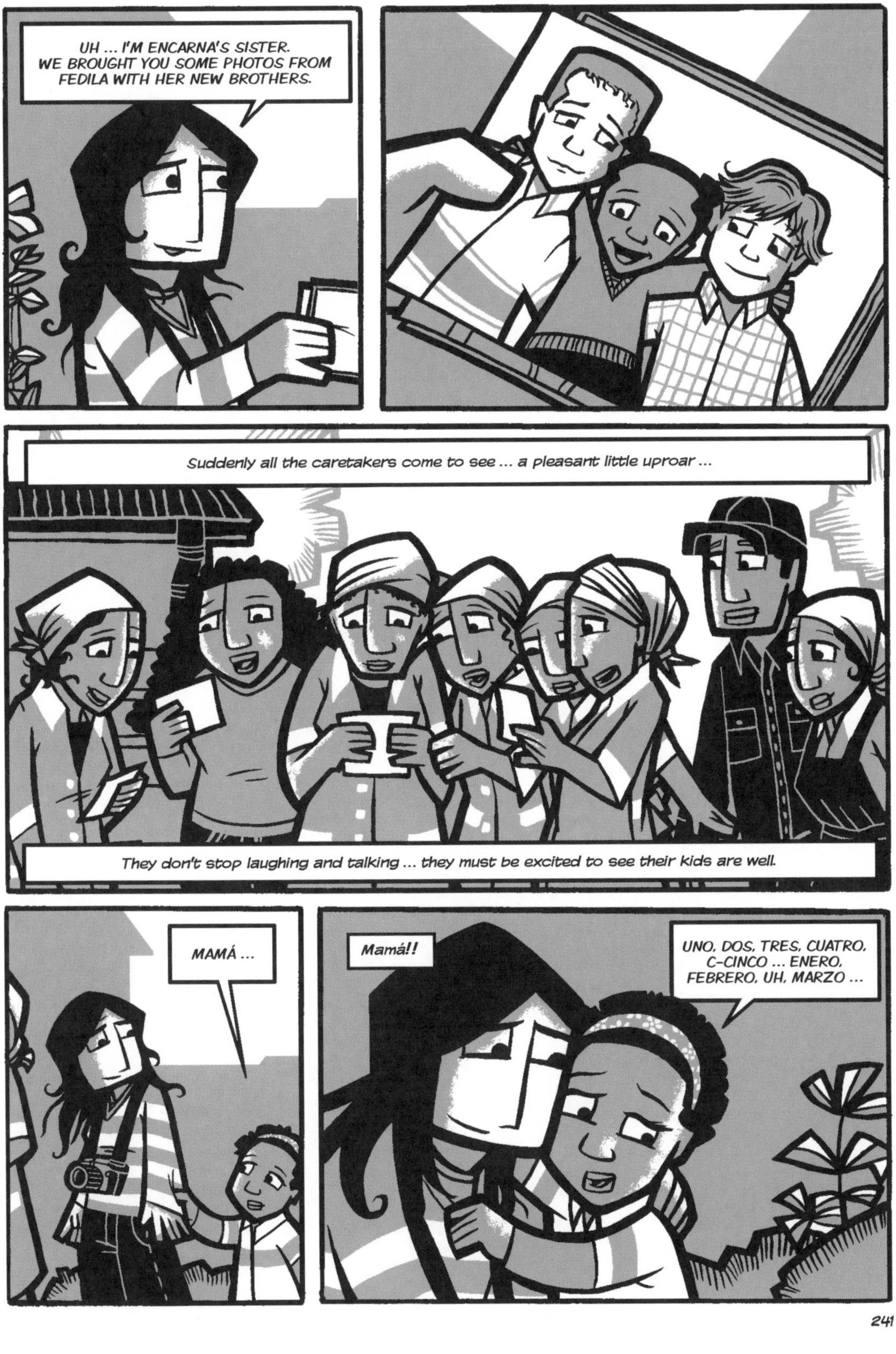
UH ... I'M ENCARNA'S SISTER. WE BROUGHT YOU SOME PHOTOS FROM FEDILA WITH HER NEW BROTHERS.
Suddenly all the caretakers come to see ... a pleasant little uproar ...
They don't stop laughing and talking ... they must be excited to see their kids are well.
MAMÁ ...
Mamá!!
UNO, DOS, TRES, CUATRO, C-CINCO ... ENERO, FEBRERO, UH, MARZO ...

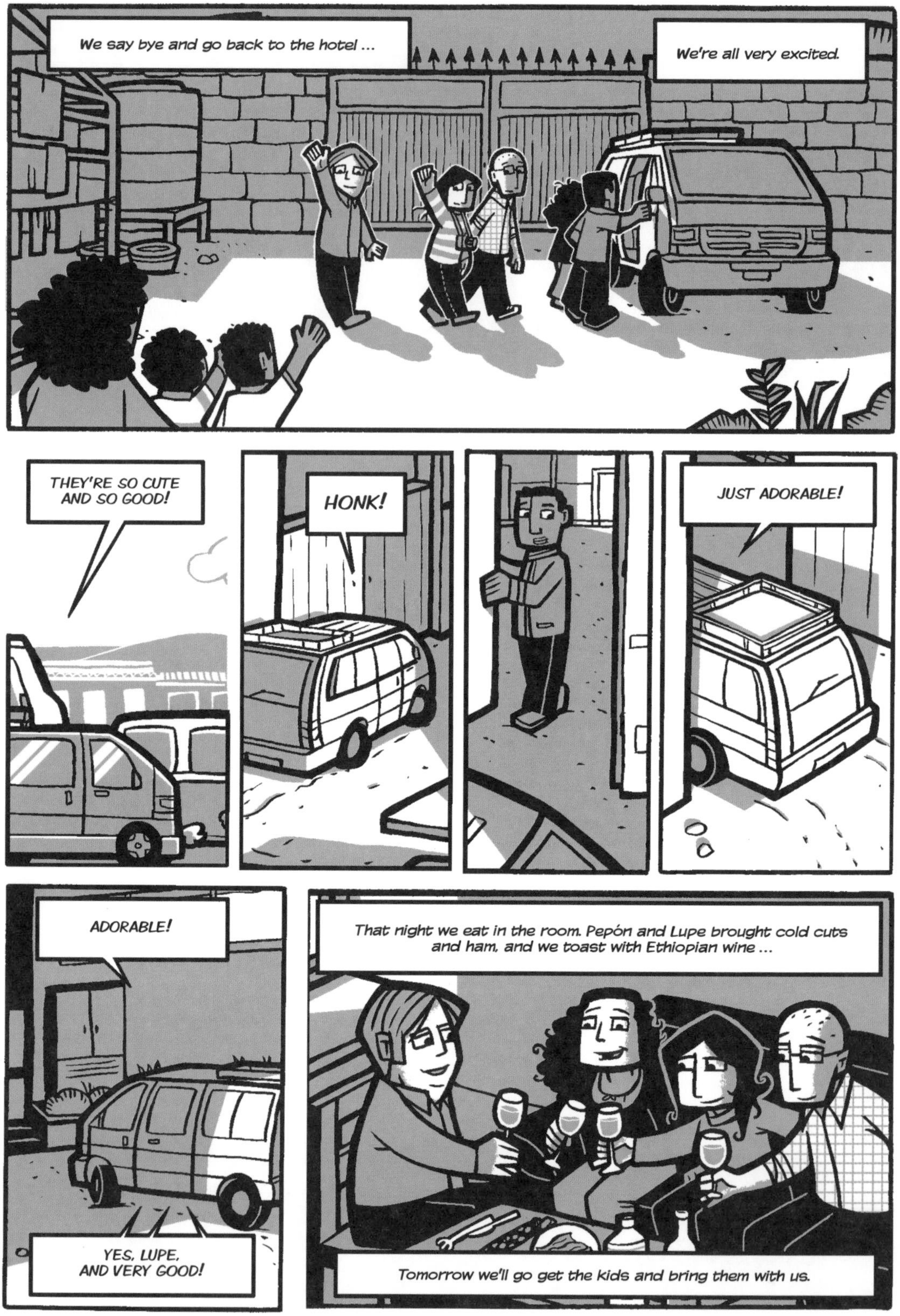
We say bye and go back to the hotel ...
We're all very excited.
THEY'RE SO CUTE AND SO GOOD!
HONK!
JUST ADORABLE!
ADORABLE!
YES, LUPE, AND VERY GOOD!
That night we eat in the room. Pepón and Lupe brought cold cuts and ham, and we toast with Ethiopian wine ...
Tomorrow we'll go get the kids and bring them with us.

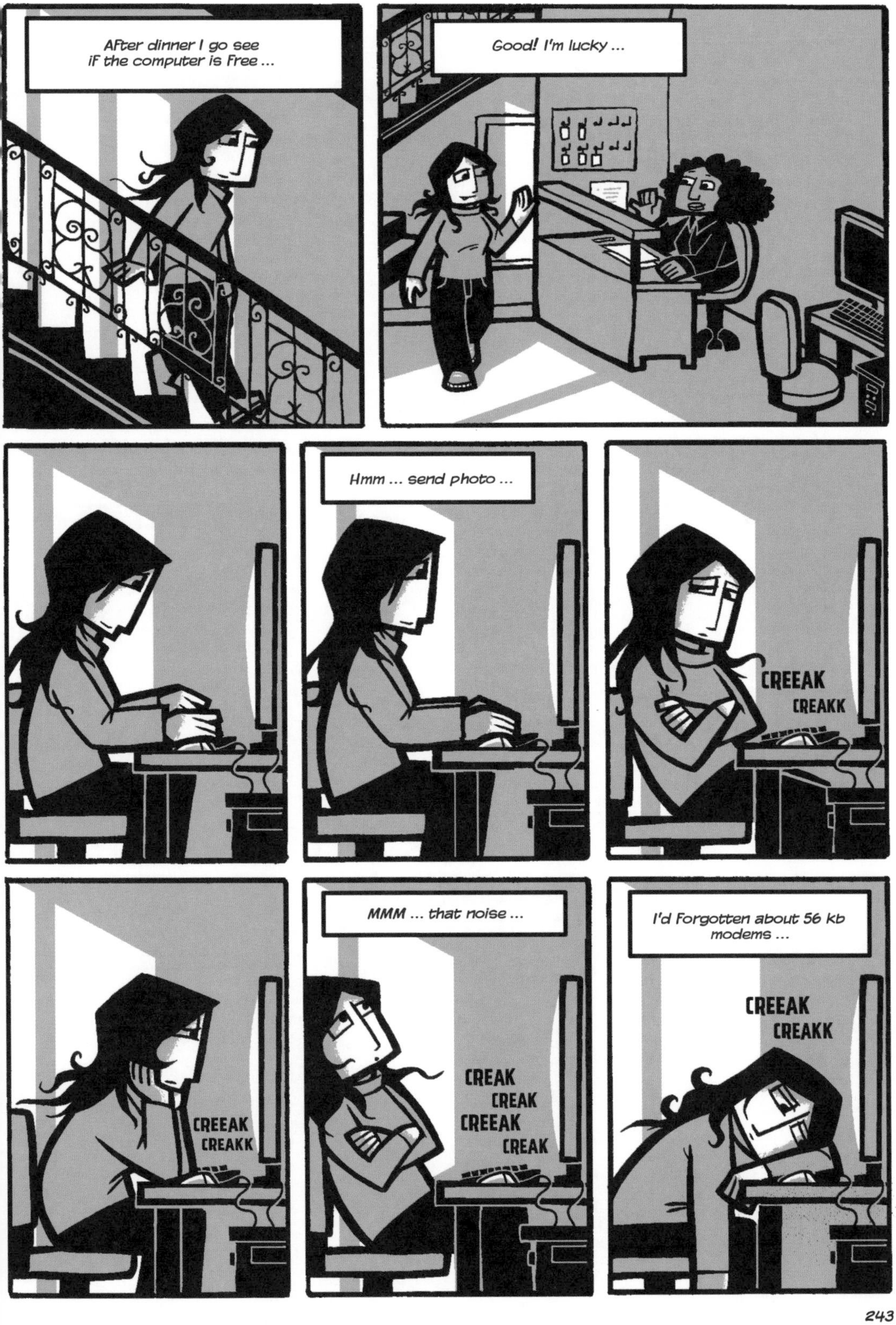
After dinner I go see if the computer is free ...
Good! I'm lucky ...
Hmm ... send photo ...
CREEAK
CREAKK
CREEAK
CREAKK
MMM ... that noise ...
CREAK
CREAK
CREEAK
CREAK
I'd forgotten about 56 kb modems ...
CREEAK
CREAKK

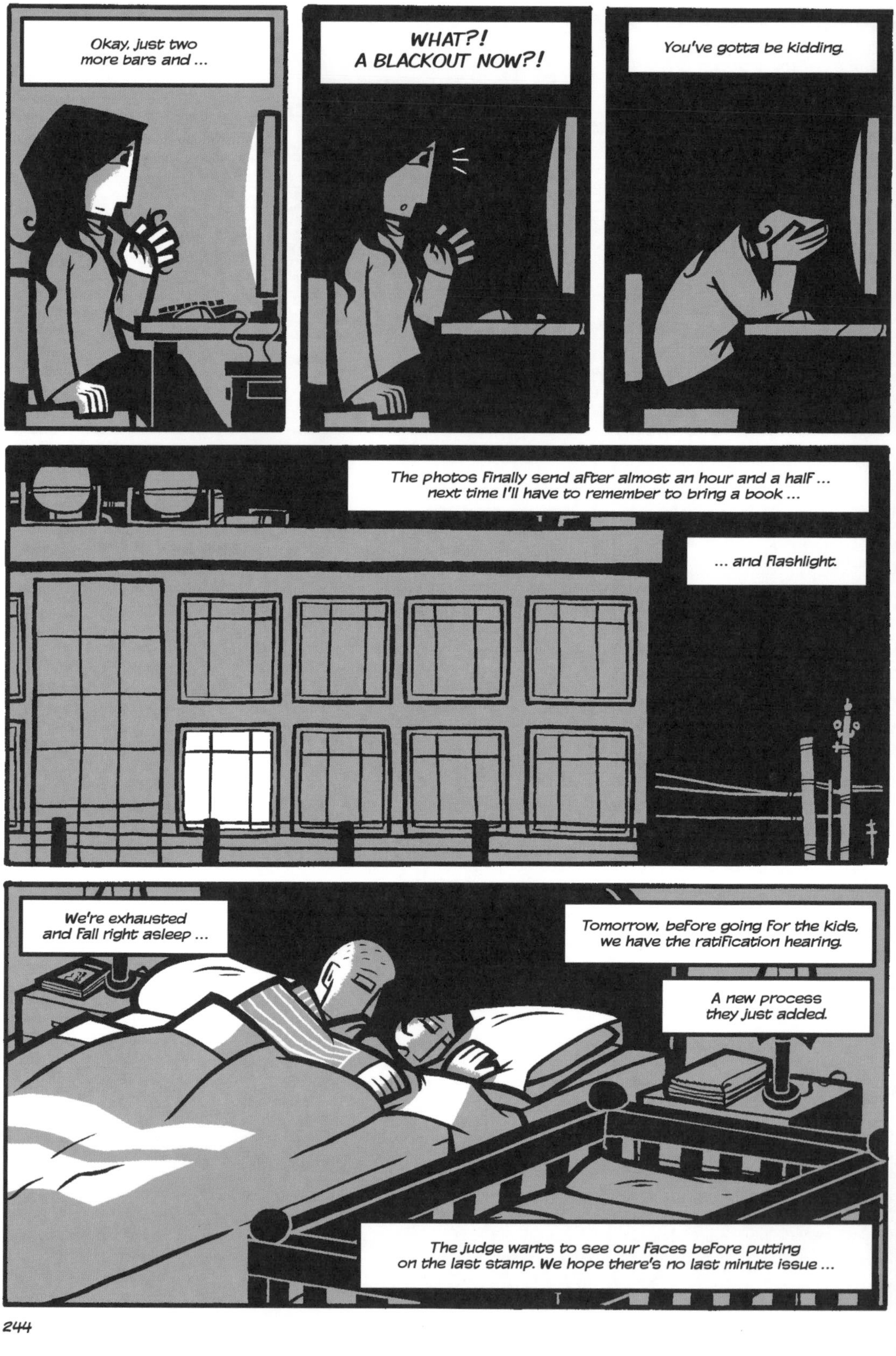
Okay, just two more bars and ...
WHAT?! A BLACKOUT NOW?!
You've gotta be kidding.
The photos finally send after almost an hour and a half ... next time I'll have to remember to bring a book ...
... and flashlight.
We're exhausted and fall right asleep ...
Tomorrow, before going for the kids, we have the ratification hearing.
A new process they just added.
The judge wants to see our faces before putting on the last stamp. We hope there's no last minute issue ...

Chapter 7
THE RATIFICATION

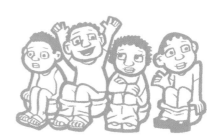

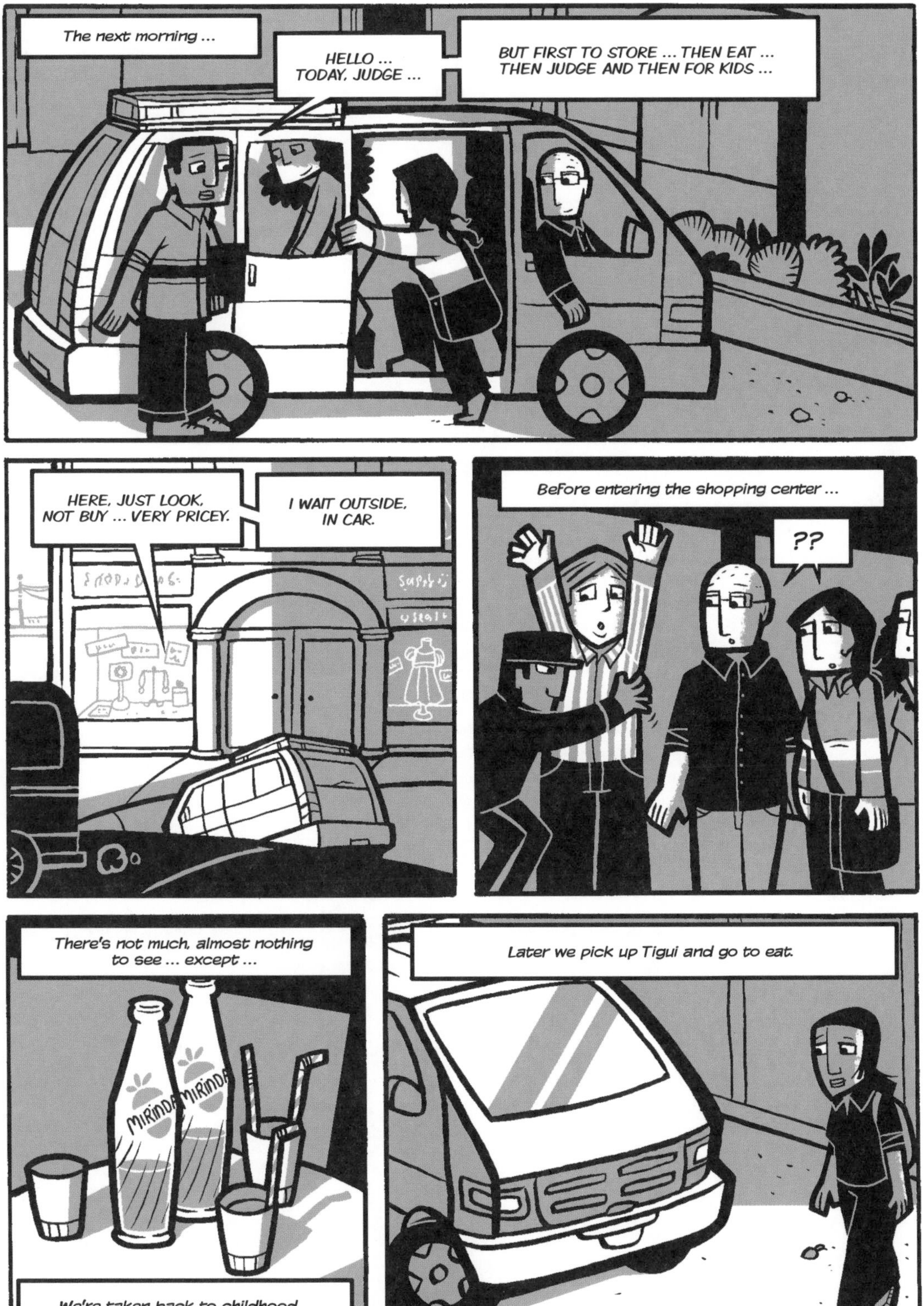
The next morning ...
HELLO ... TODAY, JUDGE ...
BUT FIRST TO STORE ... THEN EAT ... THEN JUDGE AND THEN FOR KIDS ...
HERE, JUST LOOK, NOT BUY ... VERY PRICEY.
I WAIT OUTSIDE, IN CAR.
Before entering the shopping center ...
??
There's not much, almost nothing to see ... except ...
MIRINDA
MIRINDA
We're taken back to childhood ...
Later we pick up Tigui and go to eat.

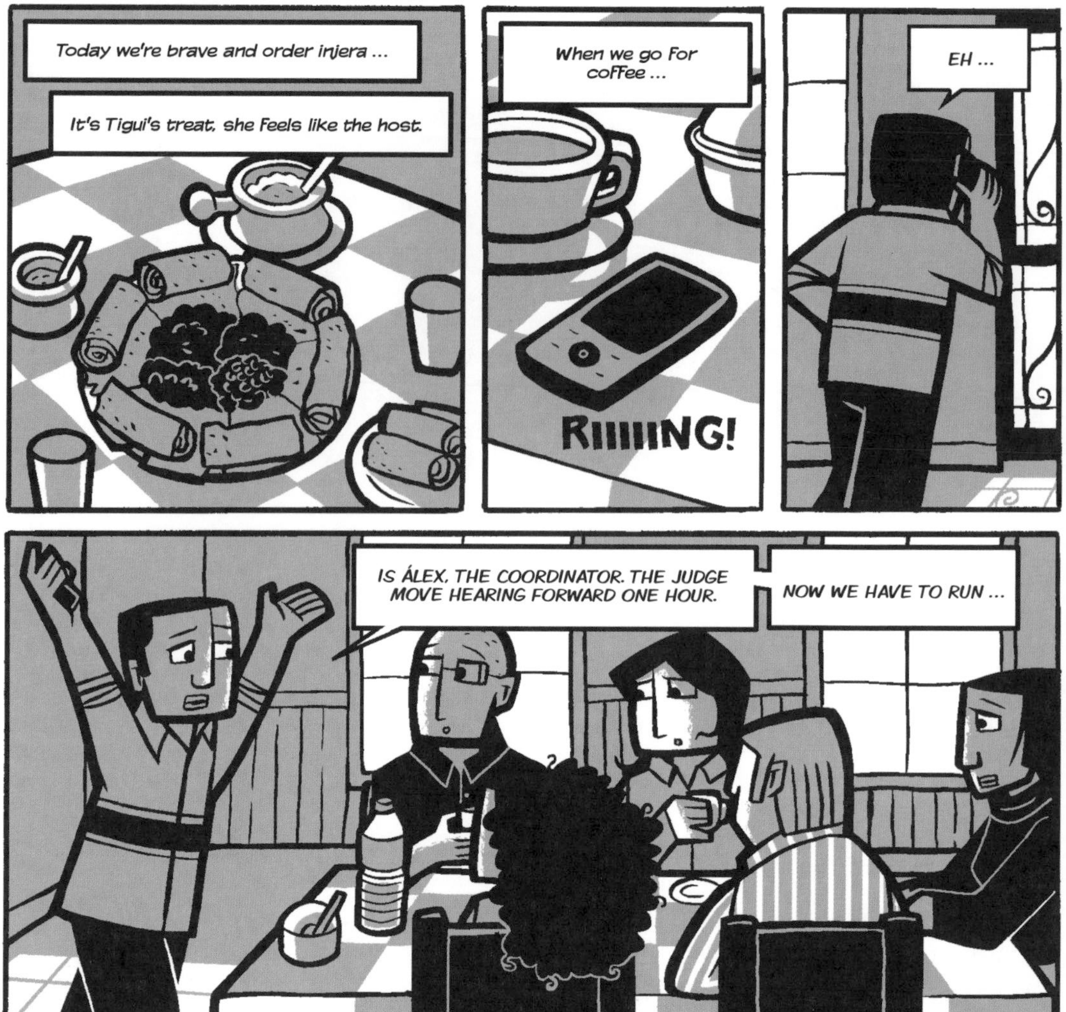
Today we're brave and order injera ...
It's Tigui's treat, she feels like the host.
When we go for coffee ...
RIIIIING!
EH ...
IS ÁLEX, THE COORDINATOR. THE JUDGE MOVE HEARING FORWARD ONE HOUR.
NOW WE HAVE TO RUN ...

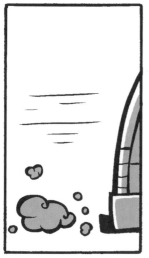

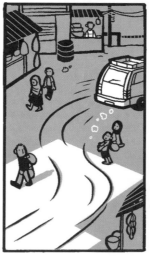

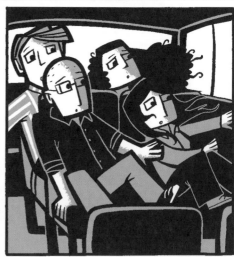

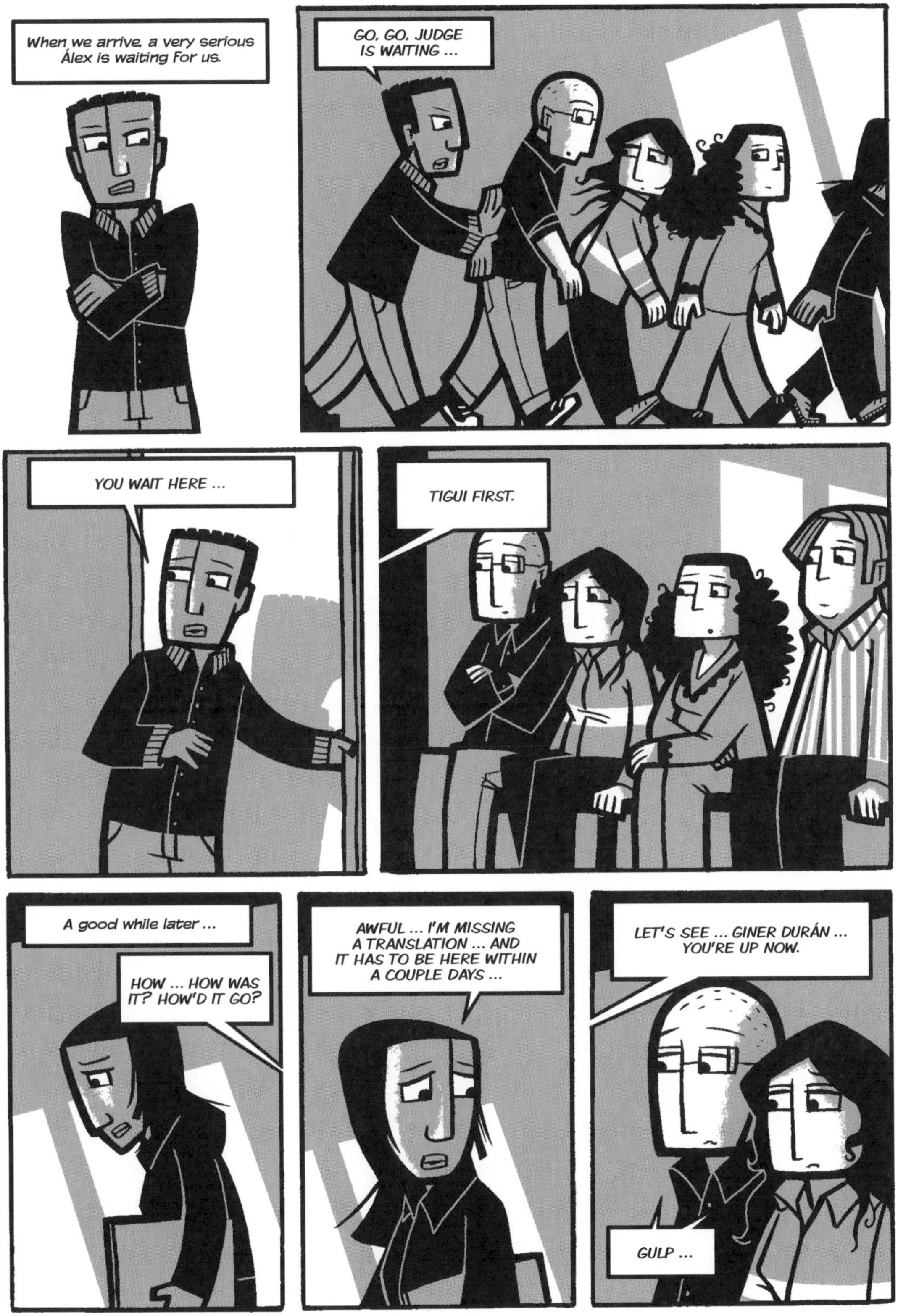
When we arrive, a very serious Álex is waiting for us.
GO, GO, JUDGE IS WAITING ...
YOU WAIT HERE ...
TIGUI FIRST.
A good while later ...
HOW ... HOW WAS IT? HOW'D IT GO?
AWFUL ... I'M MISSING A TRANSLATION ... AND IT HAS TO BE HERE WITHIN A COUPLE DAYS ...
LET'S SEE ... GINER DURÁN ... YOU'RE UP NOW.
GULP ...

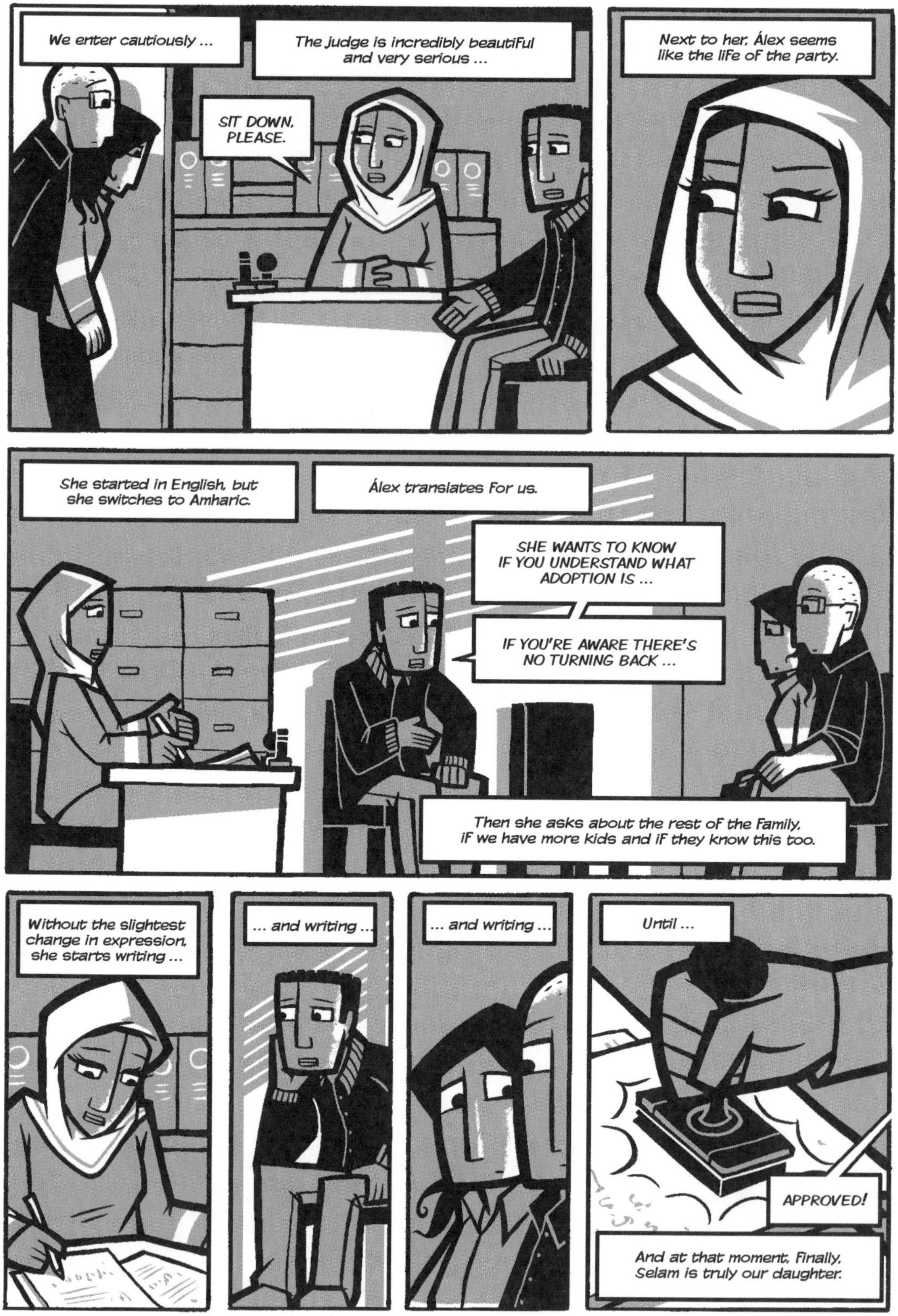
We enter cautiously ...
The judge is incredibly beautiful and very serious ...
SIT DOWN, PLEASE.
Next to her, Álex seems like the life of the party.
She started in English, but she switches to Amharic.
Álex translates for us.
SHE WANTS TO KNOW IF YOU UNDERSTAND WHAT ADOPTION IS ...
IF YOU'RE AWARE THERE'S NO TURNING BACK ...
Then she asks about the rest of the family, if we have more kids and if they know this too.
Without the slightest change in expression, she starts writing ...
... and writing ...
... and writing ...
Until ...
APPROVED!
And at that moment, finally, Selam is truly our daughter.

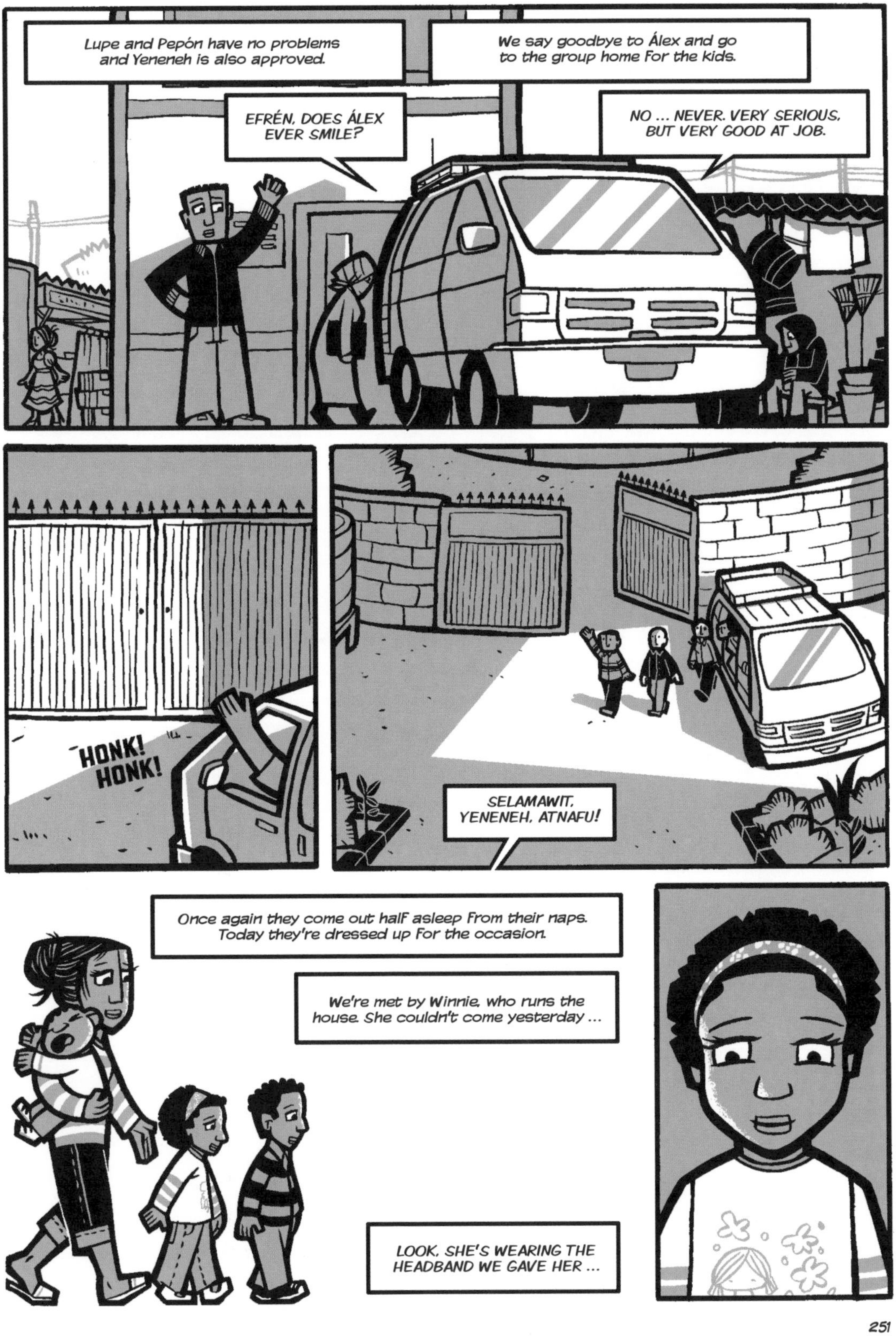
Lupe and Pepón have no problems and Yeneneh is also approved.
We say goodbye to Álex and go to the group home for the kids.
EFRÉN, DOES ÁLEX EVER SMILE?
NO ... NEVER. VERY SERIOUS, BUT VERY GOOD AT JOB.
HONK! HONK!
SELAMAWIT, YENENEH, ATNAFU!
Once again they come out half asleep from their naps. Today they're dressed up for the occasion.
We're met by Winnie, who runs the house. She couldn't come yesterday ...
LOOK, SHE'S WEARING THE HEADBAND WE GAVE HER ...

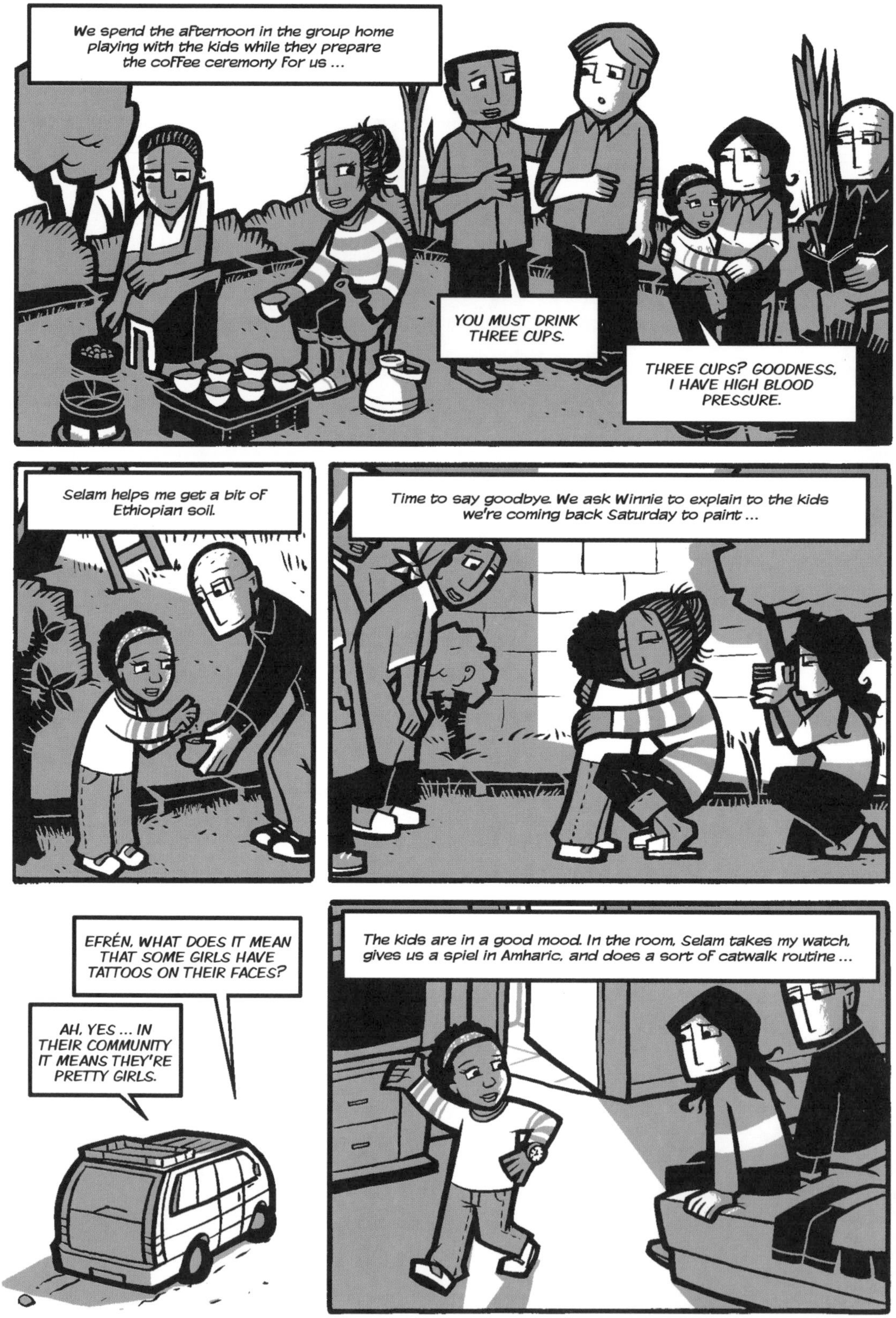
We spend the afternoon in the group home playing with the kids while they prepare the coffee ceremony for us ...
YOU MUST DRINK THREE CUPS.
THREE CUPS? GOODNESS, I HAVE HIGH BLOOD PRESSURE.
Selam helps me get a bit of Ethiopian soil.
Time to say goodbye. We ask Winnie to explain to the kids we're coming back Saturday to paint ...
EFRÉN, WHAT DOES IT MEAN THAT SOME GIRLS HAVE TATTOOS ON THEIR FACES?
AH, YES ... IN THEIR COMMUNITY IT MEANS THEY'RE PRETTY GIRLS.
The kids are in a good mood. In the room, Selam takes my watch, gives us a spiel in Amharic, and does a sort of catwalk routine ...

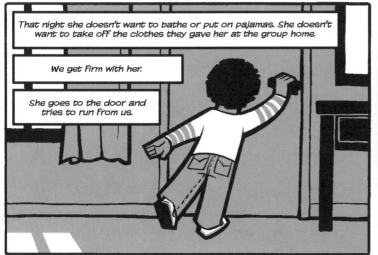

That night she doesn't want to bathe or put on pajamas. She doesn't want to take off the clothes they gave her at the group home.

We get firm with her.

She goes to the door and tries to run from us.

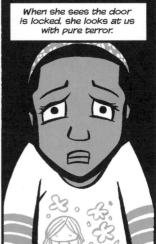

When she sees the door is locked, she looks at us with pure terror.

We realize it's not the time and place to be firm.

After all, we're just two strangers to her.

It's time to show her affection and calm ... there will be time for rules later.

We don't bathe her or put on her pajamas, and let her sleep on the sofa.

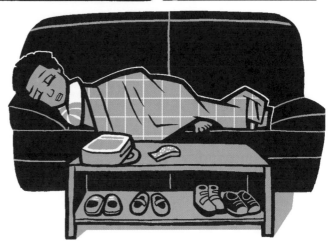

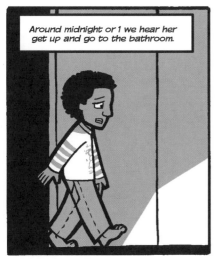

Around midnight or 1 we hear her get up and go to the bathroom.

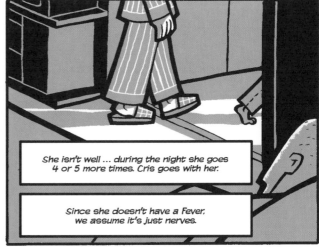

She isn't well ... during the night she goes 4 or 5 more times. Cris goes with her.

Since she doesn't have a fever, we assume it's just nerves.

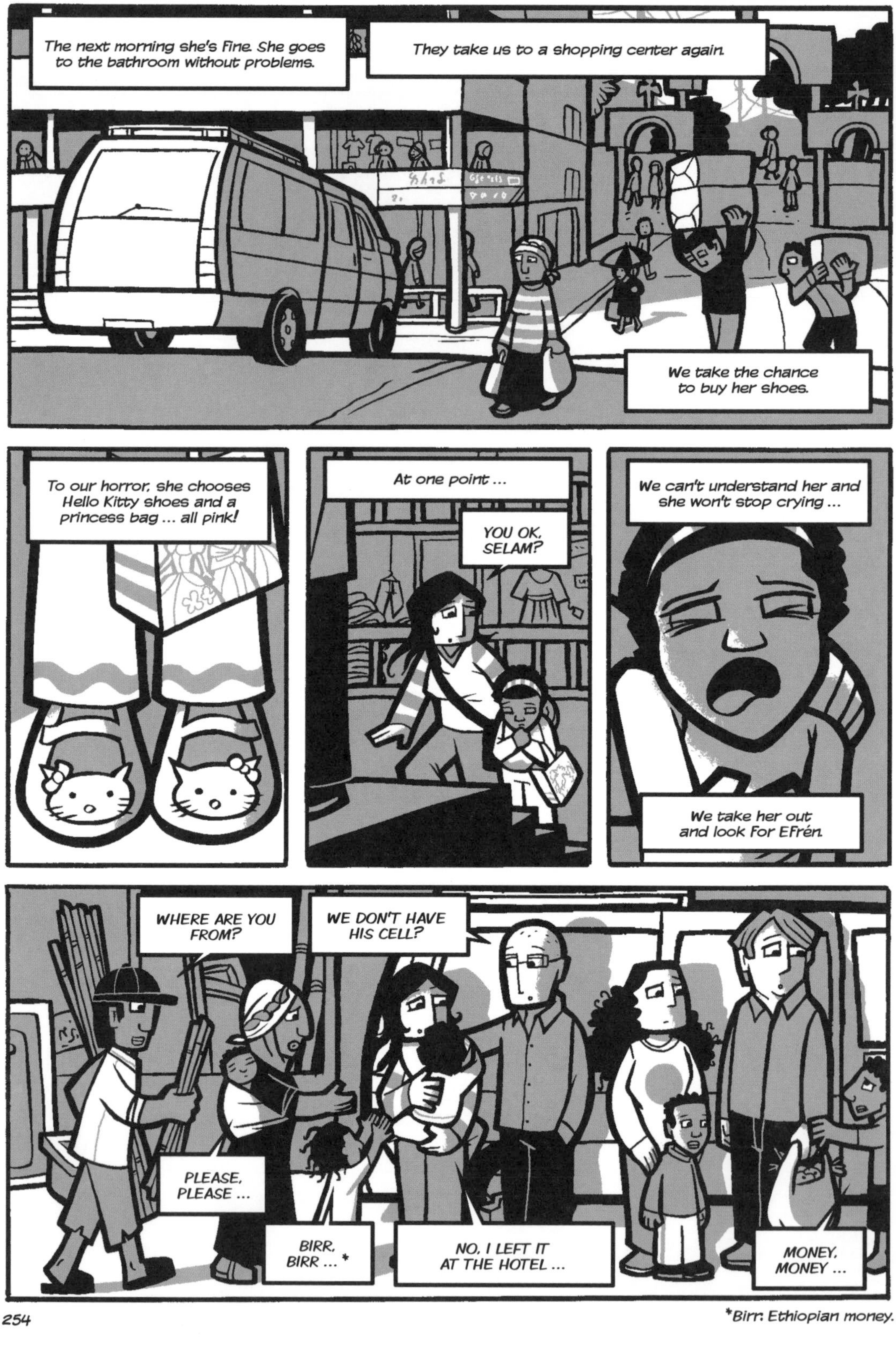
The next morning she's fine. She goes to the bathroom without problems.
They take us to a shopping center again.
We take the chance to buy her shoes.
To our horror, she chooses Hello Kitty shoes and a princess bag ... all pink!
At one point ...
YOU OK, SELAM?
We can't understand her and she won't stop crying ...
We take her out and look for Efrén.
WHERE ARE YOU FROM?
WE DON'T HAVE HIS CELL?
PLEASE, PLEASE ...
BIRR, BIRR ... *
NO, I LEFT IT AT THE HOTEL ...
MONEY, MONEY ...

*Birr: Ethiopian money.

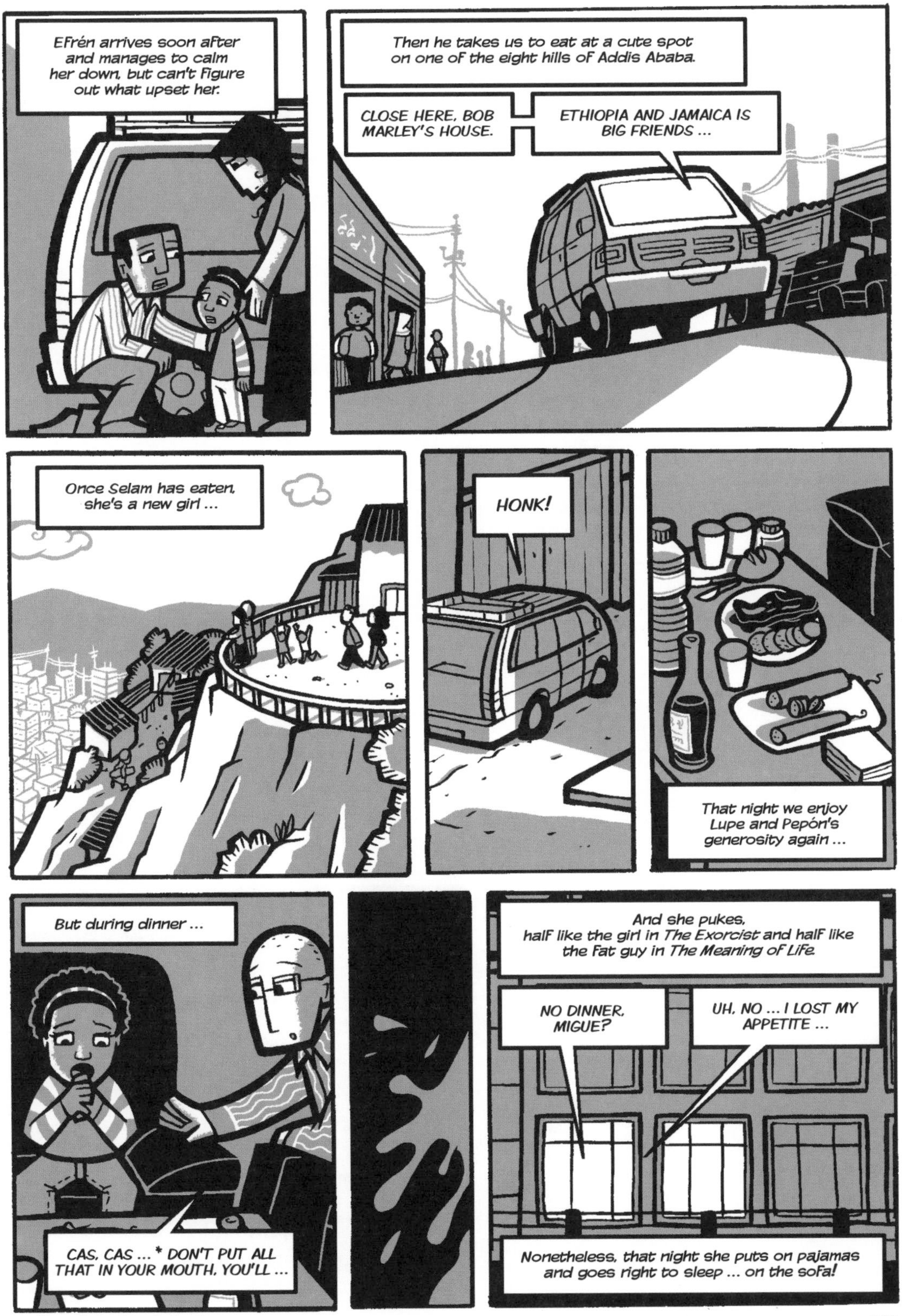
Efrén arrives soon after and manages to calm her down, but can't figure out what upset her.
Then he takes us to eat at a cute spot on one of the eight hills of Addis Ababa.
CLOSE HERE, BOB MARLEY'S HOUSE.
ETHIOPIA AND JAMAICA IS BIG FRIENDS ...
Once Selam has eaten, she's a new girl ...
HONK!
That night we enjoy Lupe and Pepón's generosity again ...
But during dinner ...
CAS, CAS ... * DON'T PUT ALL THAT IN YOUR MOUTH, YOU'LL ...
And she pukes, half like the girl in *The Exorcist* and half like the fat guy in *The Meaning of Life*.
NO DINNER, MIGUE?
UH, NO ... I LOST MY APPETITE ...
Nonetheless, that night she puts on pajamas and goes right to sleep ... on the sofa!

*Cas: "Slow" in Amharic.

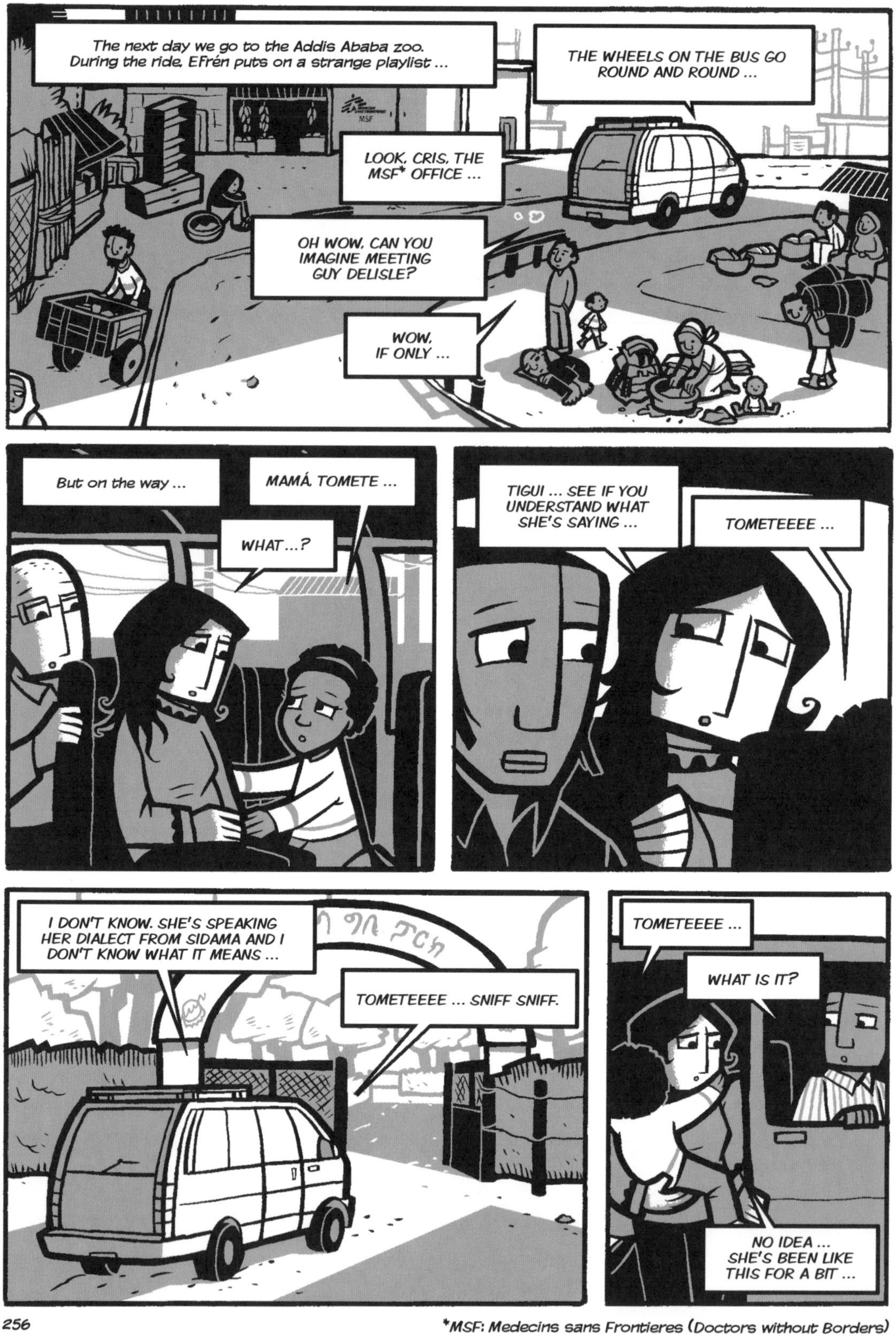
The next day we go to the Addis Ababa zoo. During the ride, Efrén puts on a strange playlist ...
THE WHEELS ON THE BUS GO ROUND AND ROUND ...
MSF
LOOK, CRIS, THE MSF* OFFICE ...
OH WOW, CAN YOU IMAGINE MEETING GUY DELISLE?
WOW, IF ONLY ...
But on the way ...
MAMÁ, TOMETE ...
WHAT ...?
TIGUI ... SEE IF YOU UNDERSTAND WHAT SHE'S SAYING ...
TOMETEEEE ...
I DON'T KNOW. SHE'S SPEAKING HER DIALECT FROM SIDAMA AND I DON'T KNOW WHAT IT MEANS ...
TOMETEEEE ... SNIFF SNIFF.
TOMETEEEE ...
WHAT IS IT?
NO IDEA ... SHE'S BEEN LIKE THIS FOR A BIT ...

*MSF: Medecins sans Frontieres (Doctors without Borders)

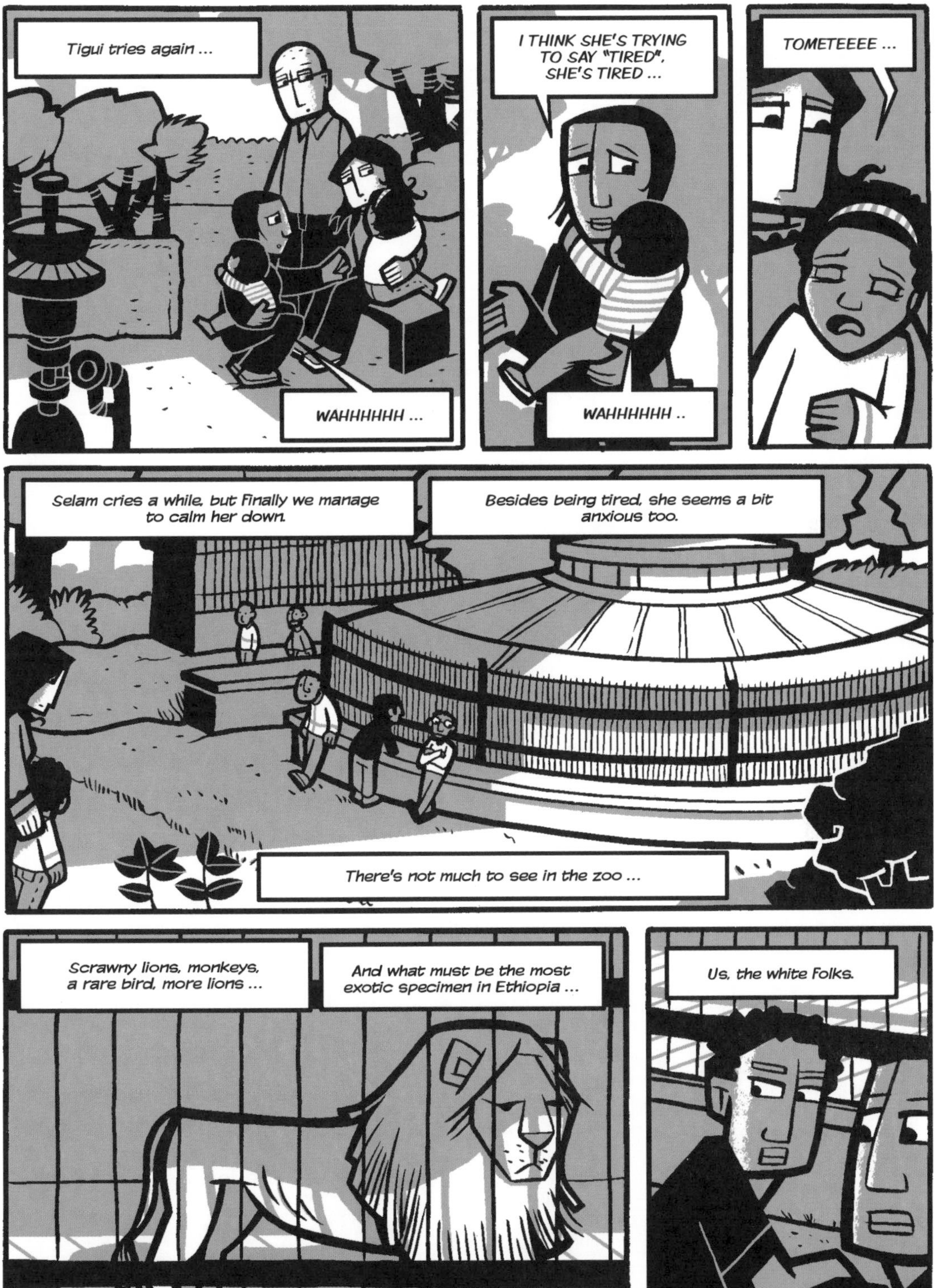
Tigui tries again ...
WAHHHHHH ...
I THINK SHE'S TRYING TO SAY "TIRED", SHE'S TIRED ...
WAHHHHHH ..
TOMETEEEE ...
Selam cries a while, but finally we manage to calm her down.
Besides being tired, she seems a bit anxious too.
There's not much to see in the zoo ...
Scrawny lions, monkeys, a rare bird, more lions ...
And what must be the most exotic specimen in Ethiopia ...
Us, the white folks.

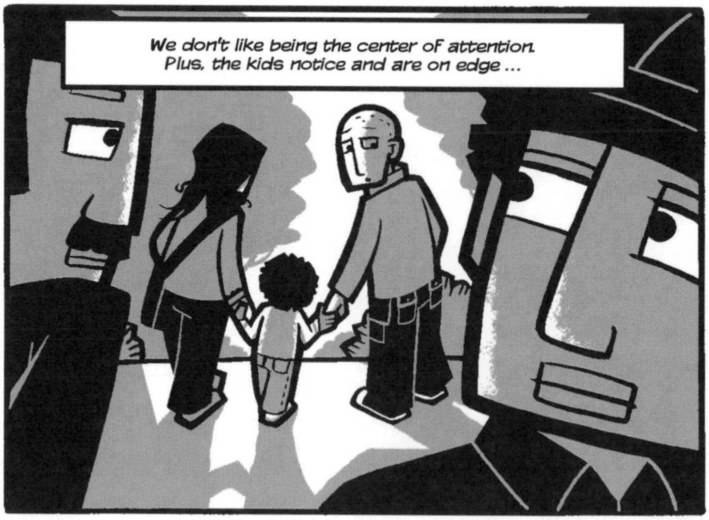
We don't like being the center of attention. Plus, the kids notice and are on edge ...

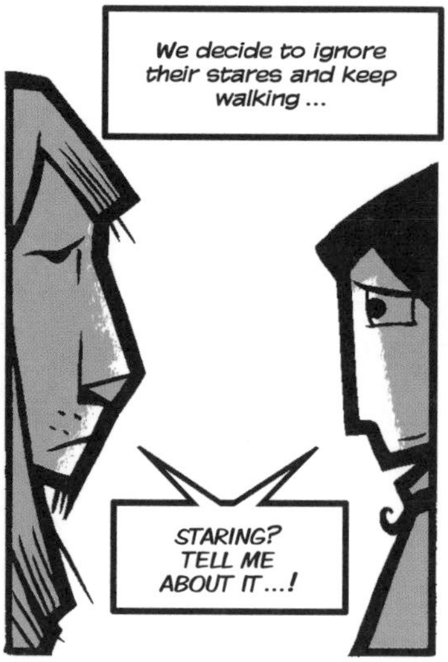
We decide to ignore their stares and keep walking ...
STARING? TELL ME ABOUT IT ...!

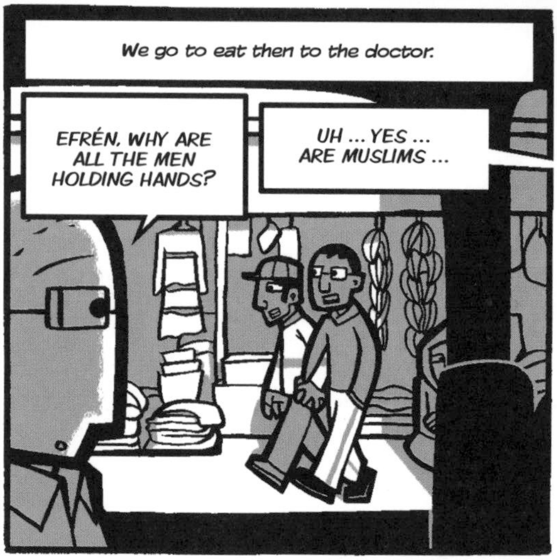
We go to eat then to the doctor.
EFRÉN, WHY ARE ALL THE MEN HOLDING HANDS?
UH ... YES ... ARE MUSLIMS ...

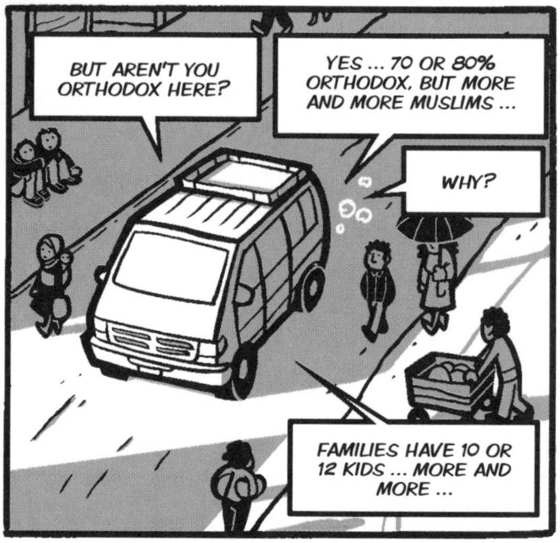
BUT AREN'T YOU ORTHODOX HERE?
YES ... 70 OR 80% ORTHODOX, BUT MORE AND MORE MUSLIMS ...
WHY?
FAMILIES HAVE 10 OR 12 KIDS ... MORE AND MORE ...

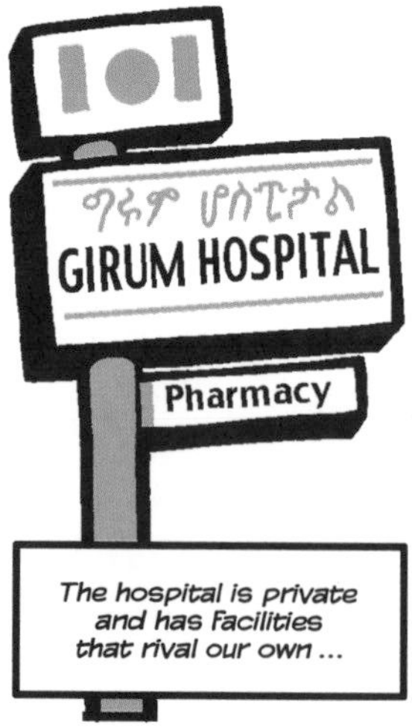
ግሩም ሆስፒታል
GIRUM HOSPITAL
Pharmacy
The hospital is private and has facilities that rival our own ...

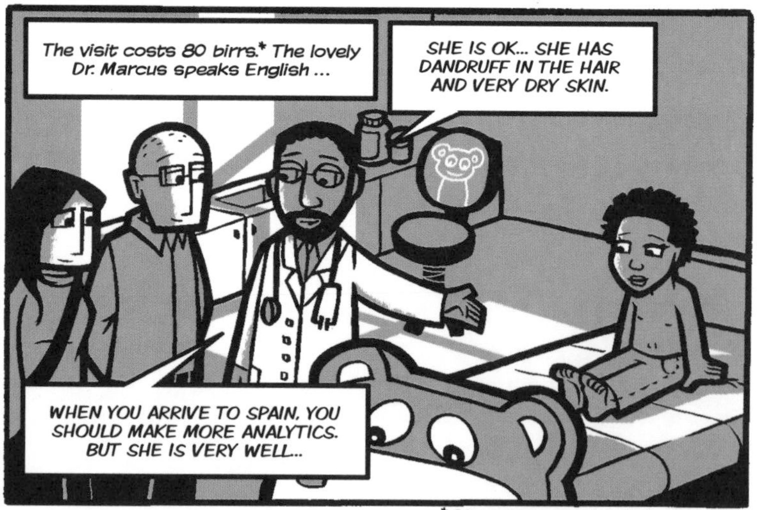
The visit costs 80 birrs.* The lovely Dr. Marcus speaks English ...
SHE IS OK... SHE HAS DANDRUFF IN THE HAIR AND VERY DRY SKIN.
WHEN YOU ARRIVE TO SPAIN, YOU SHOULD MAKE MORE ANALYTICS. BUT SHE IS VERY WELL...

*80 birrs: around 3 dollars

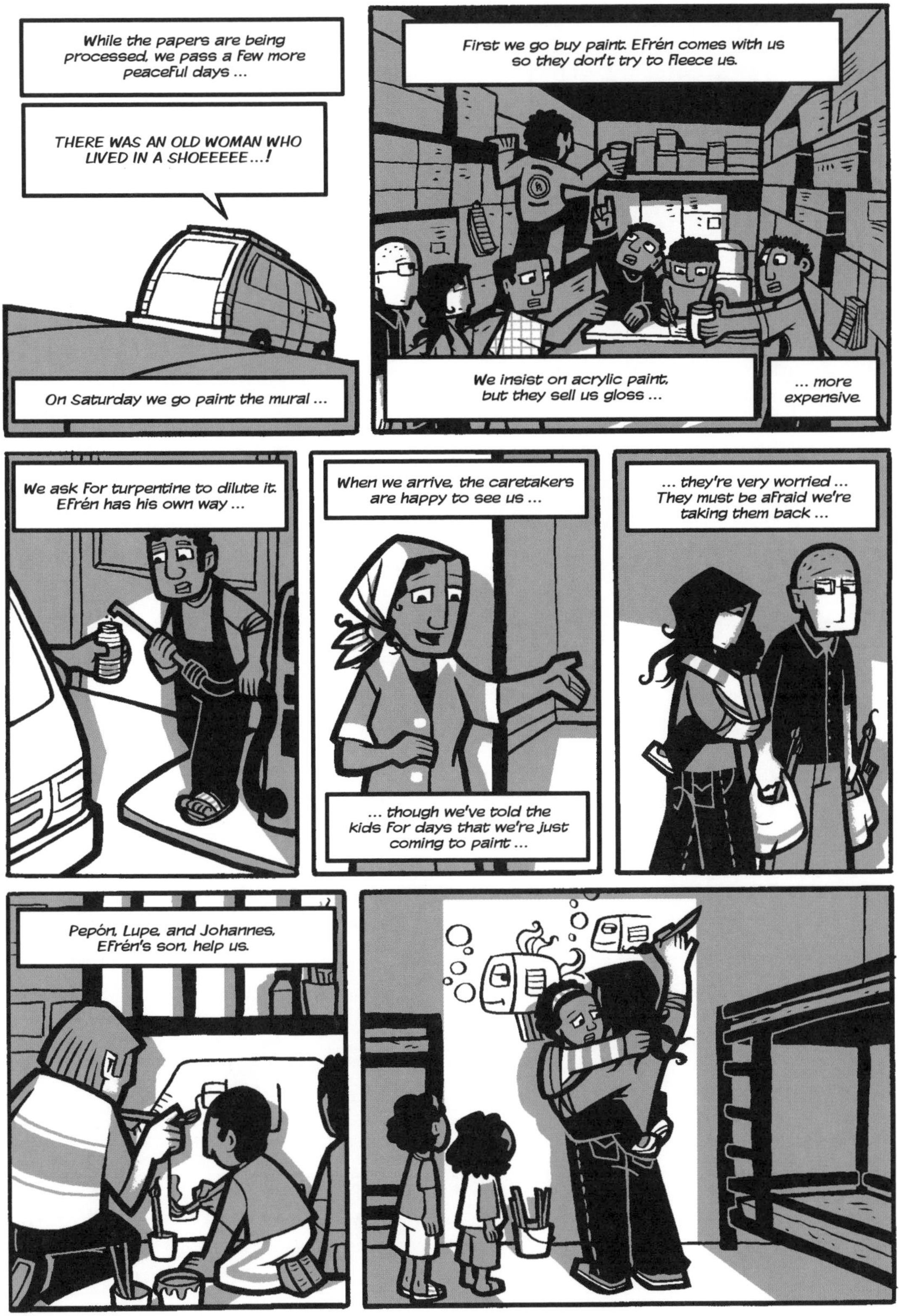
While the papers are being processed, we pass a few more peaceful days ...
THERE WAS AN OLD WOMAN WHO LIVED IN A SHOEEEEE...!
On Saturday we go paint the mural ...
First we go buy paint. Efrén comes with us so they don't try to fleece us.
We insist on acrylic paint, but they sell us gloss ...
... more expensive.
We ask for turpentine to dilute it. Efrén has his own way ...
When we arrive, the caretakers are happy to see us ...
... though we've told the kids for days that we're just coming to paint ...
... they're very worried ... They must be afraid we're taking them back ...
Pepón, Lupe, and Johannes, Efrén's son, help us.

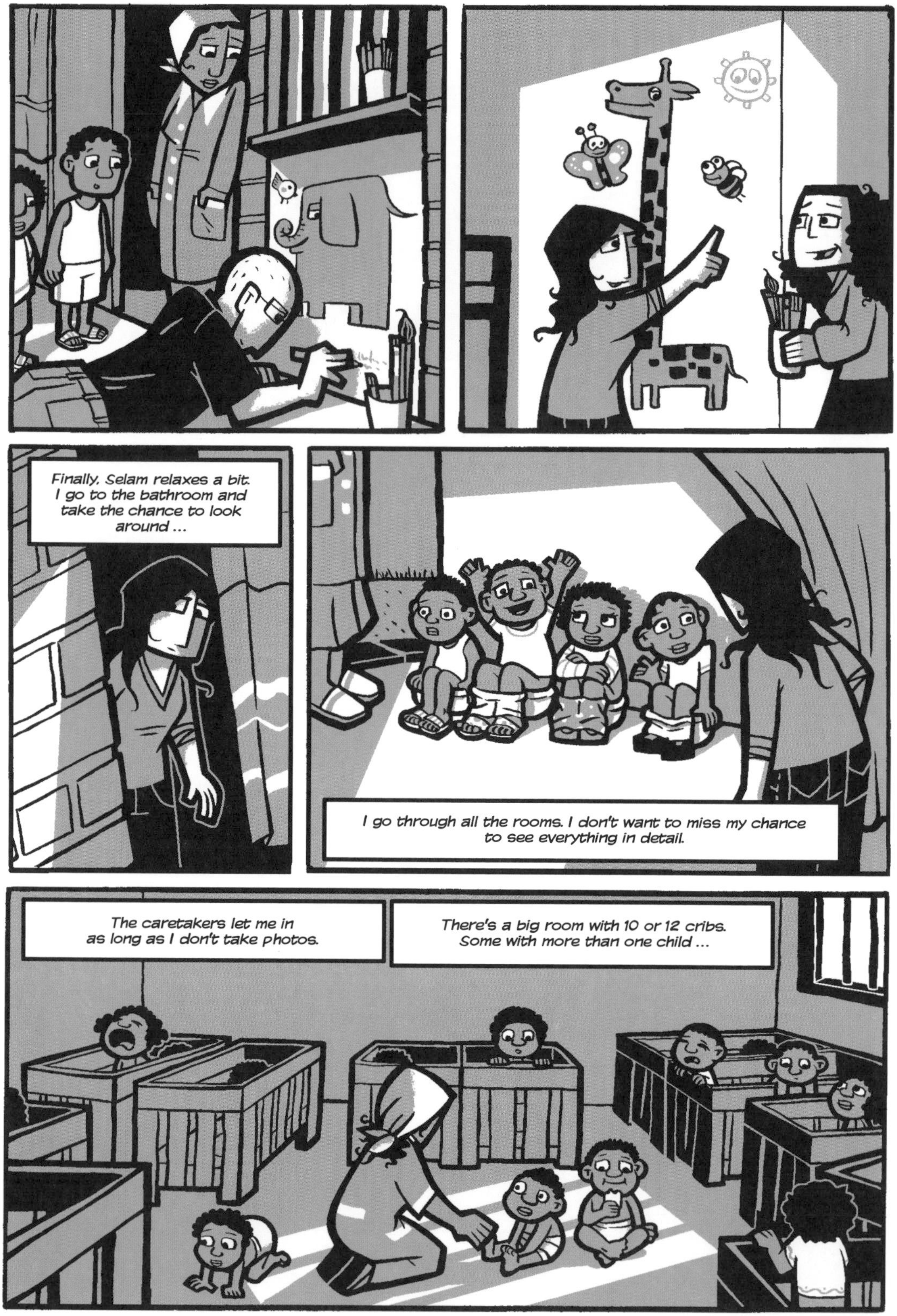
Finally, Selam relaxes a bit. I go to the bathroom and take the chance to look around ...
I go through all the rooms. I don't want to miss my chance to see everything in detail.
The caretakers let me in as long as I don't take photos.
There's a big room with 10 or 12 cribs. Some with more than one child ...

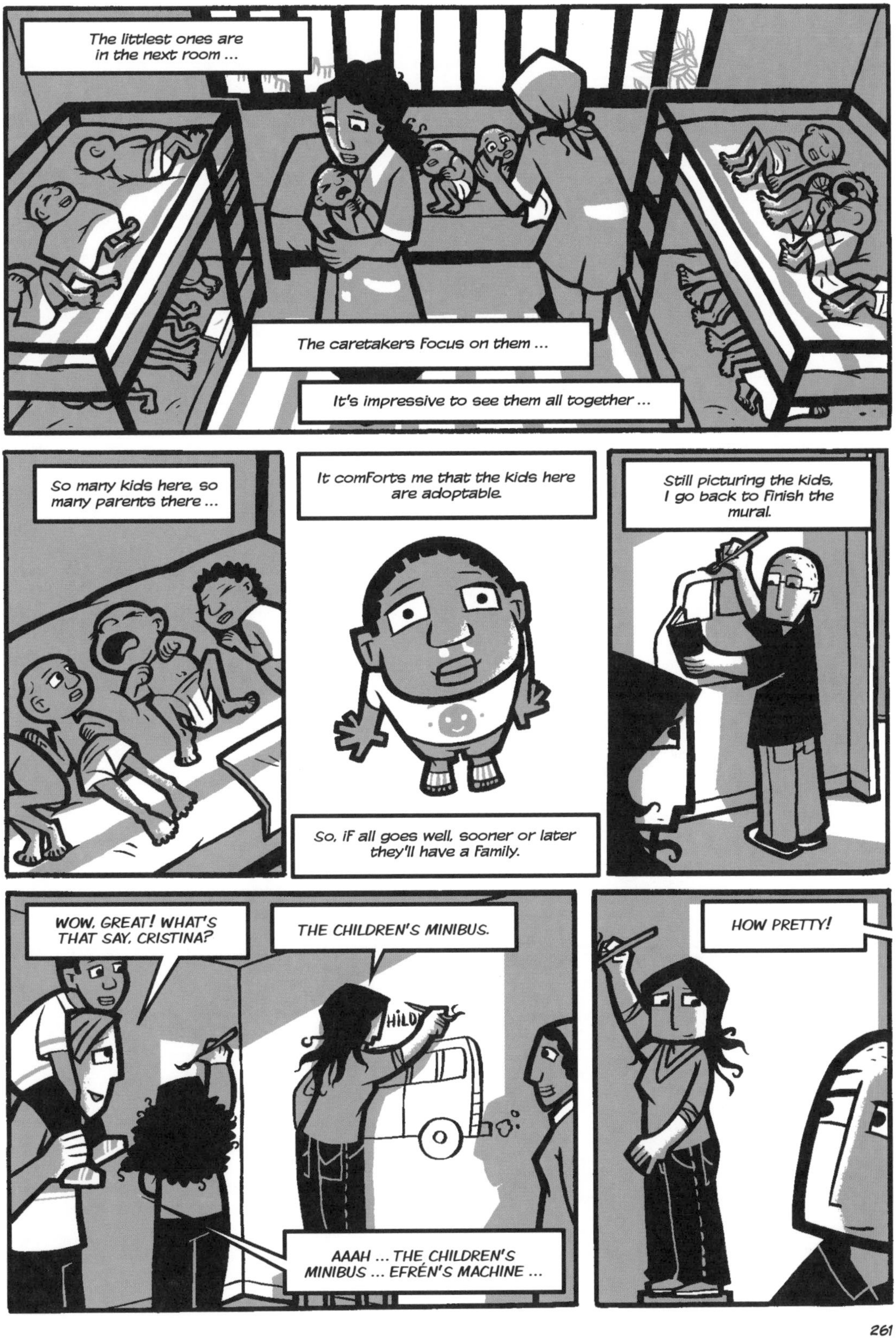
The littlest ones are in the next room ...
The caretakers focus on them ...
It's impressive to see them all together ...
So many kids here, so many parents there ...
It comforts me that the kids here are adoptable.
So, if all goes well, sooner or later they'll have a family.
Still picturing the kids, I go back to finish the mural.
WOW, GREAT! WHAT'S THAT SAY, CRISTINA?
THE CHILDREN'S MINIBUS.
AAAH ... THE CHILDREN'S MINIBUS ... EFRÉN'S MACHINE ...
HOW PRETTY!

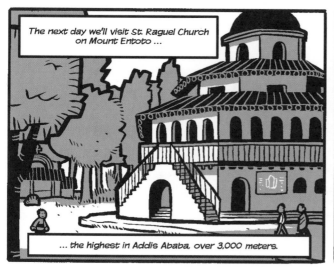

The next day we'll visit St. Raguel Church on Mount Entoto ...

... the highest in Addis Ababa, over 3,000 meters.

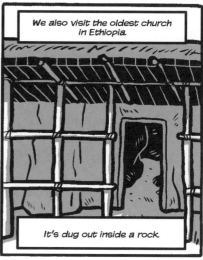

We also visit the oldest church in Ethiopia.

It's dug out inside a rock.

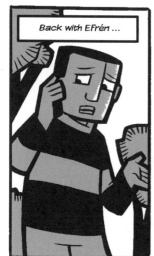

Back with Efrén ...

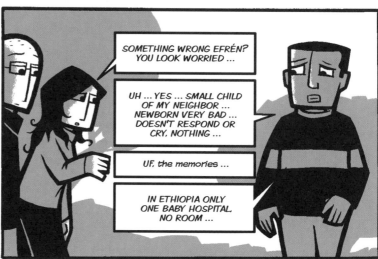

SOMETHING WRONG EFRÉN? YOU LOOK WORRIED ...

UH ... YES ... SMALL CHILD OF MY NEIGHBOR ... NEWBORN VERY BAD ... DOESN'T RESPOND OR CRY, NOTHING ...

UF, the memories ...

IN ETHIOPIA ONLY ONE BABY HOSPITAL, NO ROOM ...

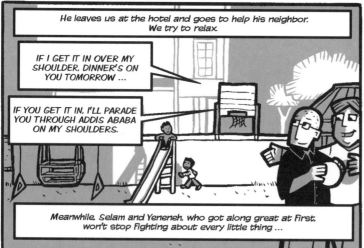

He leaves us at the hotel and goes to help his neighbor. We try to relax.

IF I GET IT IN OVER MY SHOULDER, DINNER'S ON YOU TOMORROW ...

IF YOU GET IT IN, I'LL PARADE YOU THROUGH ADDIS ABABA ON MY SHOULDERS.

Meanwhile, Selam and Yeneneh, who got along great at first, won't stop fighting about every little thing ...

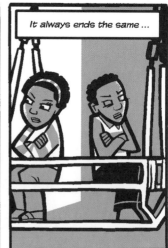

It always ends the same ...

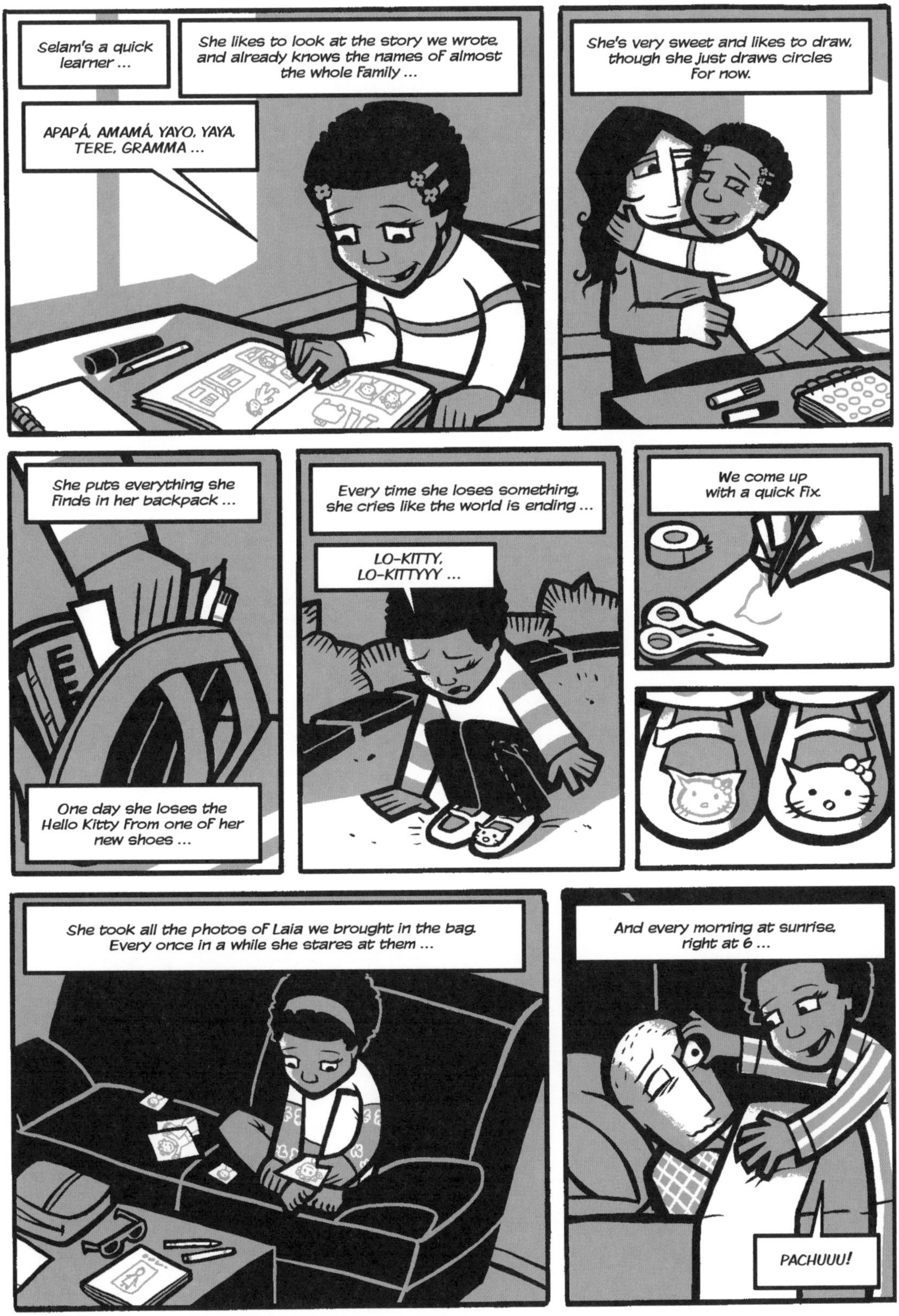
Selam's a quick learner ...
She likes to look at the story we wrote, and already knows the names of almost the whole family ...
APAPÁ, AMAMÁ, YAYO, YAYA, TERE, GRAMMA ...
She's very sweet and likes to draw, though she just draws circles for now.
She puts everything she finds in her backpack ...
One day she loses the Hello Kitty from one of her new shoes ...
Every time she loses something, she cries like the world is ending ...
LO-KITTY, LO-KITTYYY ...
We come up with a quick fix.
She took all the photos of Laia we brought in the bag. Every once in a while she stares at them ...
And every morning at sunrise, right at 6 ...
PACHUUU!

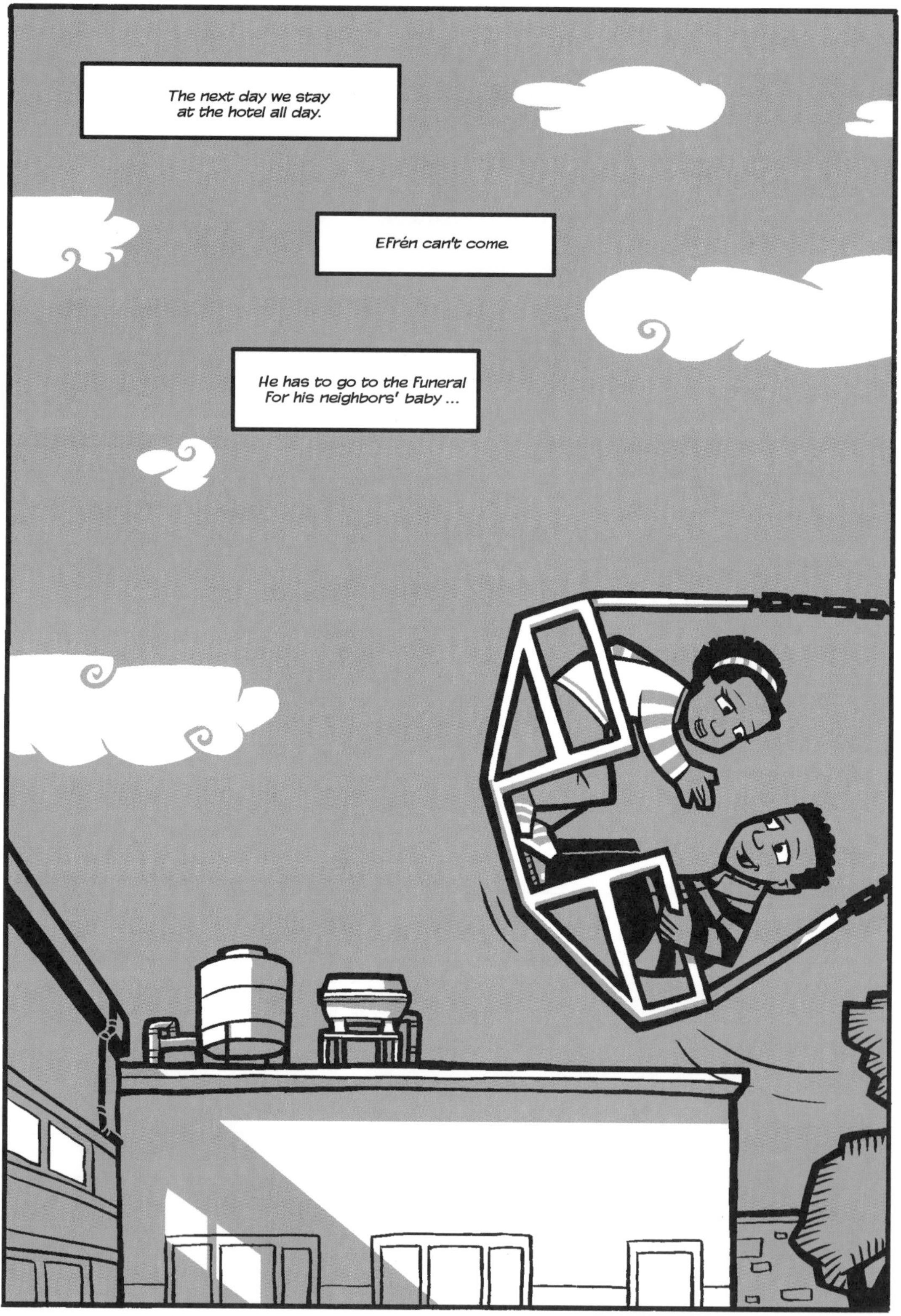
The next day we stay
at the hotel all day.
Efrén can't come.
He has to go to the funeral
for his neighbors' baby ...

Chapter 8
THE RETURN

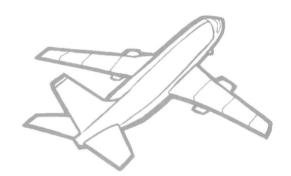

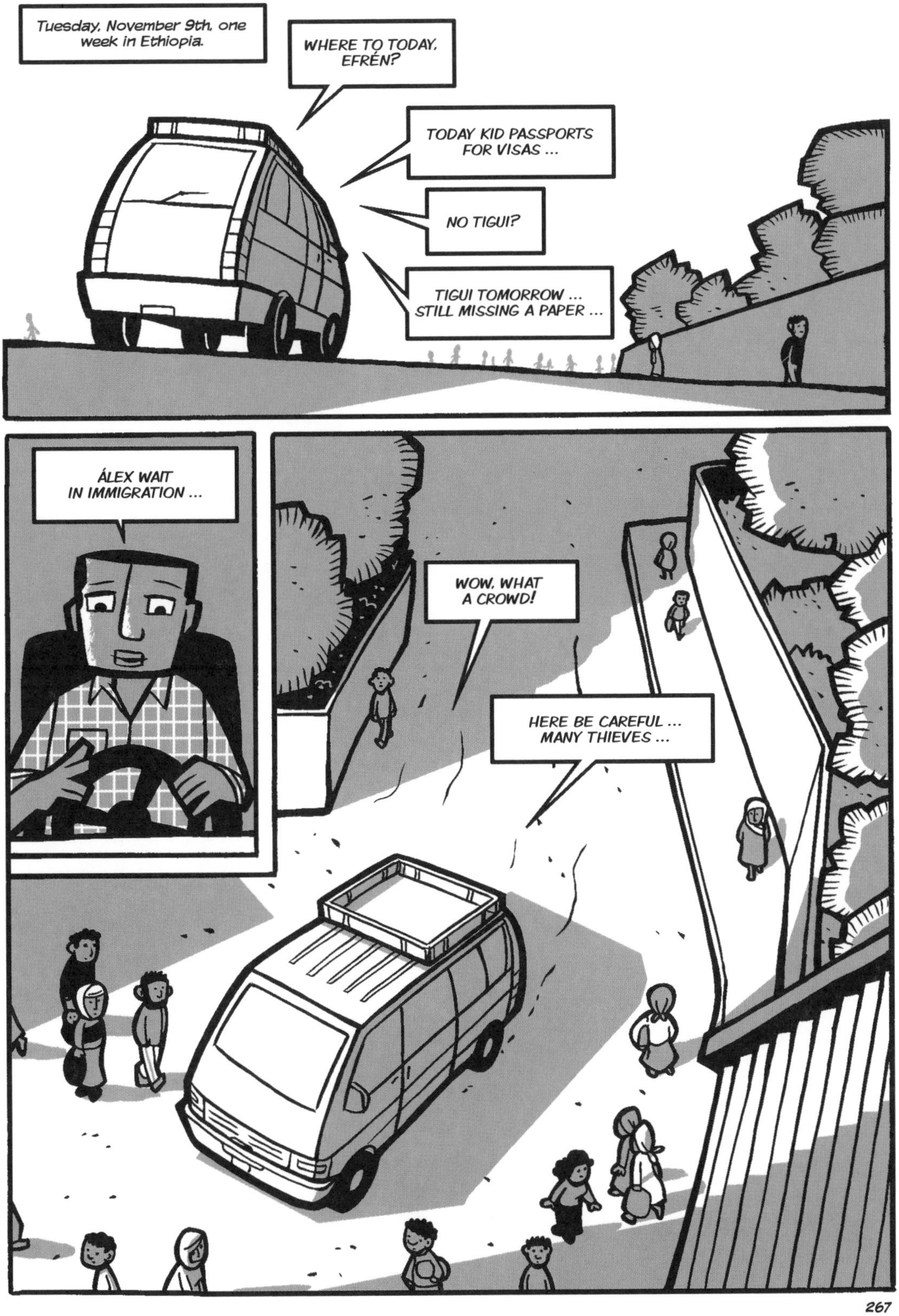
Tuesday, November 9th, one week in Ethiopia.
WHERE TO TODAY, EFRÉN?
TODAY KID PASSPORTS FOR VISAS ...
NO TIGUI?
TIGUI TOMORROW ... STILL MISSING A PAPER ...
ÁLEX WAIT IN IMMIGRATION ...
WOW, WHAT A CROWD!
HERE BE CAREFUL ... MANY THIEVES ...

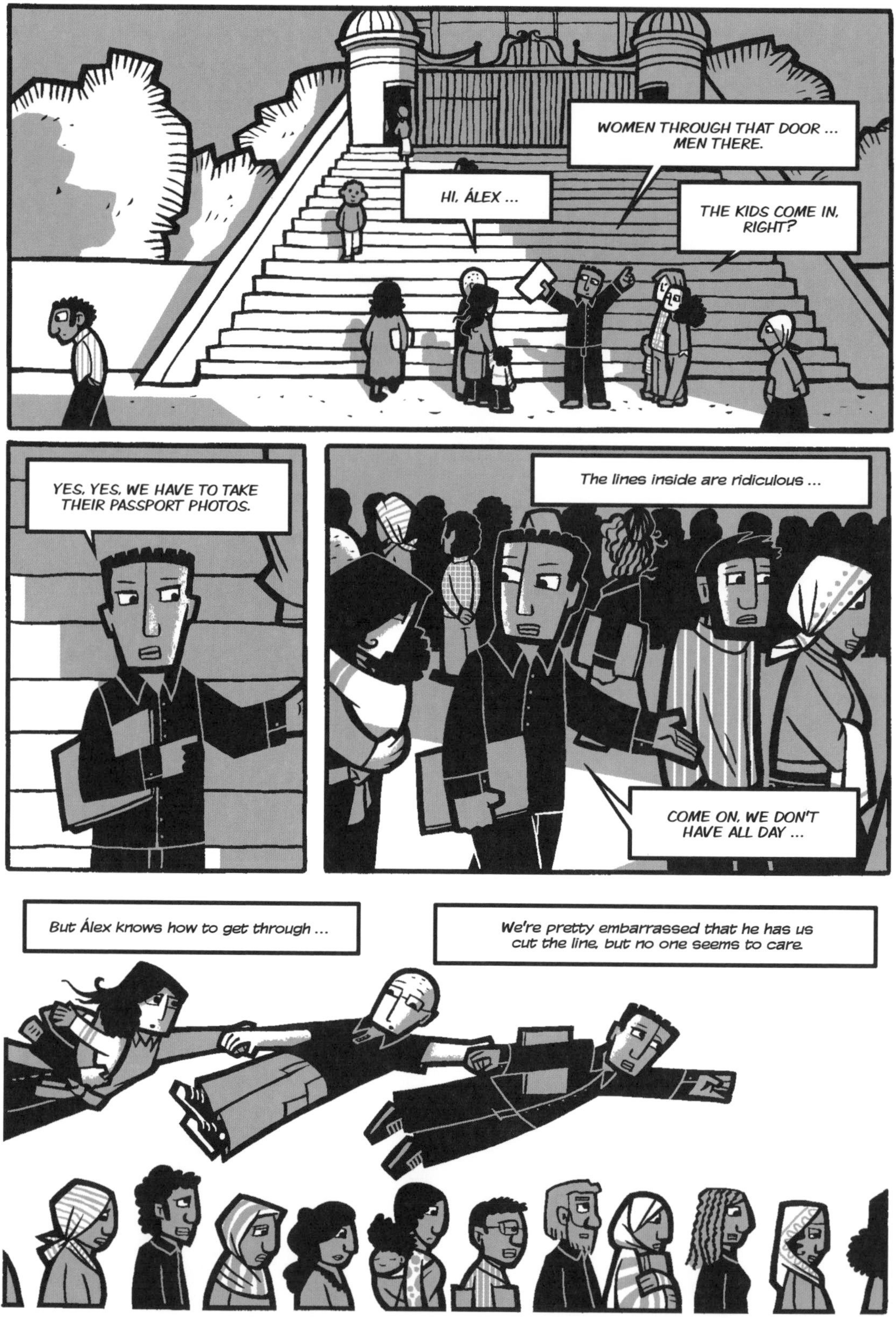
HI, ÁLEX ...
WOMEN THROUGH THAT DOOR ... MEN THERE.
THE KIDS COME IN, RIGHT?
YES, YES, WE HAVE TO TAKE THEIR PASSPORT PHOTOS.
The lines inside are ridiculous ...
COME ON, WE DON'T HAVE ALL DAY ...
But Álex knows how to get through ...
We're pretty embarrassed that he has us cut the line, but no one seems to care.

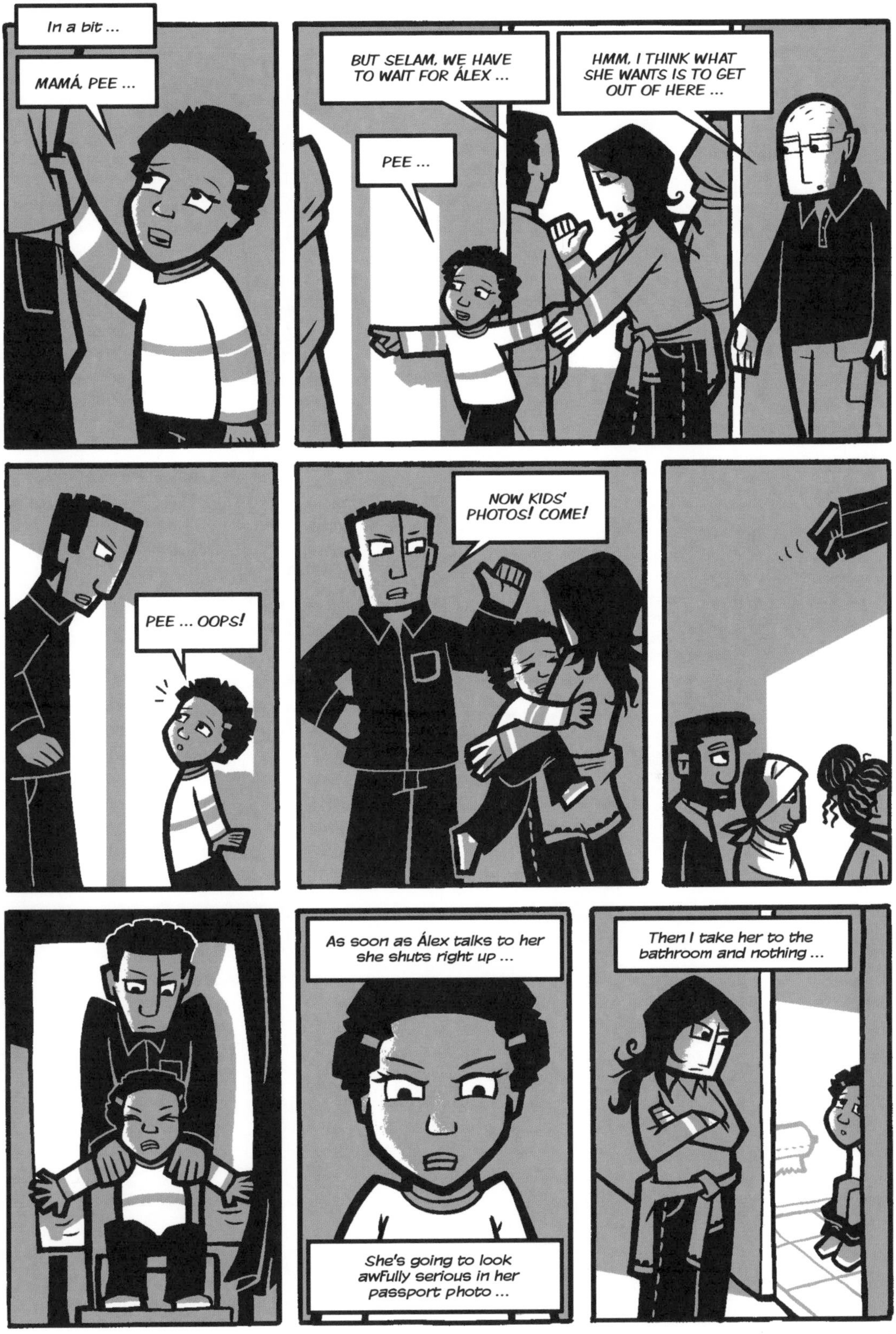
In a bit ...
MAMÁ, PEE ...
BUT SELAM, WE HAVE TO WAIT FOR ÁLEX ...
PEE ...
HMM, I THINK WHAT SHE WANTS IS TO GET OUT OF HERE ...
PEE ... OOPS!
NOW KIDS' PHOTOS! COME!
As soon as Álex talks to her she shuts right up ...
She's going to look awfully serious in her passport photo ...
Then I take her to the bathroom and nothing ...

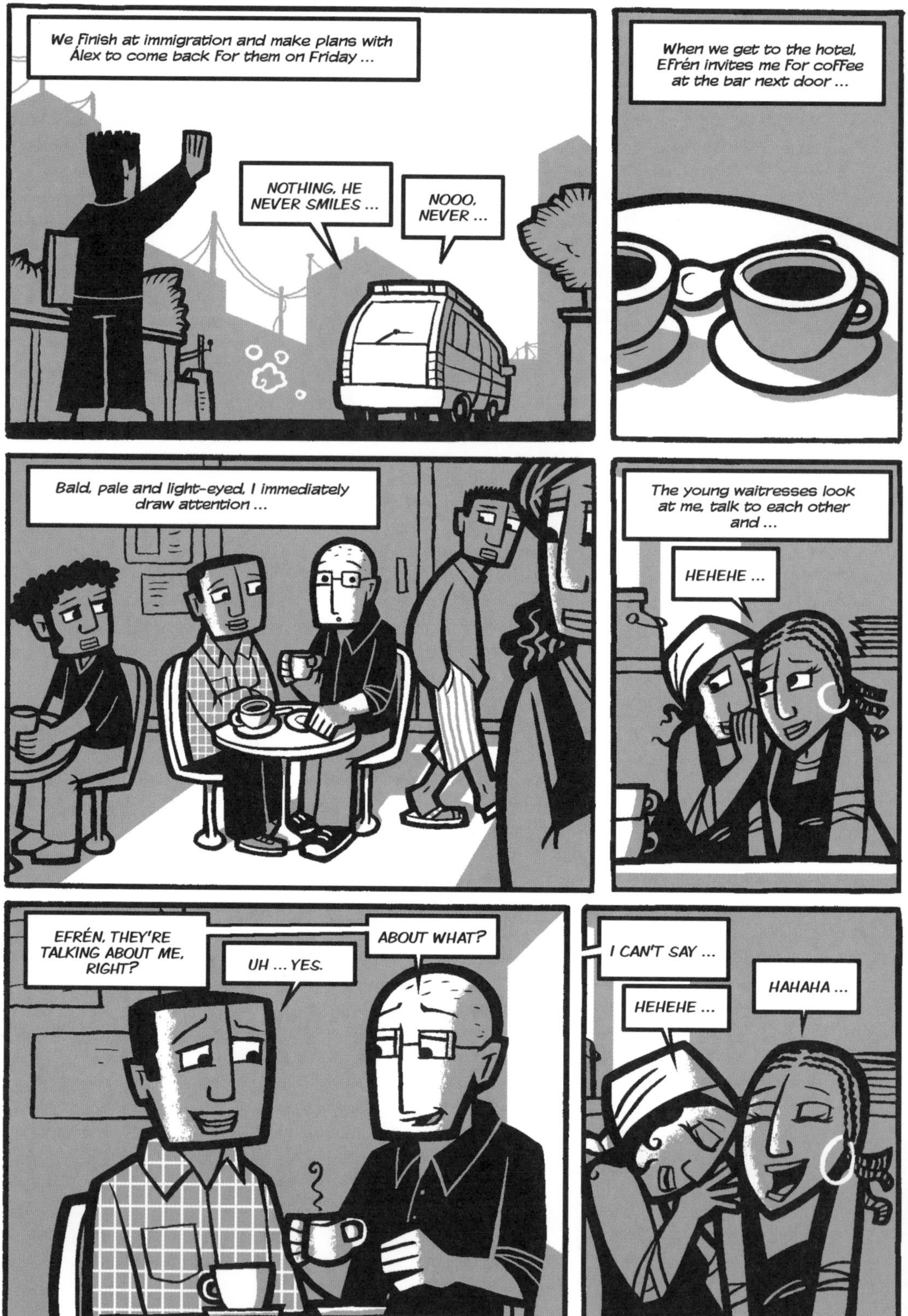
We finish at immigration and make plans with Álex to come back for them on Friday ...
NOTHING, HE NEVER SMILES ...
NOOO, NEVER ...
When we get to the hotel, Efrén invites me for coffee at the bar next door ...
Bald, pale and light-eyed, I immediately draw attention ...
The young waitresses look at me, talk to each other and ...
HEHEHE ...
EFRÉN, THEY'RE TALKING ABOUT ME, RIGHT?
UH ... YES.
ABOUT WHAT?
I CAN'T SAY ...
HEHEHE ...
HAHAHA ...

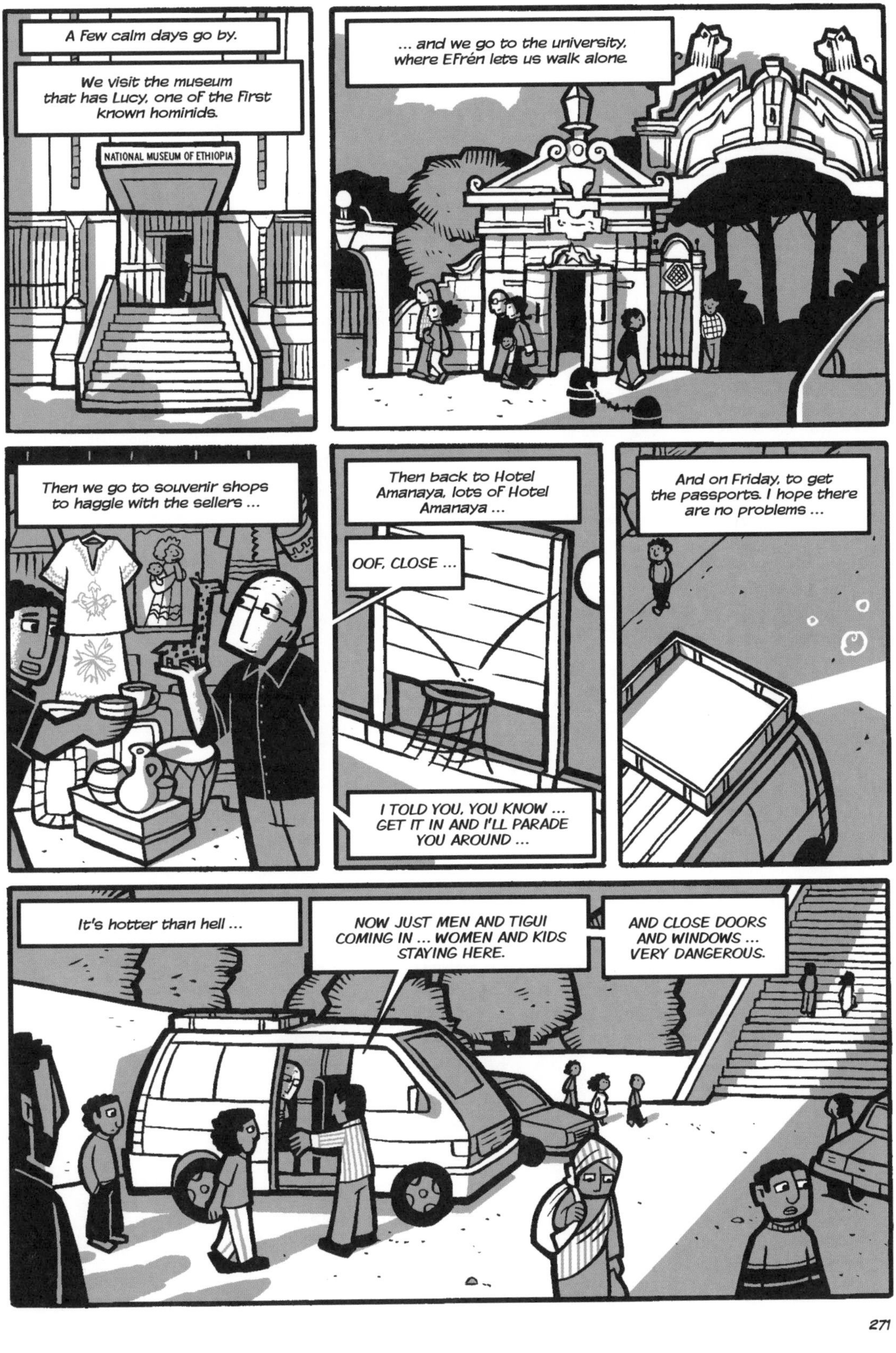
A Few calm days go by.
We visit the museum that has Lucy, one of the first known hominids.
NATIONAL MUSEUM OF ETHIOPIA
... and we go to the university, where Efrén lets us walk alone.
Then we go to souvenir shops to haggle with the sellers ...
Then back to Hotel Amanaya, lots of Hotel Amanaya ...
OOF, CLOSE ...
I TOLD YOU, YOU KNOW ... GET IT IN AND I'LL PARADE YOU AROUND ...
And on Friday, to get the passports. I hope there are no problems ...
It's hotter than hell ...
NOW JUST MEN AND TIGUI COMING IN ... WOMEN AND KIDS STAYING HERE.
AND CLOSE DOORS AND WINDOWS ... VERY DANGEROUS.

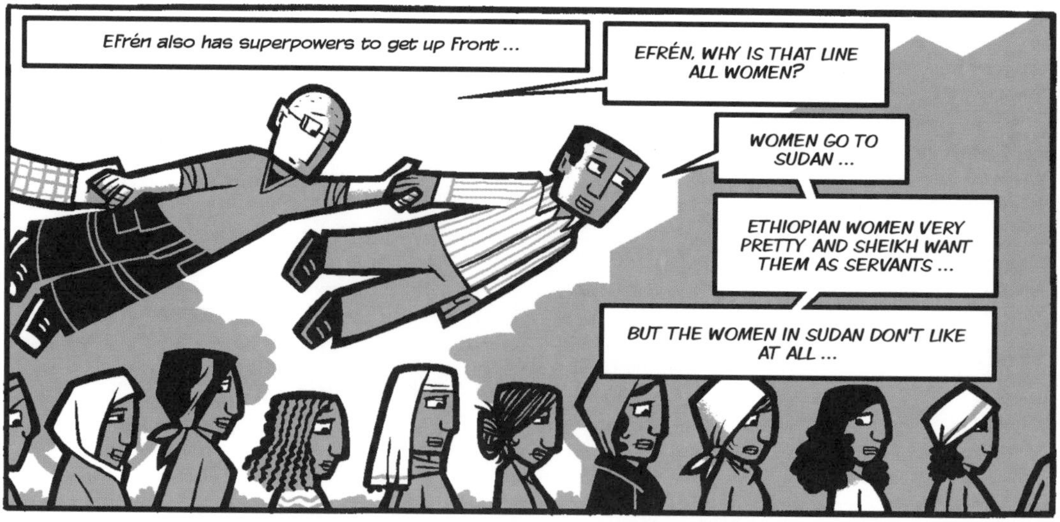
Efrén also has superpowers to get up front ...
EFRÉN, WHY IS THAT LINE ALL WOMEN?
WOMEN GO TO SUDAN ...
ETHIOPIAN WOMEN VERY PRETTY AND SHEIKH WANT THEM AS SERVANTS ...
BUT THE WOMEN IN SUDAN DON'T LIKE AT ALL ...

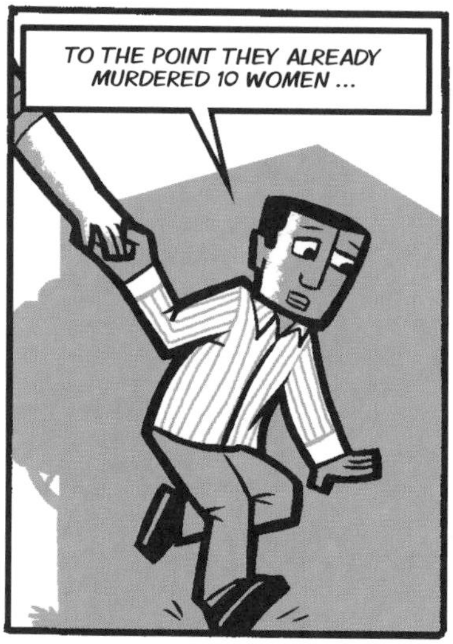
TO THE POINT THEY ALREADY MURDERED 10 WOMEN ...

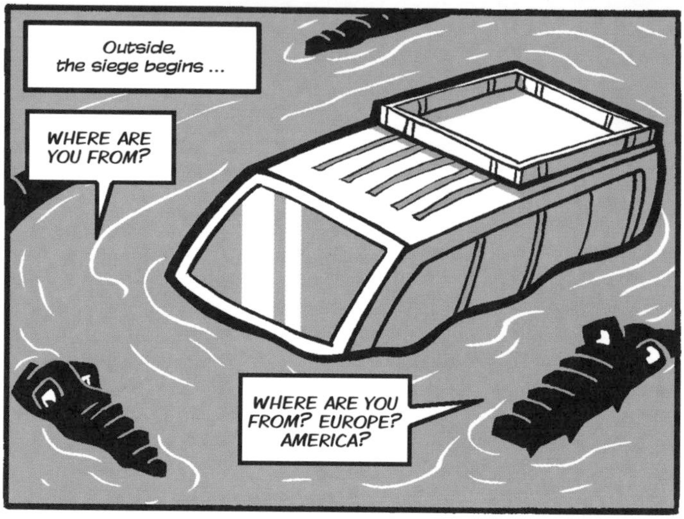
Outside, the siege begins ...
WHERE ARE YOU FROM?
WHERE ARE YOU FROM? EUROPE? AMERICA?

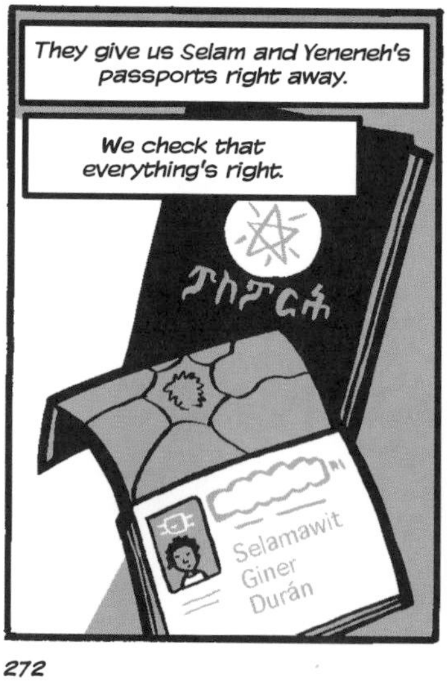
They give us Selam and Yeneneh's passports right away.
We check that everything's right.
Selamawit
Giner
Durán

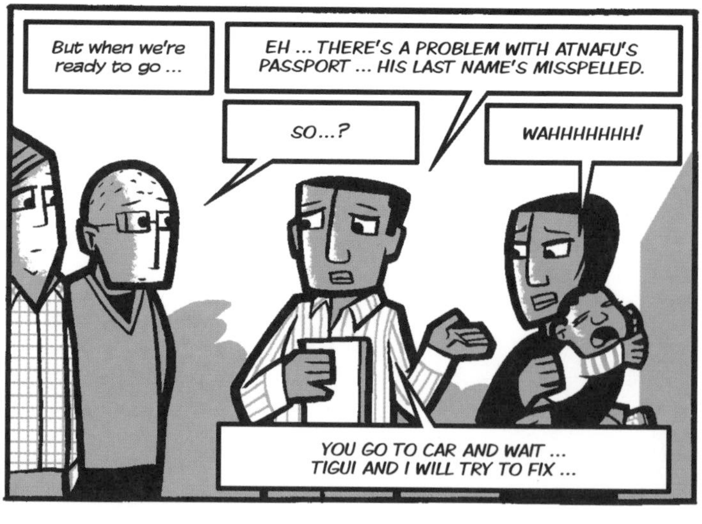
But when we're ready to go ...
EH ... THERE'S A PROBLEM WITH ATNAFU'S PASSPORT ... HIS LAST NAME'S MISSPELLED.
SO...?
WAHHHHHHH!
YOU GO TO CAR AND WAIT ... TIGUI AND I WILL TRY TO FIX ...

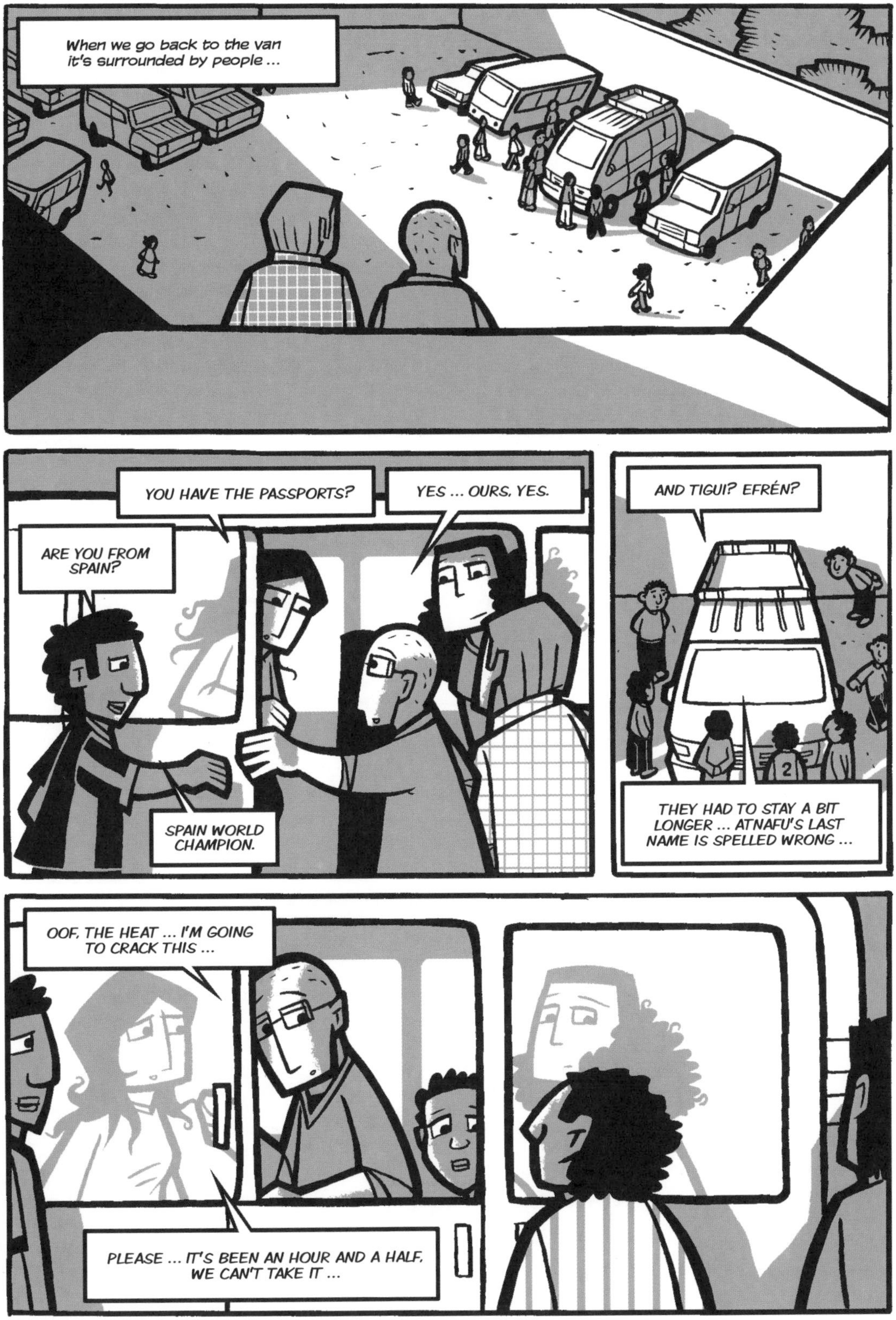
When we go back to the van it's surrounded by people ...
ARE YOU FROM SPAIN?
YOU HAVE THE PASSPORTS?
YES ... OURS, YES.
SPAIN WORLD CHAMPION.
AND TIGUI? EFRÉN?
THEY HAD TO STAY A BIT LONGER ... ATNAFU'S LAST NAME IS SPELLED WRONG ...
OOF, THE HEAT ... I'M GOING TO CRACK THIS ...
PLEASE ... IT'S BEEN AN HOUR AND A HALF, WE CAN'T TAKE IT ...

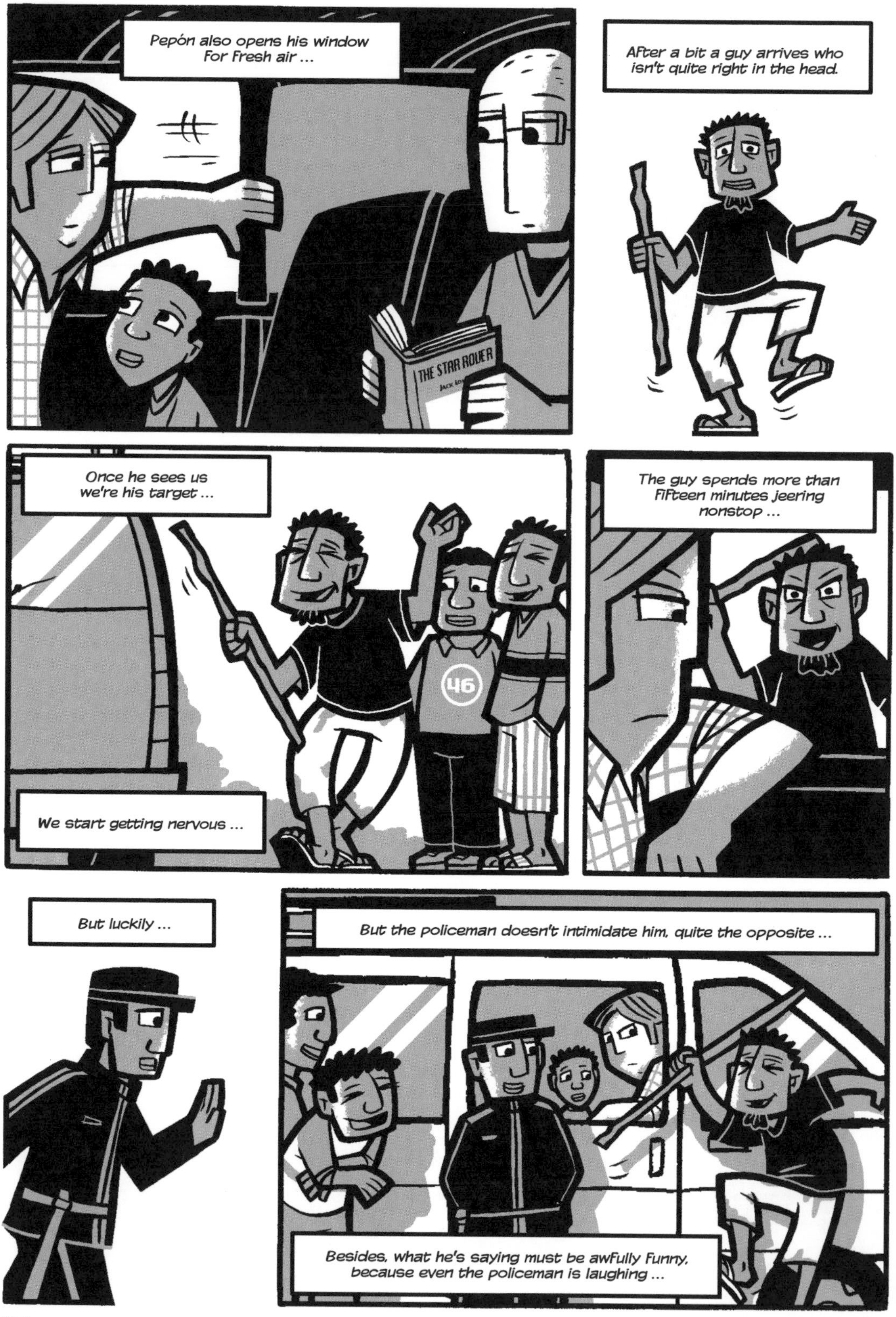
Pepón also opens his window
For fresh air ...
THE STAR ROVER
After a bit a guy arrives who
isn't quite right in the head.
Once he sees us
we're his target ...
We start getting nervous ...
46
The guy spends more than
fifteen minutes jeering
nonstop ...
But luckily ...
But the policeman doesn't intimidate him, quite the opposite ...
Besides, what he's saying must be awfully funny,
because even the policeman is laughing ...

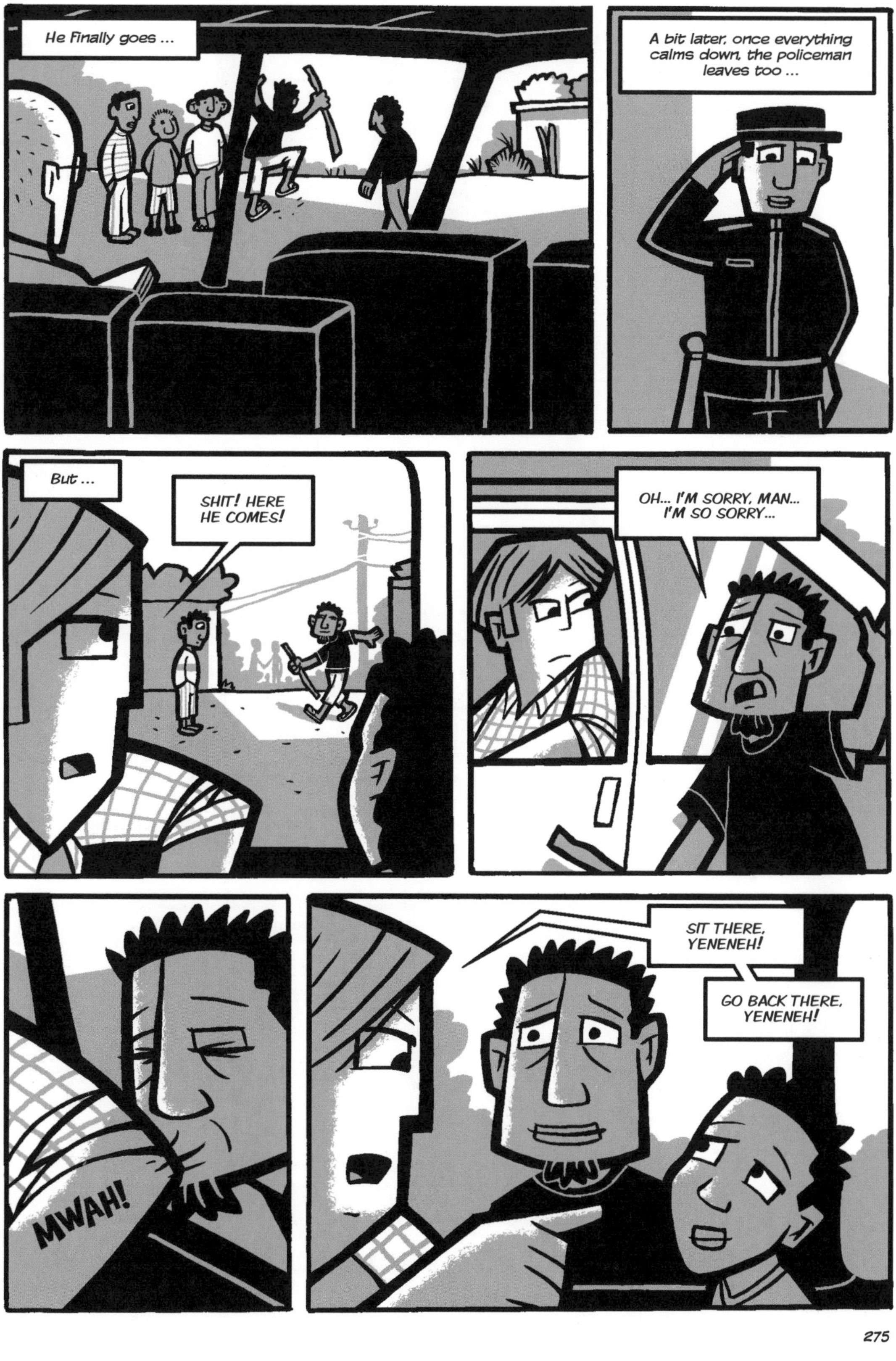
He finally goes ...
A bit later, once everything calms down, the policeman leaves too ...
But ...
SHIT! HERE HE COMES!
OH... I'M SORRY, MAN... I'M SO SORRY...
MWAH!
SIT THERE, YENENEH!
GO BACK THERE, YENENEH!

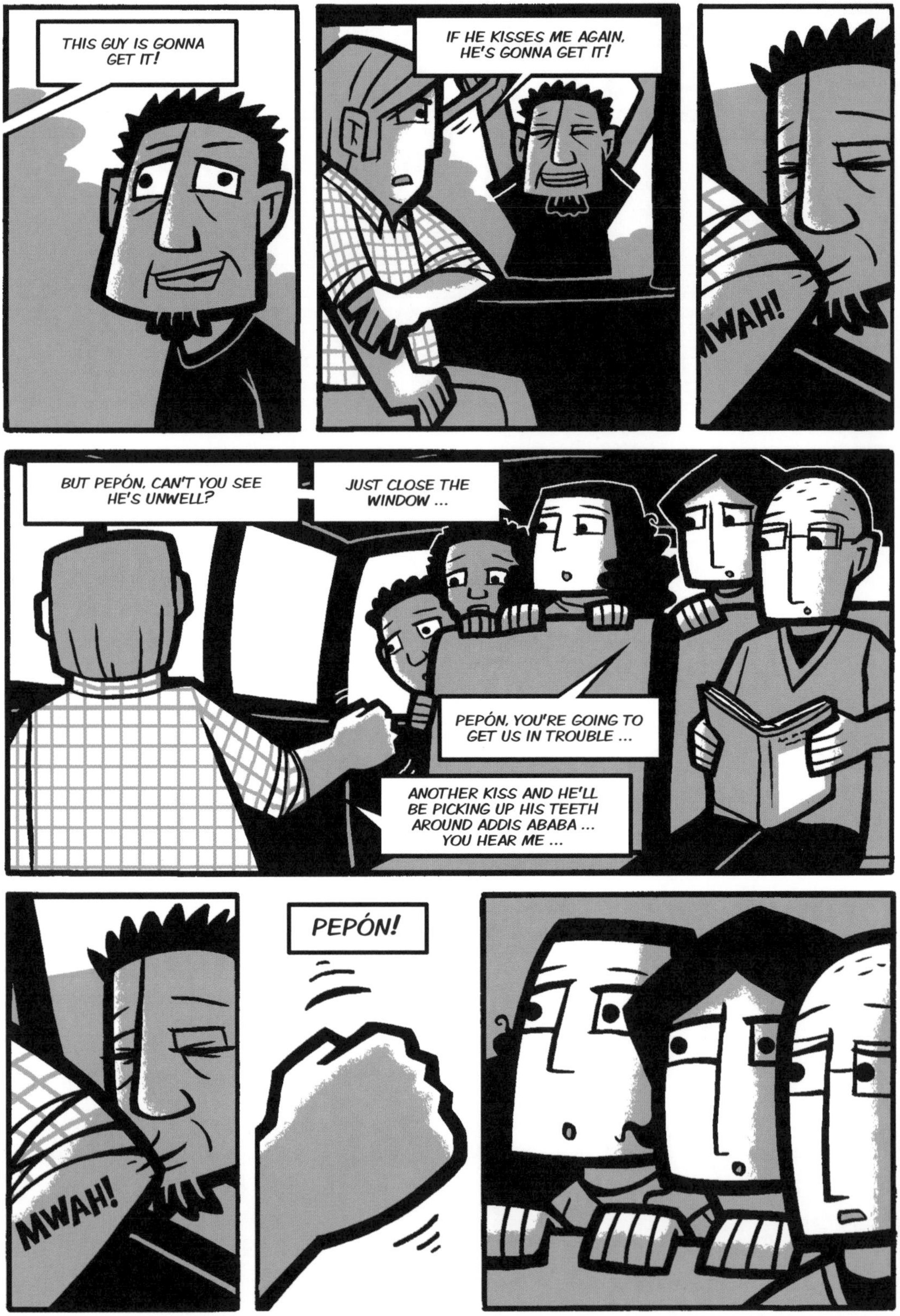
THIS GUY IS GONNA GET IT!
IF HE KISSES ME AGAIN, HE'S GONNA GET IT!
MWAH!
BUT PEPÓN, CAN'T YOU SEE HE'S UNWELL?
JUST CLOSE THE WINDOW ...
PEPÓN, YOU'RE GOING TO GET US IN TROUBLE ...
ANOTHER KISS AND HE'LL BE PICKING UP HIS TEETH AROUND ADDIS ABABA ... YOU HEAR ME ...
MWAH!
PEPÓN!

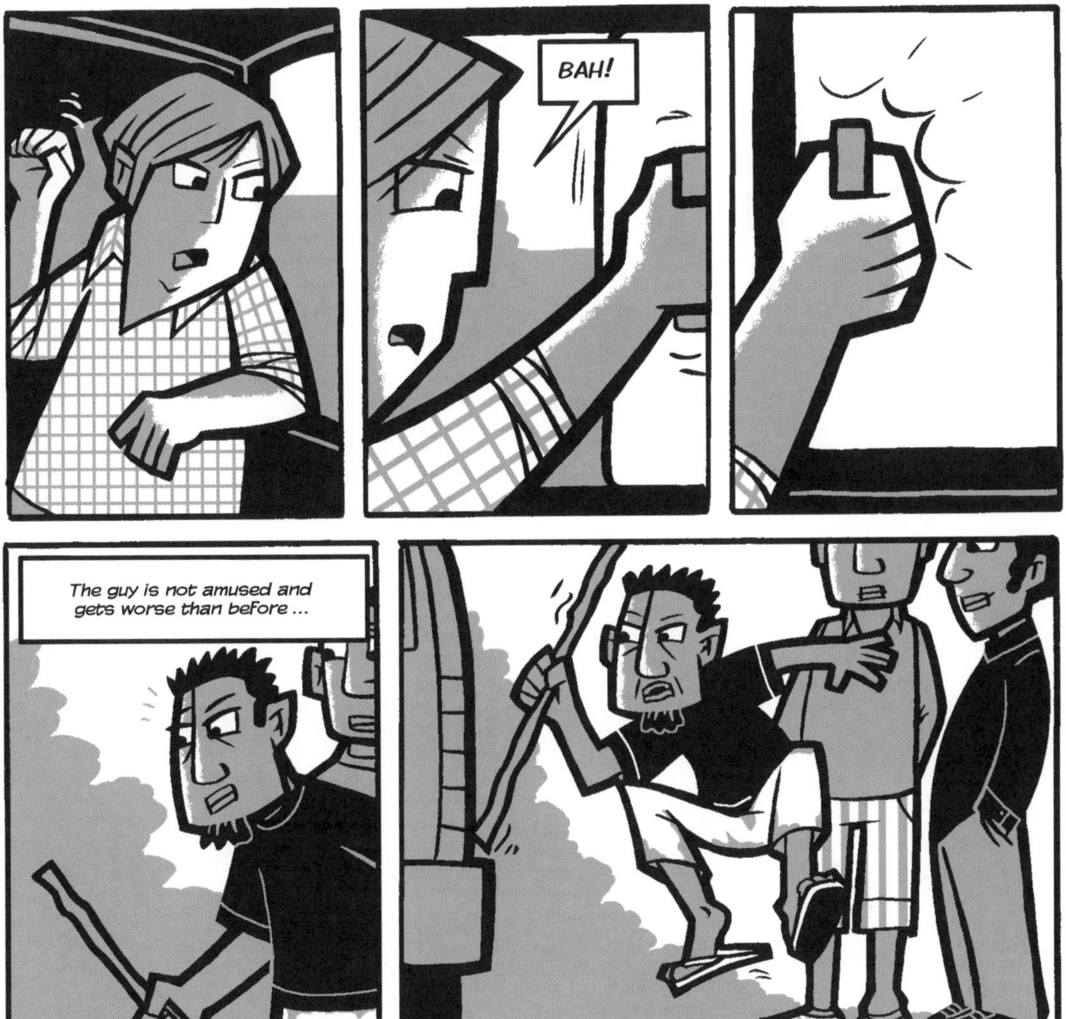
BAH!
The guy is not amused and gets worse than before ...
Finally some men decide that's enough For today, and get his attention ...
And he leaves, screaming and singing ...

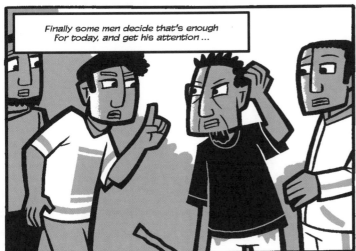

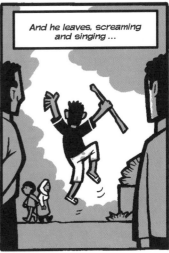

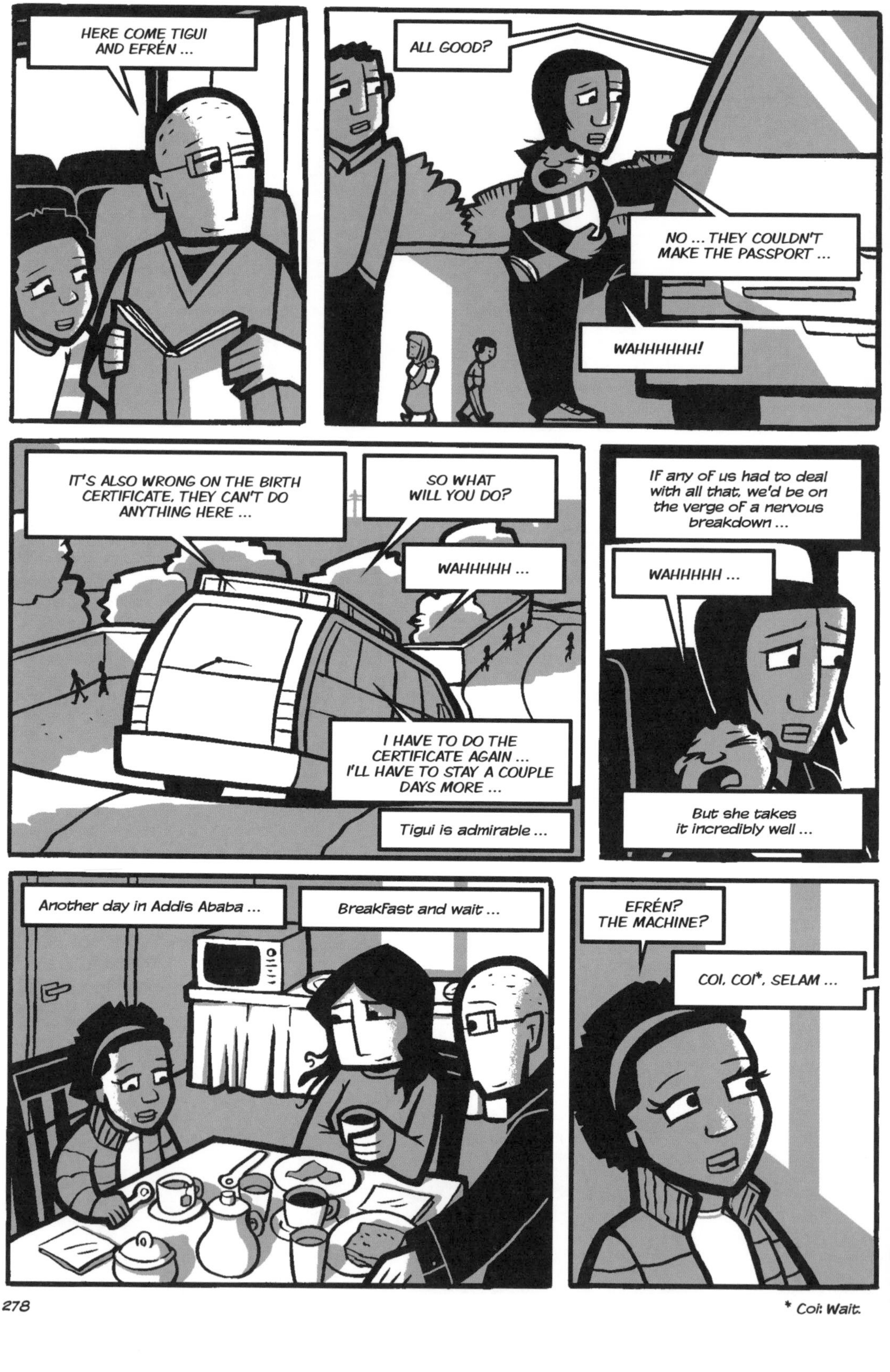
HERE COME TIGUI AND EFRÉN ...
ALL GOOD?
NO ... THEY COULDN'T MAKE THE PASSPORT ...
WAHHHHHH!
IT'S ALSO WRONG ON THE BIRTH CERTIFICATE. THEY CAN'T DO ANYTHING HERE ...
SO WHAT WILL YOU DO?
WAHHHHH ...
I HAVE TO DO THE CERTIFICATE AGAIN ... I'LL HAVE TO STAY A COUPLE DAYS MORE ...
Tigui is admirable ...
IF any of us had to deal with all that, we'd be on the verge of a nervous breakdown ...
WAHHHHH ...
But she takes it incredibly well ...
Another day in Addis Ababa ...
Breakfast and wait ...
EFRÉN? THE MACHINE?
COI, COI*, SELAM ...

* Coi: Wait.

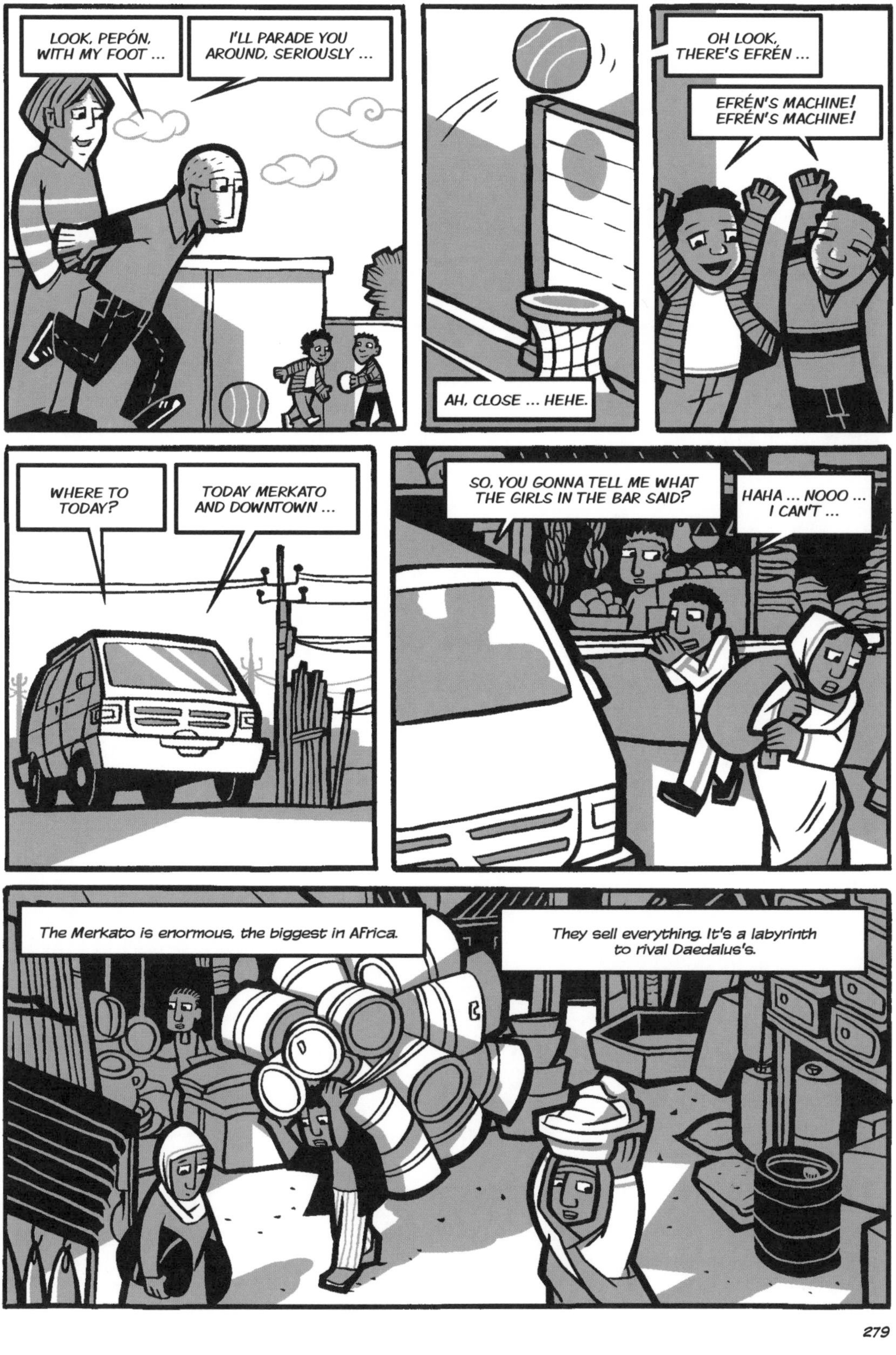
LOOK, PEPÓN, WITH MY FOOT ...
I'LL PARADE YOU AROUND, SERIOUSLY ...
AH, CLOSE ... HEHE.
OH LOOK, THERE'S EFRÉN ...
EFRÉN'S MACHINE! EFRÉN'S MACHINE!
WHERE TO TODAY?
TODAY MERKATO AND DOWNTOWN ...
SO, YOU GONNA TELL ME WHAT THE GIRLS IN THE BAR SAID?
HAHA ... NOOO ... I CAN'T ...
The Merkato is enormous, the biggest in Africa.
They sell everything. It's a labyrinth to rival Daedalus's.

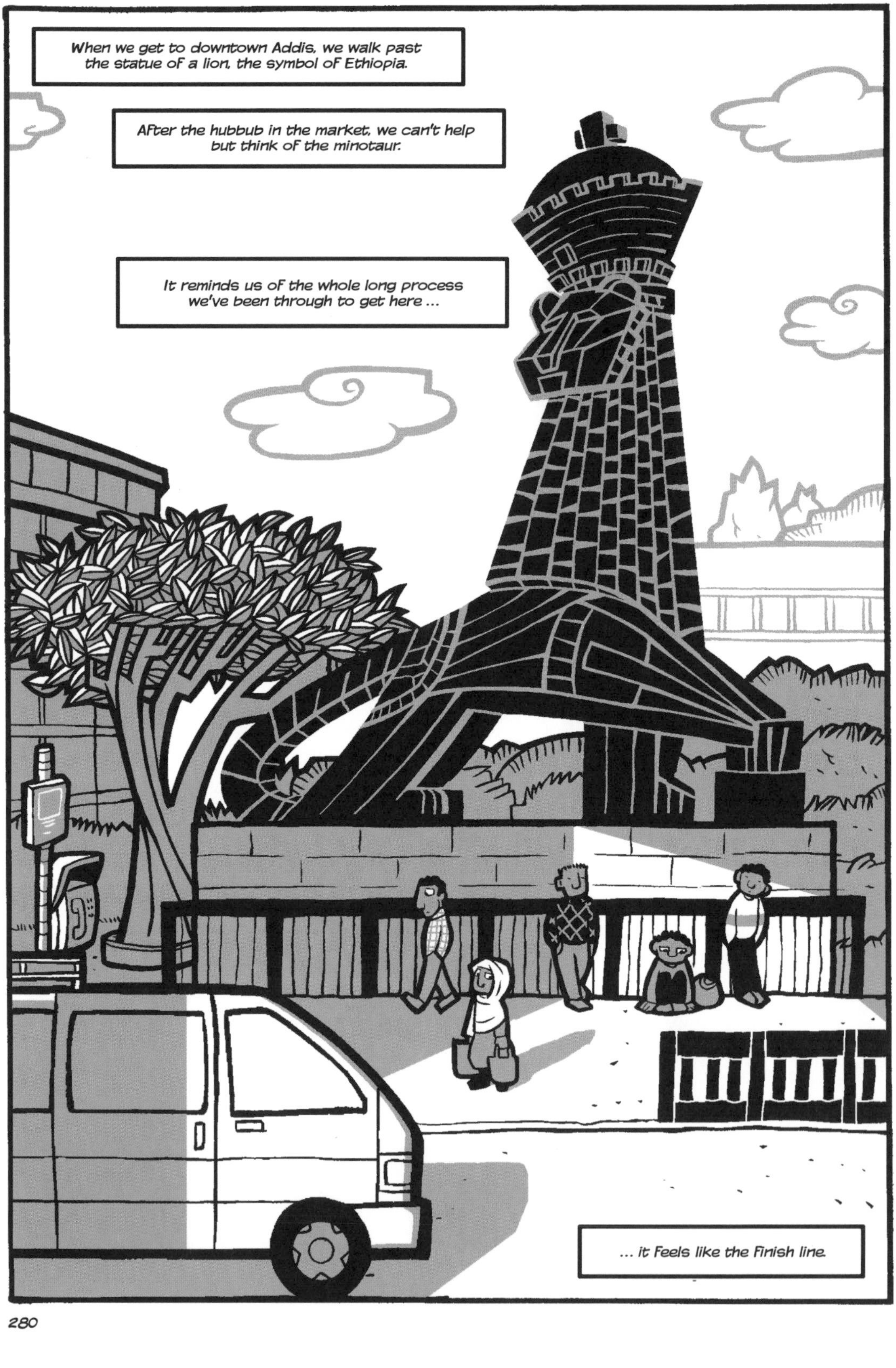
When we get to downtown Addis, we walk past the statue of a lion, the symbol of Ethiopia.
After the hubbub in the market, we can't help but think of the minotaur.
It reminds us of the whole long process we've been through to get here ...
... it feels like the finish line.

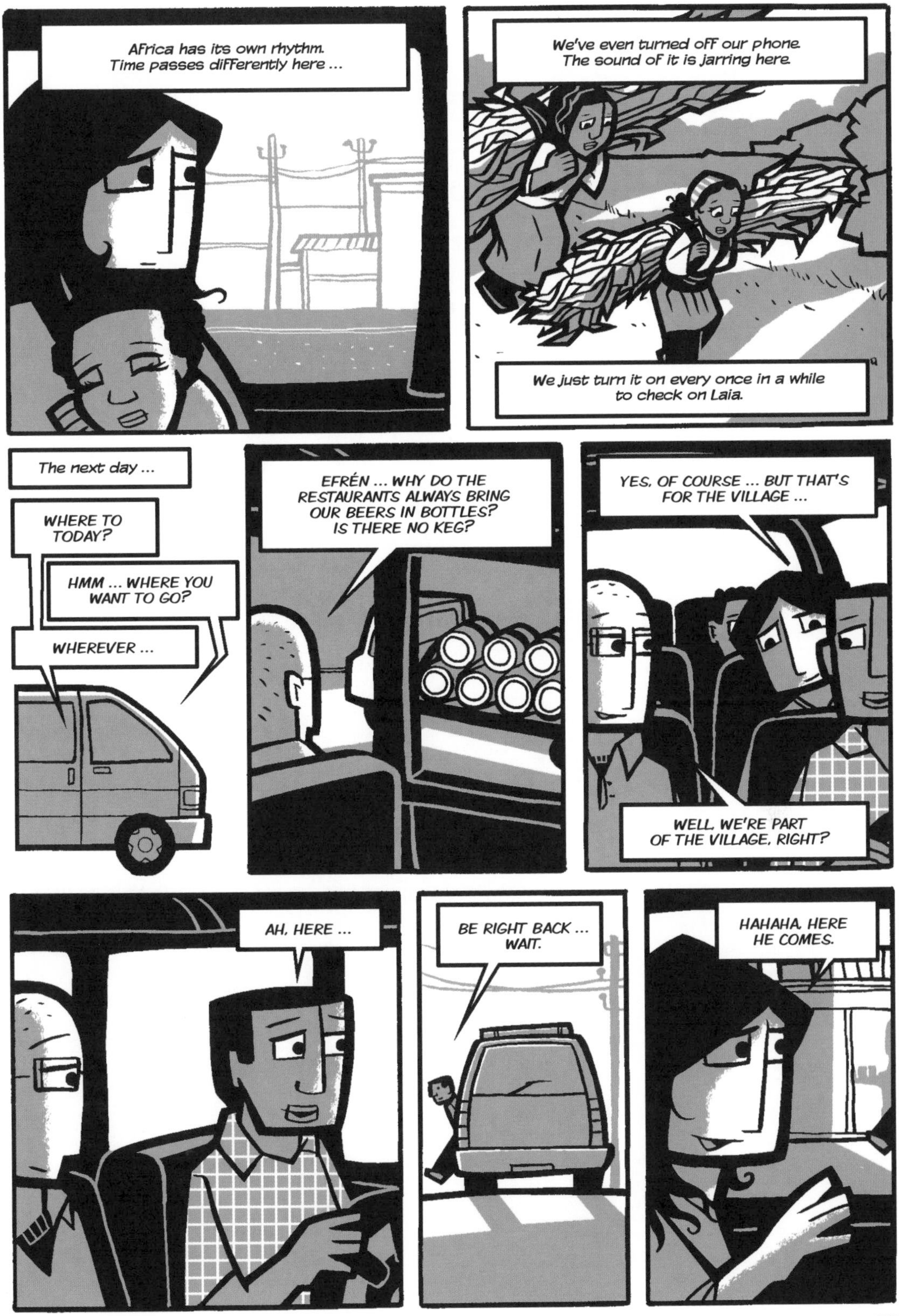
Africa has its own rhythm.
Time passes differently here ...
We've even turned off our phone.
The sound of it is jarring here.
We just turn it on every once in a while
to check on Laia.
The next day ...
WHERE TO TODAY?
HMM ... WHERE YOU WANT TO GO?
WHEREVER ...
EFRÉN ... WHY DO THE RESTAURANTS ALWAYS BRING OUR BEERS IN BOTTLES? IS THERE NO KEG?
YES, OF COURSE ... BUT THAT'S FOR THE VILLAGE ...
WELL, WE'RE PART OF THE VILLAGE, RIGHT?
AH, HERE ...
BE RIGHT BACK ... WAIT.
HAHAHA, HERE HE COMES.

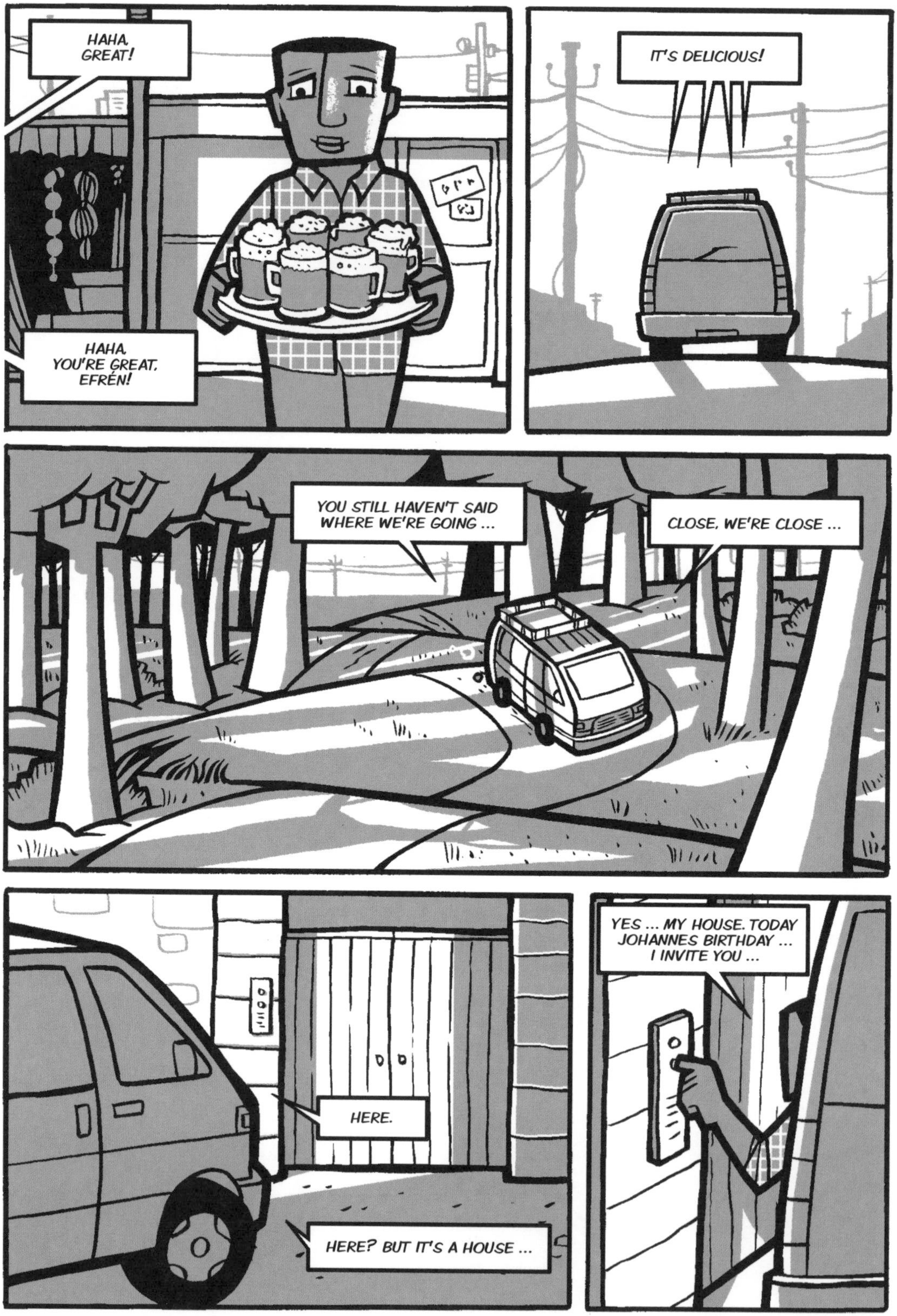
HAHA, GREAT!
HAHA, YOU'RE GREAT, EFRÉN!
IT'S DELICIOUS!
YOU STILL HAVEN'T SAID WHERE WE'RE GOING ...
CLOSE, WE'RE CLOSE ...
HERE.
HERE? BUT IT'S A HOUSE ...
YES ... MY HOUSE. TODAY JOHANNES BIRTHDAY ... I INVITE YOU ...

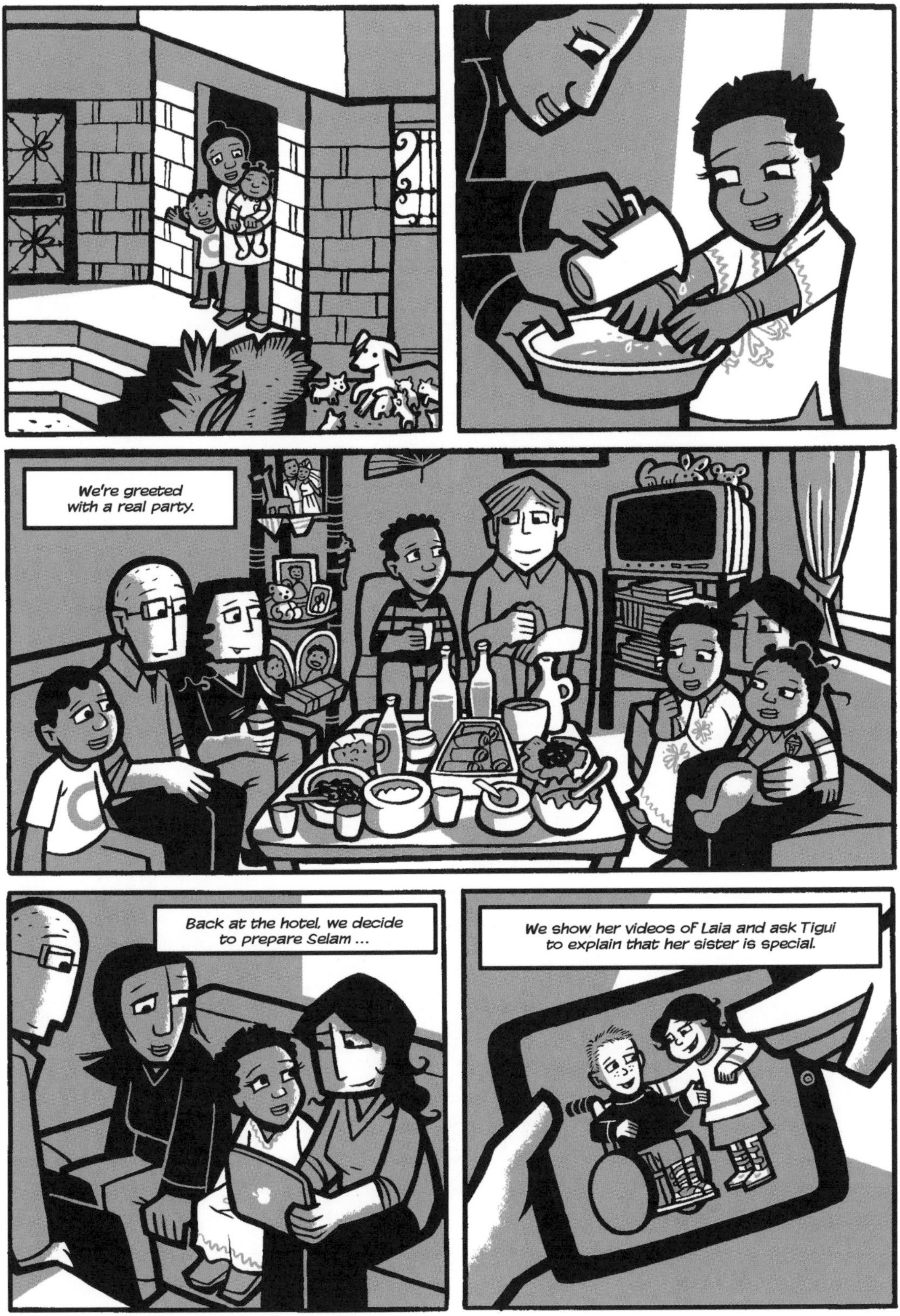
We're greeted with a real party.
Back at the hotel, we decide to prepare Selam ...
We show her videos of Laia and ask Tigui to explain that her sister is special.

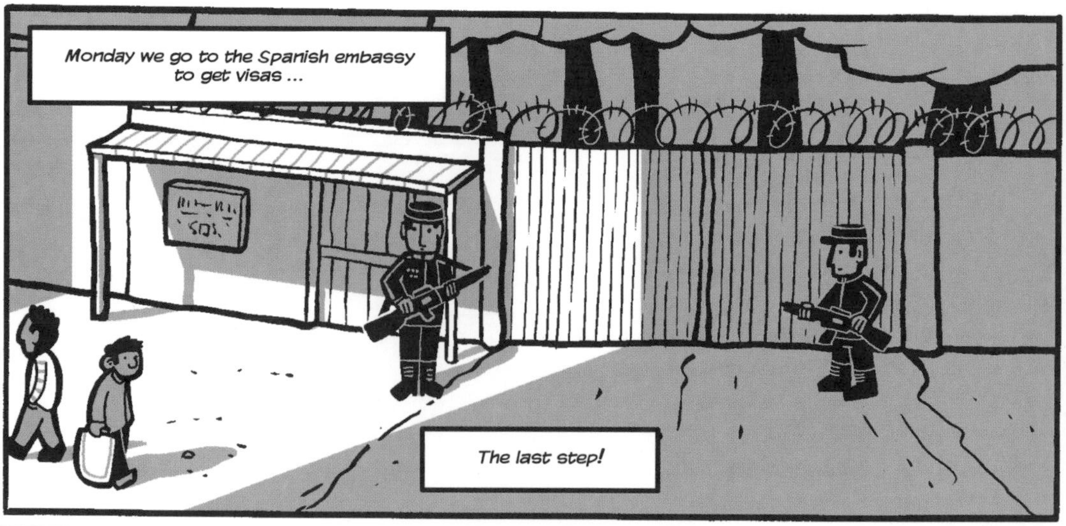
Monday we go to the Spanish embassy to get visas ...
The last step!

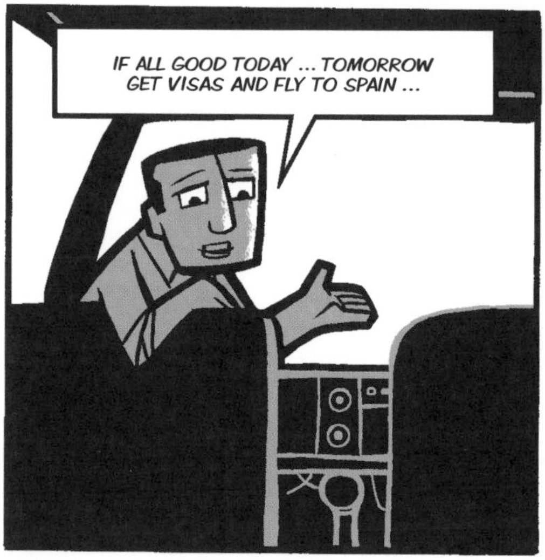
IF ALL GOOD TODAY ... TOMORROW GET VISAS AND FLY TO SPAIN ...

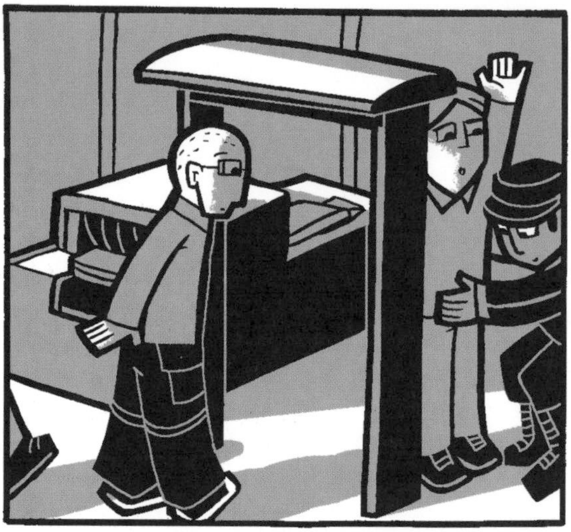

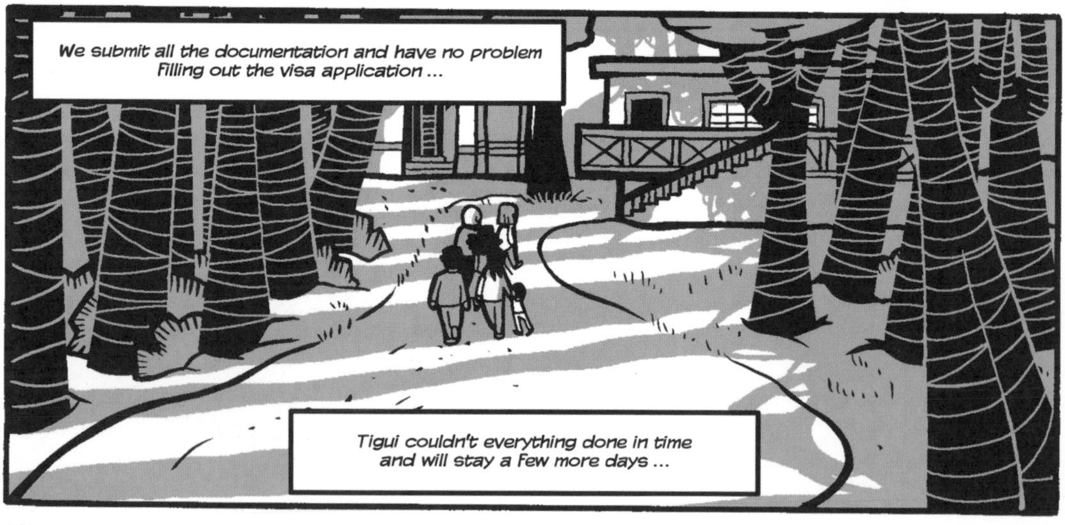
We submit all the documentation and have no problem filling out the visa application ...
Tigui couldn't everything done in time and will stay a few more days ...

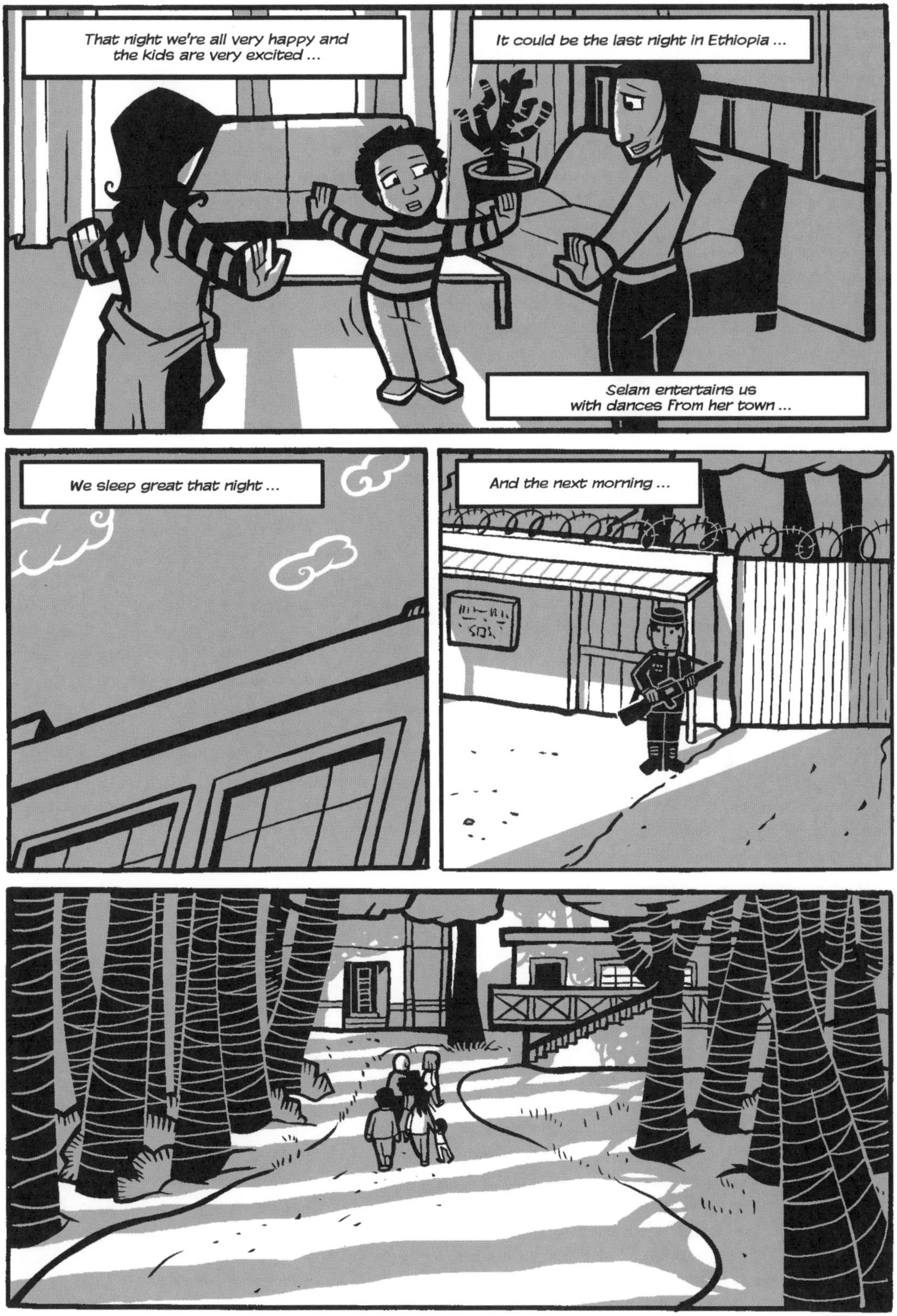
That night we're all very happy and the kids are very excited ...
It could be the last night in Ethiopia ...
Selam entertains us with dances from her town ...
We sleep great that night ...
And the next morning ...

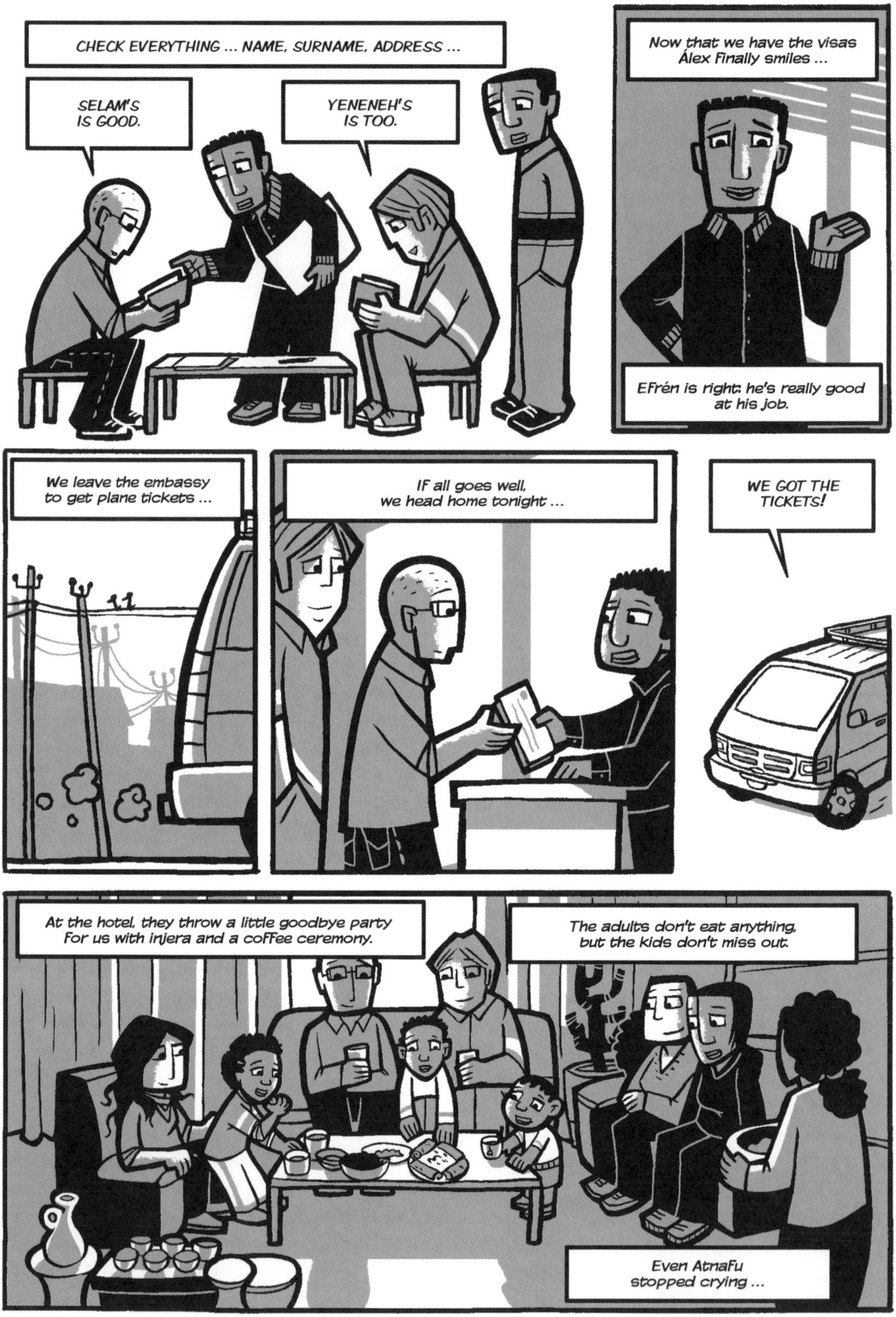
CHECK EVERYTHING ... NAME, SURNAME, ADDRESS ...
SELAM'S IS GOOD.
YENENEH'S IS TOO.
Now that we have the visas Álex finally smiles ...
Efrén is right: he's really good at his job.
We leave the embassy to get plane tickets ...
If all goes well, we head home tonight ...
WE GOT THE TICKETS!
At the hotel, they throw a little goodbye party for us with injera and a coffee ceremony.
The adults don't eat anything, but the kids don't miss out.
Even Atnafu stopped crying ...

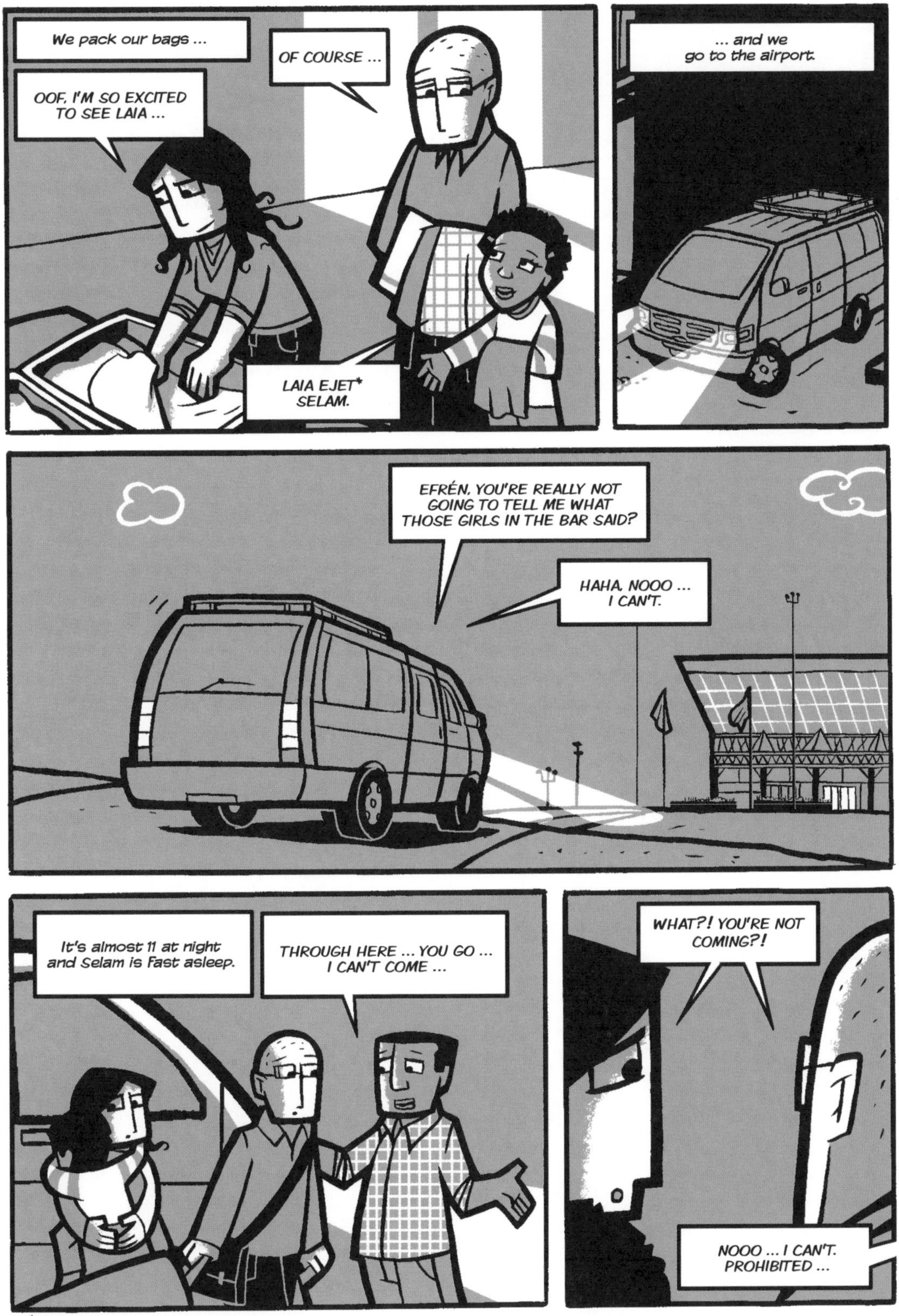
We pack our bags ...
OOF, I'M SO EXCITED TO SEE LAIA ...
OF COURSE ...
LAIA EJET* SELAM.
... and we go to the airport.
EFRÉN, YOU'RE REALLY NOT GOING TO TELL ME WHAT THOSE GIRLS IN THE BAR SAID?
HAHA, NOOO ... I CAN'T.
It's almost 11 at night and Selam is fast asleep.
THROUGH HERE ... YOU GO ... I CAN'T COME ...
WHAT?! YOU'RE NOT COMING?!
NOOO ... I CAN'T. PROHIBITED ...

*Ejet: Sister

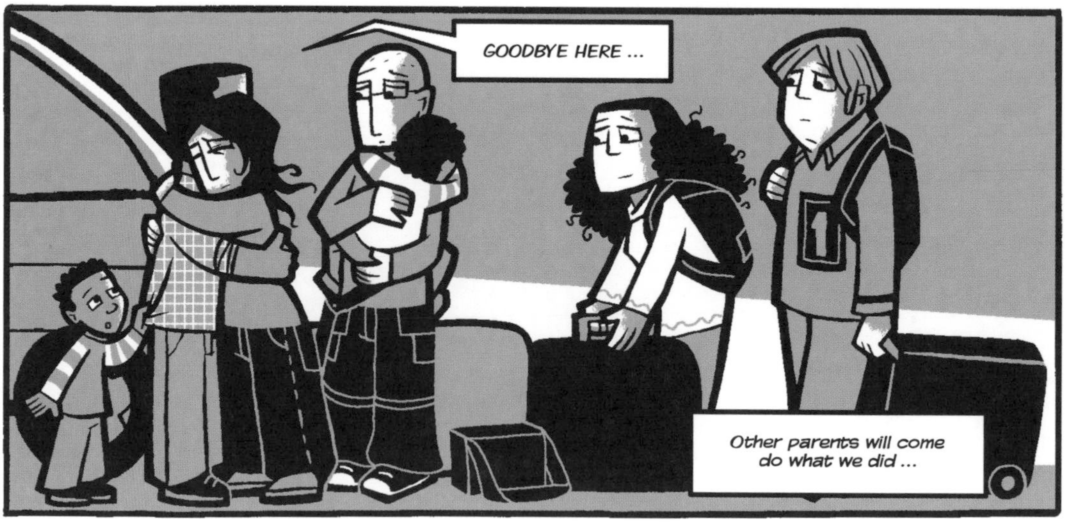
GOODBYE HERE ...
Other parents will come do what we did ...

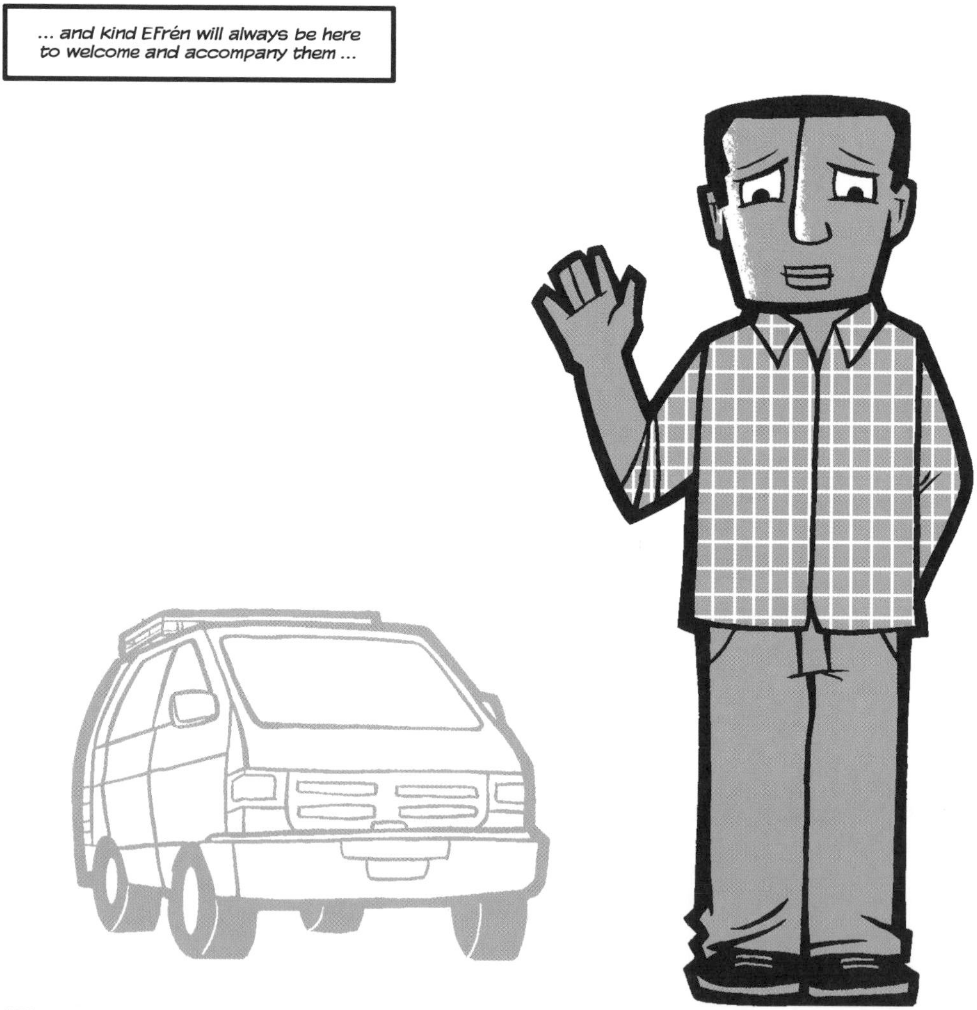
... and kind Efrén will always be here to welcome and accompany them ...

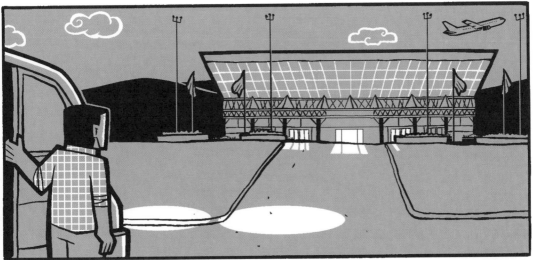

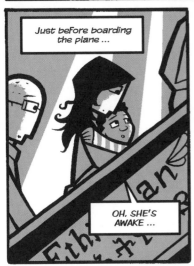

Just before boarding the plane ...

OH, SHE'S AWAKE ...

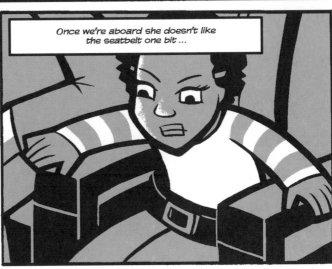

Once we're aboard she doesn't like the seatbelt one bit ...

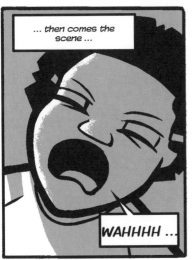

... then comes the scene ...

WAHHHH ...

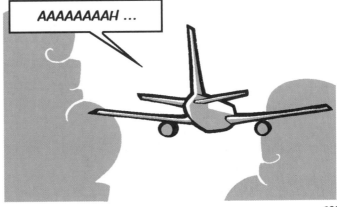

We look for an attendant to help us calm her down ... but it seems like they've vanished ...

AAAAAAAAH ...

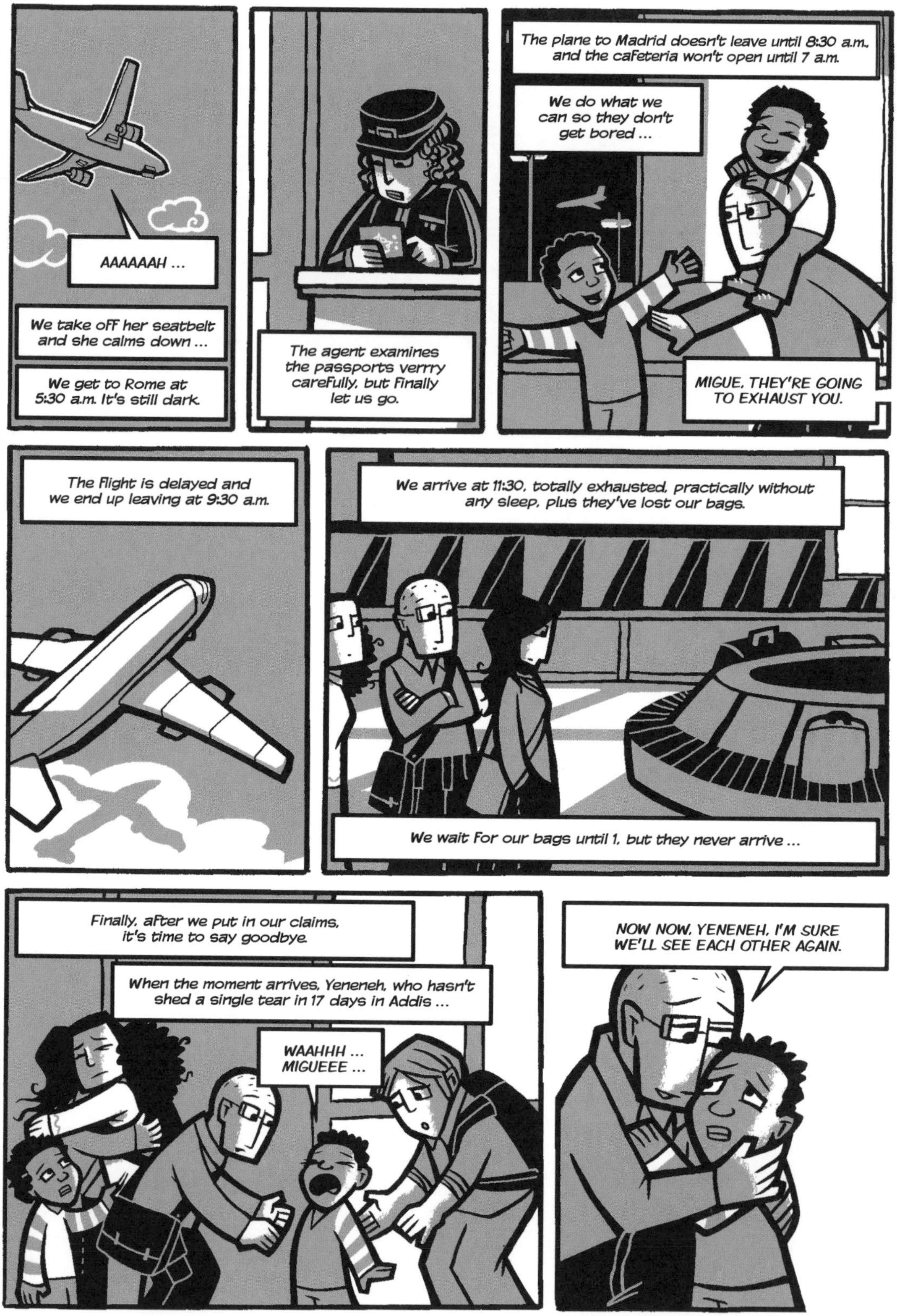
AAAAAAH ...
We take off her seatbelt and she calms down ...
We get to Rome at 5:30 a.m. It's still dark.
The agent examines the passports verrry carefully, but finally let us go.
The plane to Madrid doesn't leave until 8:30 a.m., and the cafeteria won't open until 7 a.m.
We do what we can so they don't get bored ...
MIGUE, THEY'RE GOING TO EXHAUST YOU.
The flight is delayed and we end up leaving at 9:30 a.m.
We arrive at 11:30, totally exhausted, practically without any sleep, plus they've lost our bags.
We wait for our bags until 1, but they never arrive ...
Finally, after we put in our claims, it's time to say goodbye.
When the moment arrives, Yeneneh, who hasn't shed a single tear in 17 days in Addis ...
WAAHHH ... MIGUEEE ...
NOW NOW, YENENEH, I'M SURE WE'LL SEE EACH OTHER AGAIN.

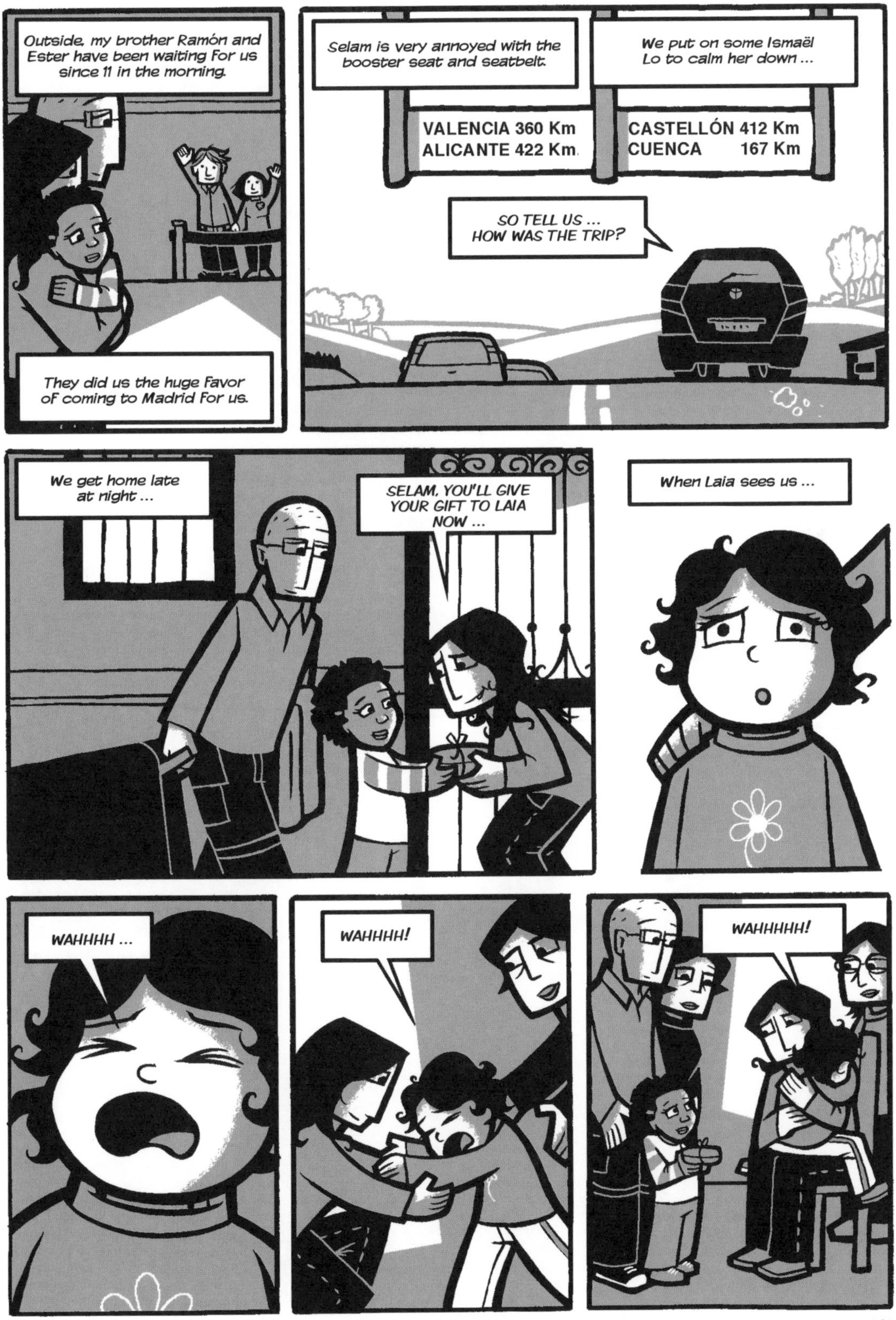
Outside, my brother Ramón and Ester have been waiting for us since 11 in the morning.
They did us the huge favor of coming to Madrid for us.
Selam is very annoyed with the booster seat and seatbelt.
We put on some Ismaël Lo to calm her down ...
VALENCIA 360 Km
ALICANTE 422 Km.
CASTELLÓN 412 Km
CUENCA 167 Km
SO TELL US ... HOW WAS THE TRIP?
We get home late at night ...
SELAM, YOU'LL GIVE YOUR GIFT TO LAIA NOW ...
When Laia sees us ...
WAHHHH ...
WAHHHH!
WAHHHHH!

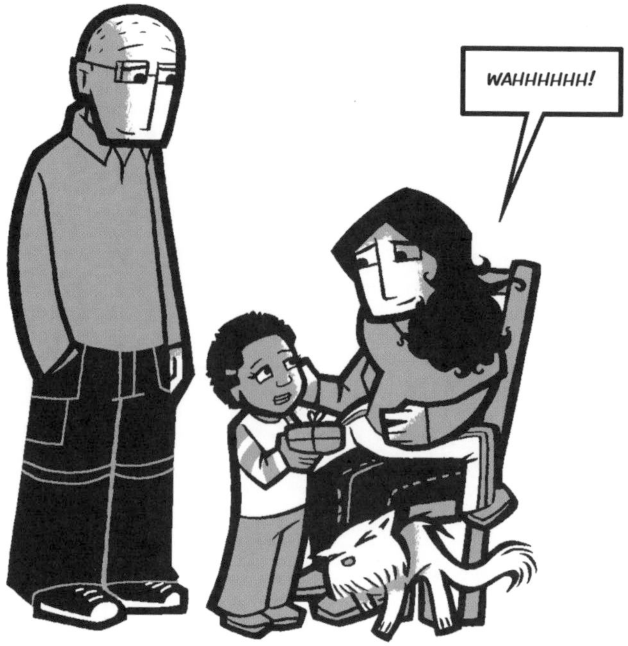
WAHHHHHH!

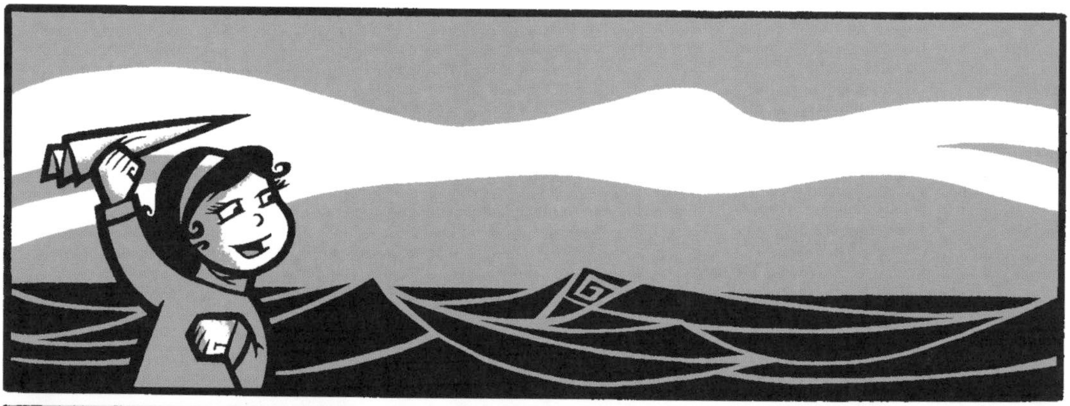

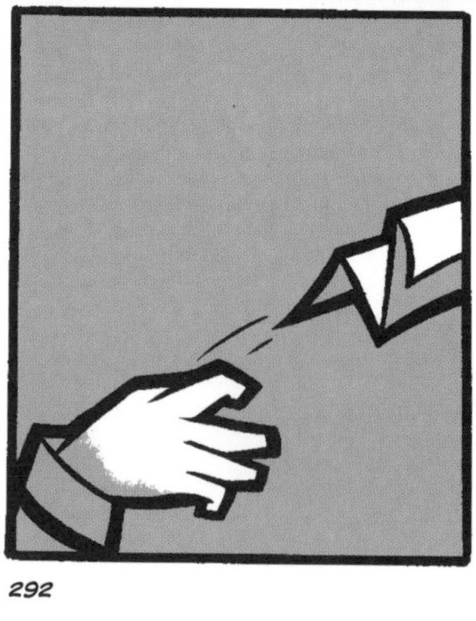

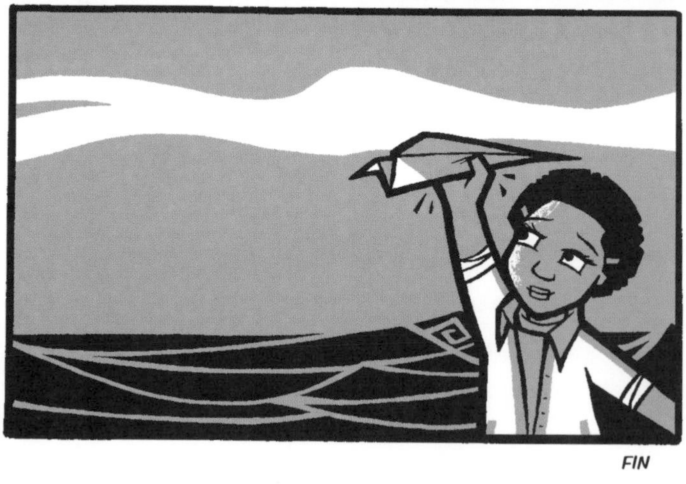

FIN

EPILOGUE

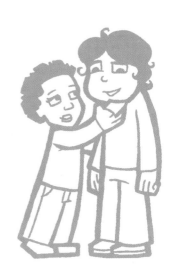

The first weeks at home are pretty intense ...

We have to be really careful adapting to the situation without losing our balance.

Sometimes Selam cries and we don't know why.

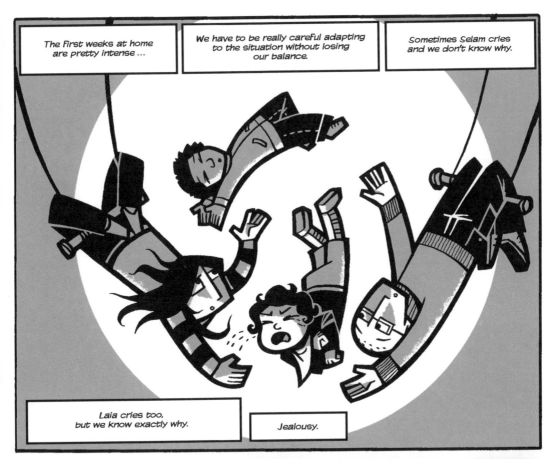

Laia cries too, but we know exactly why.

Jealousy.

Both need all our attention.

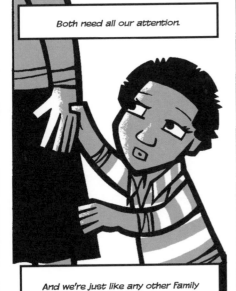

And we're just like any other family after a birth ...

... exhausted and swamped.

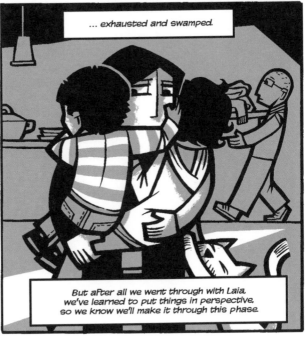

But after all we went through with Laia, we've learned to put things in perspective, so we know we'll make it through this phase.

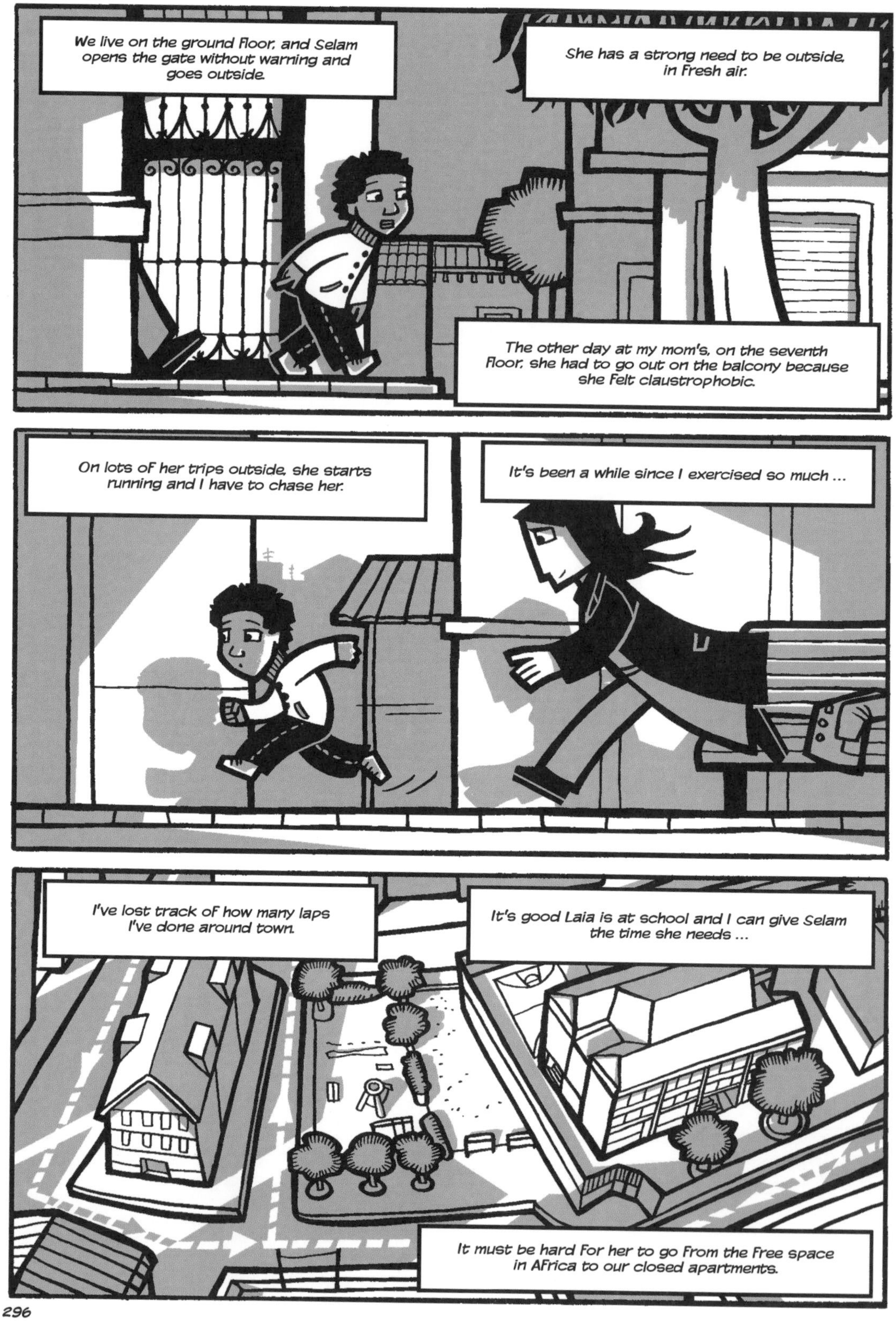
We live on the ground floor, and Selam opens the gate without warning and goes outside.
She has a strong need to be outside, in fresh air.
The other day at my mom's, on the seventh floor, she had to go out on the balcony because she felt claustrophobic.
On lots of her trips outside, she starts running and I have to chase her.
It's been a while since I exercised so much ...
I've lost track of how many laps I've done around town.
It's good Laia is at school and I can give Selam the time she needs ...
It must be hard for her to go from the free space in Africa to our closed apartments.

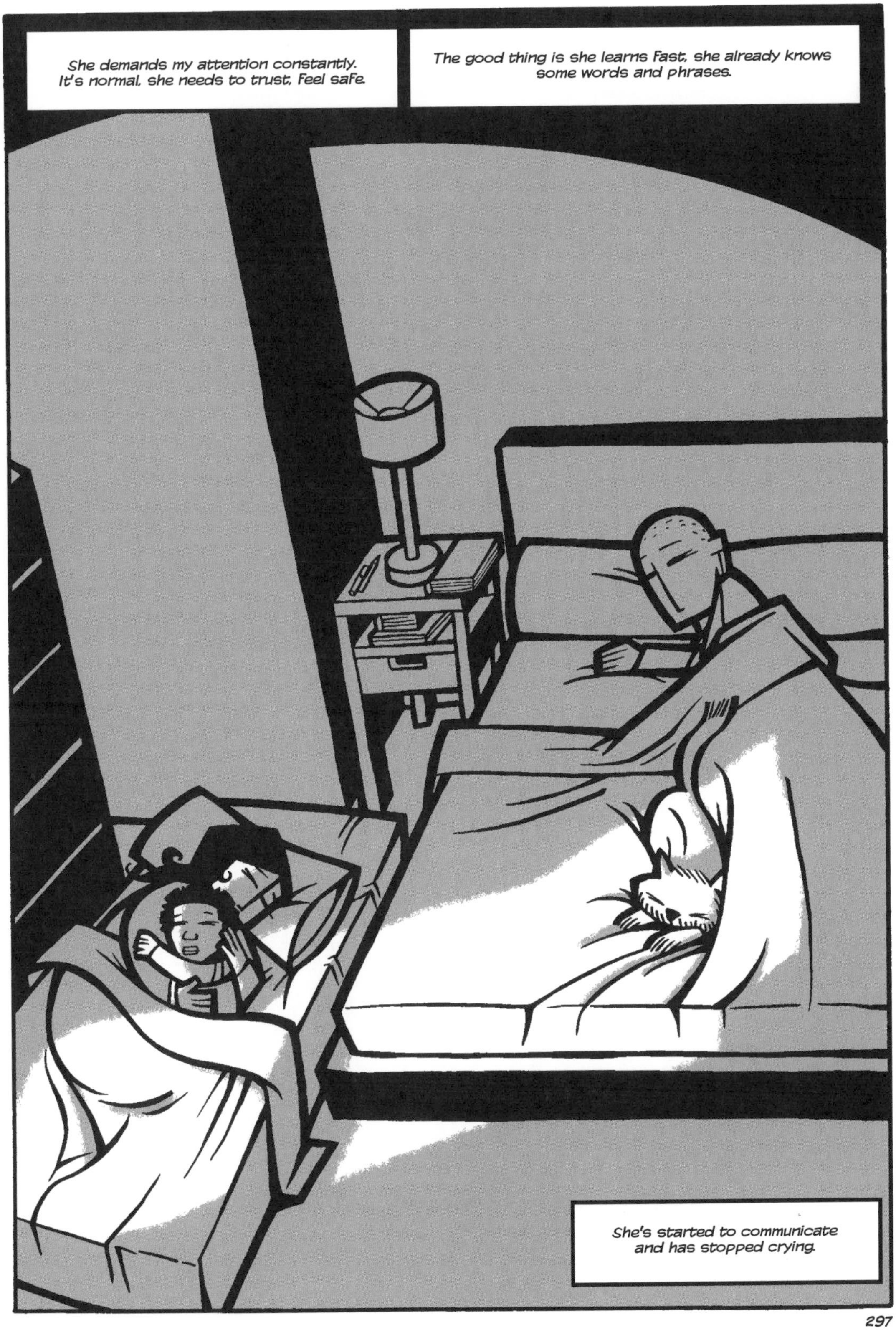
She demands my attention constantly. It's normal, she needs to trust, feel safe.
The good thing is she learns fast, she already knows some words and phrases.
She's started to communicate and has stopped crying.

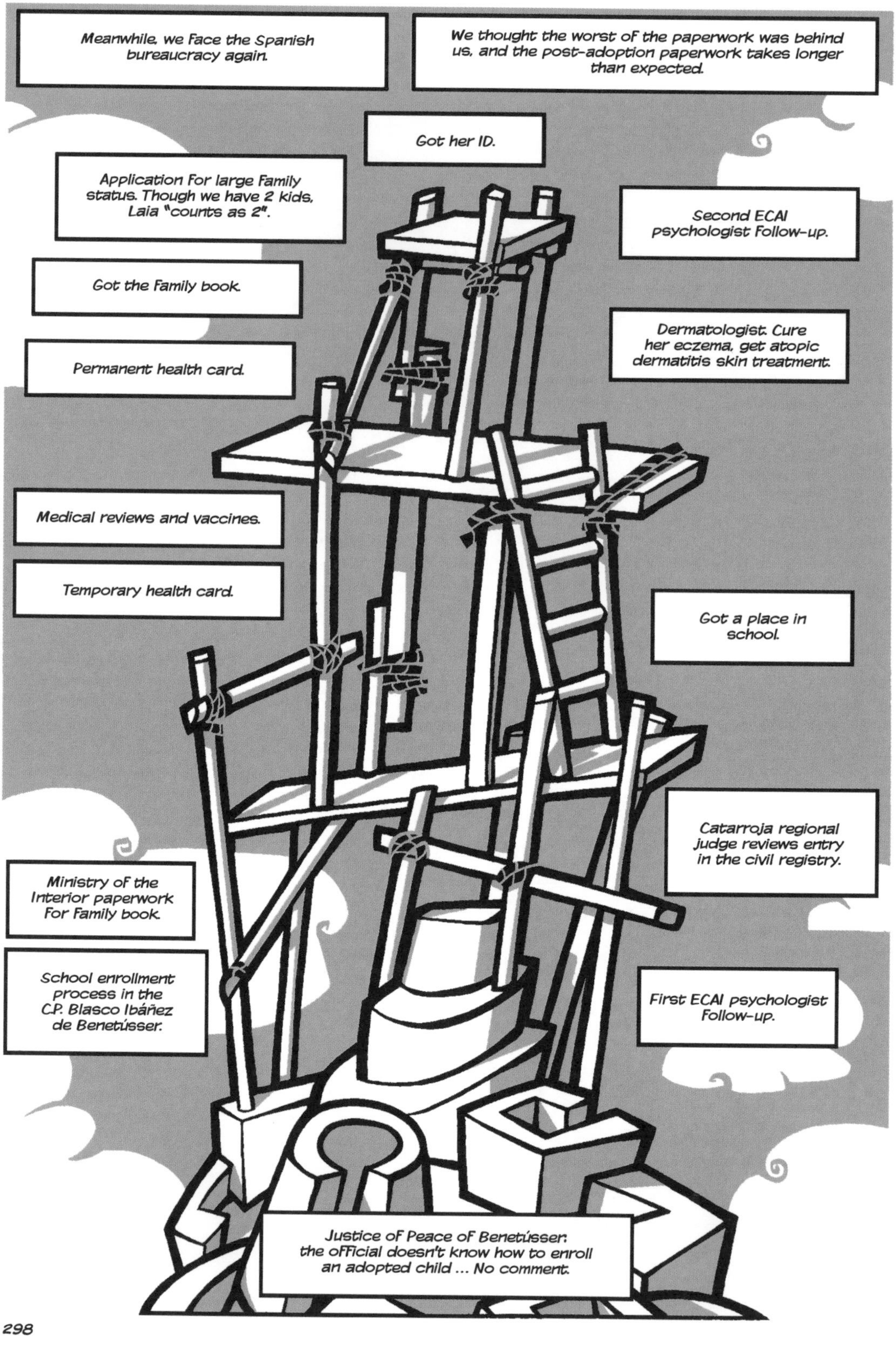

Meanwhile, we Face the Spanish bureaucracy again.
We thought the worst of the paperwork was behind us, and the post-adoption paperwork takes longer than expected.
Got her ID.
Application For large Family status. Though we have 2 kids, Laia "counts as 2".
Second ECAI psychologist Follow-up.
Got the Family book.
Dermatologist. Cure her eczema, get atopic dermatitis skin treatment.
Permanent health card.
Medical reviews and vaccines.
Temporary health card.
Got a place in school.
Catarroja regional judge reviews entry in the civil registry.
Ministry of the Interior paperwork For Family book.
School enrollment process in the C.P. Blasco Ibáñez de Benetússer.
First ECAI psychologist Follow-up.
Justice of Peace of Benetússer: the official doesn't know how to enroll an adopted child ... No comment.

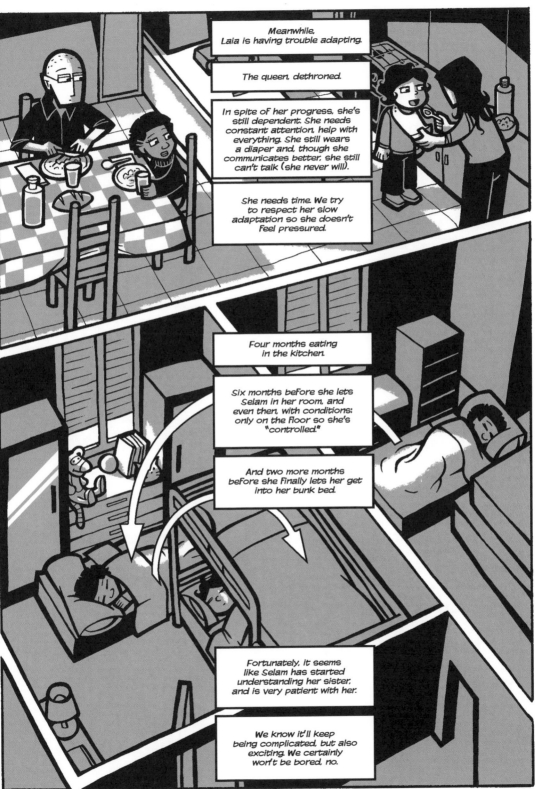

Meanwhile,
Laia is having trouble adapting.

The queen, dethroned.

In spite of her progress, she's still dependent. She needs constant attention, help with everything. She still wears a diaper and, though she communicates better, she still can't talk (she never will).

She needs time. We try to respect her slow adaptation so she doesn't feel pressured.

Four months eating in the kitchen.

Six months before she lets Selam in her room, and even then, with conditions: only on the floor so she's "controlled."

And two more months before she finally lets her get into her bunk bed.

Fortunately, it seems like Selam has started understanding her sister, and is very patient with her.

We know it'll keep being complicated, but also exciting. We certainly won't be bored, no.

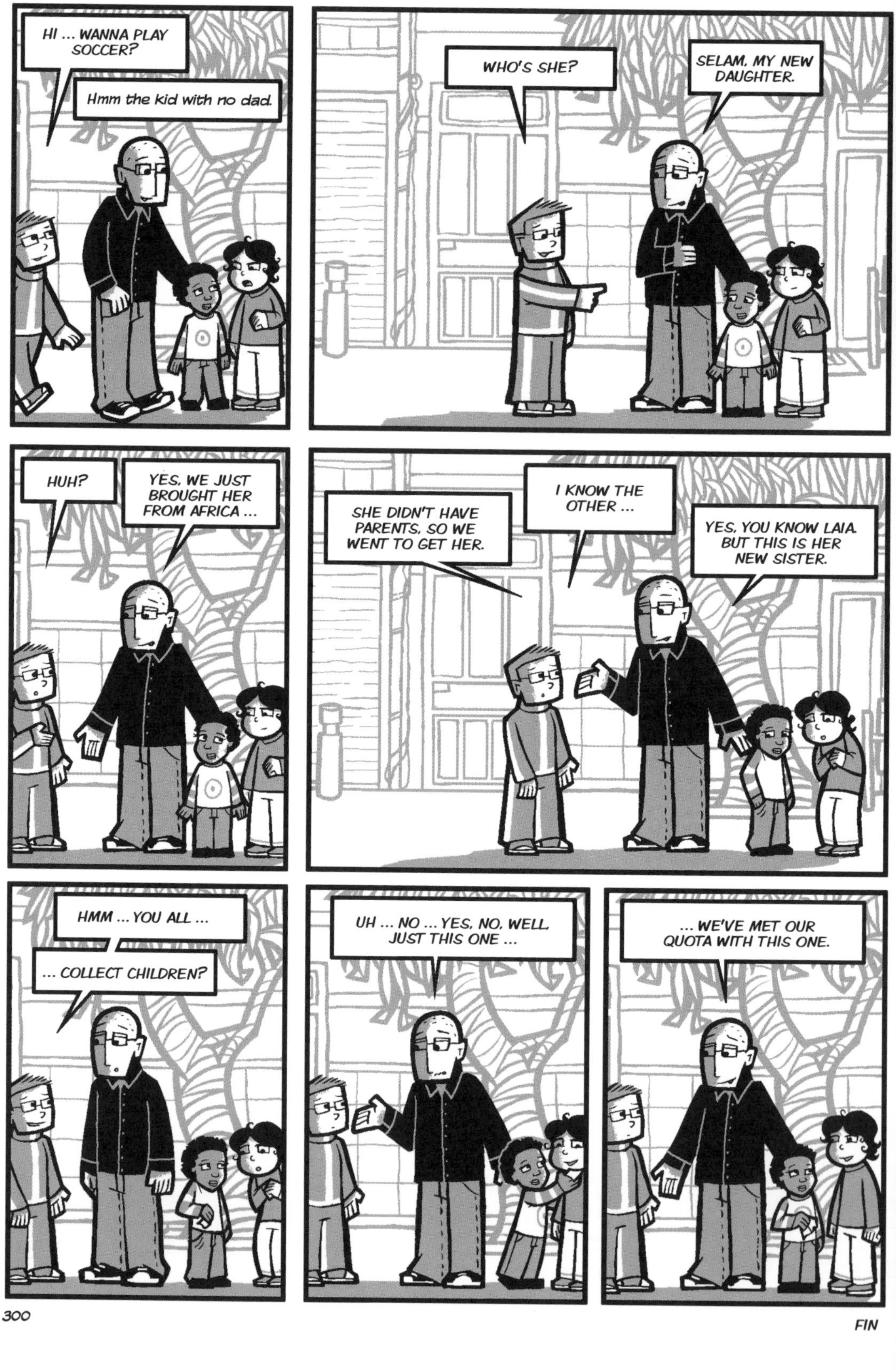
HI ... WANNA PLAY SOCCER?
Hmm the kid with no dad.
WHO'S SHE?
SELAM, MY NEW DAUGHTER.
HUH?
YES, WE JUST BROUGHT HER FROM AFRICA ...
SHE DIDN'T HAVE PARENTS, SO WE WENT TO GET HER.
I KNOW THE OTHER ...
YES, YOU KNOW LAIA. BUT THIS IS HER NEW SISTER.
HMM ... YOU ALL ...
... COLLECT CHILDREN?
UH ... NO ... YES, NO, WELL, JUST THIS ONE ...
... WE'VE MET OUR QUOTA WITH THIS ONE.

FIN

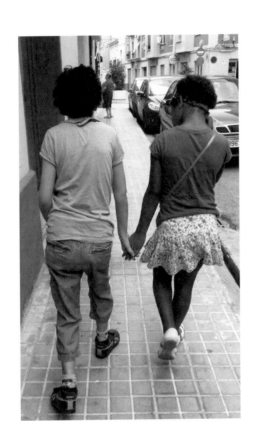

Acknowledgments

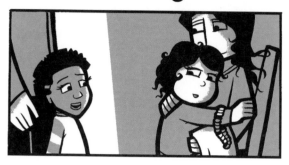

To all the healthcare staff at Hospital Doctor Peset, the Hospital Clínico Universitario, and the La Fe University Hospital of Valencia, and the Benetússer and Vilamarxant Health Center, who have treated and continue to treat Laia with so much care and affection. You don't know such magnificent people exist until life puts them right in front of you.

To Mariano and Florencio, for always being by our side, to Dr. Rafa Carrasco, to Dr. Vicente García Aymerich, to Dr. Mercedes Andrés, to Dr. Laura Uixera, Nurse Paqui, Dr. Rafa Fernández-Delgado, Dr. García Callejo, Dr. Viosca, Dr. Villar, and Rosana Fuset. And especially our friend, Dr. Ana de Gonzalo, for continuing to take care of all of us.

To everyone who was with us in Ethiopia and throughout the long adoption and post-adoption process: the staff of the ECAI Feyda, the Amanaya Guest House Hotel and the caretakers in the group home. To AVACU (Valencian Association of Consumers and Users) for the T-shirts, notebooks, and pencils for the group home. And a special thanks to Efrén, our guide.

To all the staff of the Department of Family, Minors and Adoptions of the Ministry of Social Welfare for their service, availability, and good work.

To the Parc Central Daycare, to Amamanta (Association for Breastfeeding Support), and to Avapace (Valencia Association for Cerebral Palsy Assistance). To all the staff of the CPCI Red Cross Center in Valencia and their AMPA (Parents' Association). To the Villar Palasí School in Valencia and to all the staff of the Blasco Ibáñez School in Benetússer and their AMPA.

To our colleagues who helped and advised us on both books: Paco Giménez, Carlos Ortin, Rosa Albero, Nacho Casanova, Rosa Martí, Incha, Creumont, Javi Gay, Álvaro de los Ángeles, Víctor Soler, and Sento. To Paco Bascuñán and Lupe Martínez for designing the fonts and being kind enough to give them to us. And to everyone in our studio, who have patiently supported us from the first page to the last.

To Jesús Moreno for trusting us. To Catalina Mejía for her generosity and to the entire Astiberri team for opening the doors to their home, especially to Héloïse, who was the start of it all.

Thanks to Ian Williams and Monica Lalanda for recommending our book and sending it to Kendra. And thanks a lot to Kendra Boileau and Graphic Mundi's team for their warm welcome.

To Tere, the babysitter we couldn't do without. And our families, especially our parents, who continue to support us all the time.

Fotografía: Juanjo Laudes

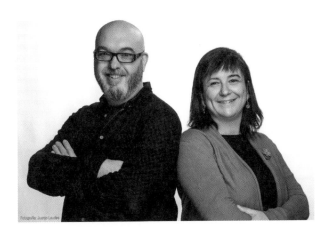

Cristina Durán (Valencia, 1970) and **Miguel Ángel Giner Bou** (Benetússer, Valencia, 1969) are graduates from the Faculty of Fine Arts in Valencia. While they were in university, they founded Equipo Grúa, which created the fanzine *No Aparcar Llamo GRUA*.

Early in their careers, they worked in animation and founded their studio, LaGRUAestudio, in 1993. They have worked on illustration and comics there ever since.

Together they have published the graphic novels *Una posibilidad entre mil* (*A One in a Thousand Chance*, Sins entido, 2009) and *La máquina de Efrén* (*Efren's Machine*, Sins entido, 2012)—joined in this comprehensive volume under the title *A Chance*—and *Cuando no sabes qué decir* (Salamandra Graphic, 2015), *El día 3* (Astiberri, 2018). They have also published other comics like *Pillada por ti* (Ministerio de Sanidad, 2011), *El siglo de oro valenciano* (Biblioteca Valenciana, 2014), *Vicente Blasco Ibáñez, Una vida apasionante* (Ayuntamiento de Valencia, 2017), and *Una niña, un perro y mil gatos* (Ayuntamiento de Valencia, 2019). They participated in the collective album *Viñetas de Vida* for Oxfam Intermón (Astiberri, 2014) and wrote short stories for *Usted está aquí*, *Arròs negre* and *Cómic 1*.

Individually, Cristina contributed to the collective album *Enjambre* (Norma, 2014) and Miguel Ángel wrote the comic books *Anna Dédalus detective: El misterio de la mansión quemada*, illustrated by Núria Tamarit y Xulia Vicente (Andana, 2015) and *Anna Dédalus detective: La paradoja de Fermi* (Andana, 2019), illustrated by Susanna Martín. And as a cartoonist, he has published *Astucia Laperla: Luna roja, corazón negro* (De Ponent, 2016) with script by Stygryt.

They have received various awards and nominations for their comics, including the Turia Award (2012), the Flash Back (2012), the Silver Badge of Culture from the Benetússer City Council (2013), the Dones Progressistes Award, and second place in the inaugural *Les BDs qui font la difference* award. In addition, *El día 3* was awarded the Premi Ciutat de Palma de Cómic (2016), the prize for best script (2018) in the Splash Sagunt Festival del Cómic, the prize for the best national work in the VIII Premios del Cómic Aragonés del Salón del Cómic de Zaragoza (2018), and the National Comic Award (2019).

Both were founders and served as presidents of the Professional Association of Illustrators of Valencia (APIV), an association that they belonged to for twenty-two years. Cristina was also a member of the board of directors for the Federación de Asociaciones de Ilustradores Profesionales (FADIP) and of the founding board of the European Illustrators Forum (EIF).

Both are teachers in the Máster Propio en Medicina Gráfica program through UNIA and the Colegio de Médicos de Málaga.

Miguel Ángel shares his passion for storytelling with the students of the Masters in Design and Illustration program at the Facultad de Bellas Artes de Valencia (Universitat Politècnica de València) where he teaches screenwriting. He is currently president of the Asociación Profesional de Guionistas de Cómic, ARGH!, and editorial director of Andana Gráfica, a line of graphic novels from Andana Editorial.

Song lyrics on pages 3, 17, 40, 63, 87 are reprinted with permission and loosely translated here.

1.
Se aprende en la cuna,
se aprende en la cama,
se aprende en la puerta
de un hospital.

Se aprende de golpe,
se aprende de a poco
y a veces se aprende recién al final.

We learn in our cradles,
we learn in our beds,
we learn in the doorway
of a hospital.

We learn all of the sudden,
we learn little by little,
and sometimes we only learn at the end.

   "Polvo de estrellas" ("Star Dust"),
   Jorge Drexler

2.
Jo tinc, per a tu, un niu
en el meu arbre
¡un núvol blanc, penjat
d'alguna branca.

I have, for you, a nest
in my tree
and a white cloud
hanging from a branch.

   "Un núvol blanc" ("A White Cloud"),
   Lluís Llach

3.
Terra para o pé, firmeza
Terra para a mão, carícia

Earth to the foot, solidity
Earth to the hand, caress

   "Terra" ("Earth"),
   Caetano Veloso

4.
Lo más terrible se aprende enseguida
y lo hermoso nos cuesta la vida.

We learn the worst right away,
while the beauty takes our whole life.

   "Canción del elegido" ("Song of the Chosen One"),
   Silvio Rodríguez

5.
É melhor ser alegre que
ser triste.
Alegria é la melhor coisa
que existe.

It's better to be happy than
to be sad.
Happiness is the best thing
in the world.

   "Samba da bênçâo" ("Samba Blessing"),
   Vinicius de Moraes and Baden Powell

Library of Congress Cataloging-in-Publication Data

Names: Durán, Cristina, 1970– author, illustrator. | Giner Bou, Miguel, author, illustrator. | Rucker, Katherine, translator.
Title: A chance / by Cristina Durán and Miguel Giner Bou ; translated by Katherine Rucker.
Other titles: Posibilidad. English
Description: University Park, Pennsylvania : Graphic Mundi, [2021] | Originally published under the title "Una posibilidad: edición integral" by Astiberri in 2017.
Summary: "A narrative, in graphic novel format, following Cristina Durán and Miguel Giner Bou as they rebuild and reinvent themselves after their daughter Laia is born with cerebral palsy. Their story continues through the arduous process of adopting their second daughter, Selam, from Ethiopia"—Provided by publisher.
Identifiers: LCCN 2021018929 | ISBN 9781637790038 (hardback)
Subjects: LCSH: Durán, Cristina, 1970——Comic books, strips, etc. | Giner Bou, Miguel—Comic books, strips, etc. | Cerebral palsied children—Comic books, strips, etc. | Cerebral palsy—Comic books, strips, etc. | Adopted children—Comic books, strips, etc. | Intercountry adoption—Comic books, strips, etc. | Courage—Comic books, strips, etc. | LCGFT: Graphic novels.
Classification: LCC RJ496.C4 D87 2021 | DDC 618.92/836—dc23
LC record available at https://lccn.loc.gov/2021018929

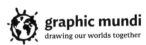

Graphic Mundi is an imprint of The Pennsylvania State University Press.

Translated by Katherine Rucker

Text and Illustrations © 2017 by Miguel Giner Bou and Cristina Durán.
Lettering for cover, book 1, and book 2 titles © Paco Bascuñán.
Typography ("Cristina Durán") © Fernando Fuentes.
All rights reserved.
Originally published as Una posibilidad: edición integral by agreement with Astiberri ediciones, www.astiberri.com

The Pennsylvania State University Press is a member of the Association of University Presses.

It is the policy of The Pennsylvania State University Press to use acid-free paper. Publications on uncoated stock satisfy the minimum requirements of American National Standard for Information Sciences—Permanence of Paper for Printed Library Material, ANSI Z39.48–1992.

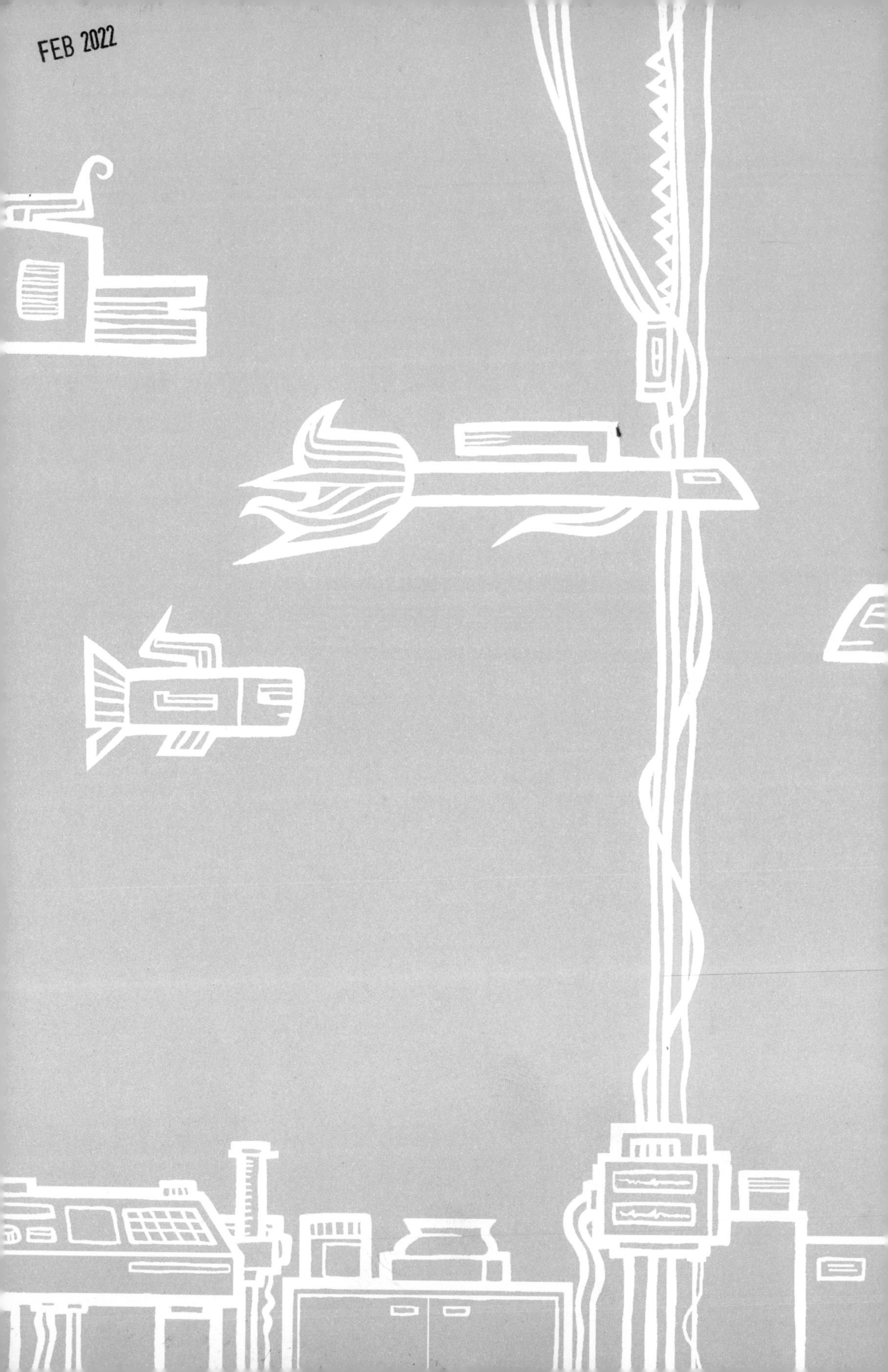